John Hunter

A Treatise on the Venereal Disease

John Hunter

A Treatise on the Venereal Disease

ISBN/EAN: 9783742819437

Manufactured in Europe, USA, Canada, Australia, Japa

Cover: Foto ©Lupo / pixelio.de

Manufactured and distributed by brebook publishing software
(www.brebook.com)

John Hunter

A Treatise on the Venereal Disease

TREATISE

ON

THE VENEREAL DISEASE.

By JOHN HUNTER.

LONDON,
SOLD AT No. 13, CASTLE-STREET, LEICESTER-SQUARE.
MDCCLXXXVI.

TO

SIR GEORGE BAKER, BART.

PHYSICIAN TO HER MAJESTY,

PRESIDENT OF THE COLLEGE OF PHYSICIANS,

AND

FELLOW OF THE ROYAL SOCIETY,

THIS WORK

IS INSCRIBED

AS A MARK OF ESTEEM,

BY HIS FRIEND, AND

HUMBLE SERVANT,

JOHN HUNTER.

LEICESTER-SQUARE,
MARCH, 30, 1786.

THE

CONTENTS.

INTRODUCTION.

PART I.

THE CONTENTS.

PART II.

CHAP. V.

THE CONTENTS.

PART III.

Chap. II.

THE CONTENTS.

CHAP. IX.

THE CONTENTS.

PART IV.

PART V.

Sect. VI.

vi

THE CONTENTS.

PART VI.

Sect. I.

PART VII.

INTRODUCTION.

INTRODUCTION.

I Am induced by two motives to publiſh the following treatiſe: in the firſt place, I am in hopes, that ſeveral new obſervations contained in it will be deemed worthy of the public attention; in the next place, I am deſirous to have an opportunity of aſſerting my right to ſome opinions, that have made their way into the world under other names.

There are many opinions reſpecting the animal œconomy peculiar to myſelf, which are frequently referred to in the courſe of the work. It is therefore neceſſary to give a ſhort explanation of ſome of them, that the terms made uſe of may be better underſtood.

I. OF SYMPATHY.

I Divide ſympathy into two kinds; *univerſal*, and *partial*.

Univerſal ſympathy is, when the whole conſtitution ſympathiſes with ſome ſenſation or action. Partial ſympathy is, when one or more diſtinct parts ſympathiſe with ſome local ſenſation, or action.

The univerſal Sympathies are various in different diſeaſes; but thoſe that we have in the venereal diſeaſe are principally two; the ſymptomatic fever, and the hectic fever. The ſymptomatic fever is an immediate effect of ſome local injury, and ſeldom takes place in the venereal diſeaſe in any great degree under any of its forms, except in the caſe of a ſwelled teſticle, which is itſelf an inſtance of a partial ſympathy; the ſymptomatic fever here, therefore, is an univerſal ſympathy ariſing from a partial one. The hectic fever is an univerſal ſympathy with a local diſeaſe, which the conſtitution is not able to overcome. This takes place oftener and in a greater degree in the *lues venerea* than in any other form of the diſeaſe.

Partial ſympathy I divide into three kinds; the *remote*, the *contiguous*, and the *continuous*. The remote is, where there appears to be no viſible connection of parts that can account for ſuch effects, as the pain of the ſhoulder in an inflammation of the liver. The contiguous is, that which appears to have no other connection than what ariſes from vicinity or contact of ſeparate parts; an inſtance of which we have, in the ſtomach and inteſtines ſympathiſing with the integuments of the abdomen. The continuous is, where there is no interruption of parts, and the ſympathy runs along from the irritating point, as from a centre, which is the moſt common of all the Sympathies; and we have an example of it in the ſpreading of inflammation.

II. OF DISEASED ACTIONS BEING INCOMPATIBLE WITH EACH OTHER.

THE venereal diſeaſe is not only ſuſpected to be preſent in many caſes, where the nature of the diſorder is not well marked, but it is ſuppoſed that it can be combined with other diſeaſes, ſuch as the itch and the ſcurvy: thus we hear of *pocky* itch, and of ſcurvy and the venereal diſeaſe combined; but this ſuppoſition appears to me to be founded in ignorance. I have never ſeen any ſuch caſes, nor do they ſeem to be conſiſtent with the principles of diſeaſed action in the animal œconomy. It appears to me, beyond a doubt, that no two actions can take place in the ſame conſtitution, nor in the ſame part, at one and the ſame time. No two different fevers can exiſt in the ſame conſtitution, nor two local diſeaſes in the ſame part at the ſame time; yet as the venereal diſeaſe, when it attacks the ſkin, is very ſimilar to thoſe diſeaſes which are vulgarly called ſcorbutic, they are often ſuppoſed to be mixed and to exiſt in the ſame part.

What has been called a ſcorbutic conſtitution, is no more than a conſtitution very ſuſceptible of an action producing eruptions on the ſkin, whenever an immediate cauſe ſhall take place; and there are ſome parts of the body more ſuſceptible of this than others, in which therefore a ſlighter immediate cauſe is ſufficient to excite the action; but the circumſtance of a conſtitution's being ſuſceptible of one diſeaſe, does not hinder it from being ſuſceptible

ſuſceptible of others. A man may have the lues and the ſmall pox at the ſame time; that is, parts of his body may have been contaminated by the venereal poiſon, and the ſmall pox may take place, and both may appear together, but not in the ſame parts. If both were conſequences of fever, and each followed the fever nearly about the ſame time, then it would be impoſſible for both to have their reſpective eruptions, even in different parts, at the ſame time; for it is impoſſible for the preceding fevers to have been coexiſtent.

From this principle, I think I may fairly put the following queries. Does not the failure of inoculation, and the power of reſiſting many infections, ariſe from the perſon's having, at the ſame time, ſome other diſeaſe, and therefore being incapable of a new action? Does not the great difference in the time, from the application of the cauſe, to the appearance of the diſeaſe, in many caſes, depend upon the ſame principle? For inſtance, a perſon is inoculated, and the puncture does not inflame for fourteen days, which I have ſeen; and is it not becauſe there is another diſeaſe in the conſtitution at the time of inoculation? Does not the cure of ſome diſeaſes depend upon the ſame principle, as the ſuſpenſion, or cure of a gonorrhœa by a fever?

Let me illuſtrate this principle ſtill further, by one of many caſes which have come under my own obſervation. On Thurſday, the ſixteenth of March, one thouſand ſeven hundred and ſeventy-five, I inoculated a gentleman's child; it was obſerved, that I made pretty large punctures. On the Sunday following, the nineteenth, he appeared to have received the infection; a ſmall inflammation or redneſs appearing round each puncture, and a ſmall tumour above the ſurface of the ſkin having taken place. On the twentieth, and the twenty-firſt, the child was feveriſh; but I declared it was not the variolous fever, as the inflammation had not at all advanced ſince the nineteenth. On the twenty-ſecond, a conſiderable eruption appeared, which was evidently the meaſles; the ſores on the arms appeared to go back, becoming leſs inflamed. On the twenty-third, he was very full of the meaſles; the punctures on the arms being in the ſame ſtate as on the preceding day. On the twenty-fifth, the meaſles began to diſappear. On the twenty-ſixth, and twenty-ſeventh, the punctures began again to look a little red. On the twenty-ninth, the inflammation increaſed, and there was a little matter formed.

formed. On the thirtieth, he was ſeized with fever. The ſmall pox appeared at the regular time, went through its uſual courſe, and terminated favourably. In like manner, it may be obſerved, that the venereal diſeaſe makes its appearance at different periods after infection. Is not this explicable on the ſame principle?

III. OF THE COMPARATIVE POWERS OF DIFFERENT PARTS OF THE BODY—FROM SITUATION—FROM STRUCTURE.

We ſhall have occaſion to obſerve, that the parts affected take on the action more readily, and go on more rapidly with it, when near to the ſource of the circulation than when far from it; for the heart exerts its influence upon the different parts of the body, in proportion to their vicinity to it; and the more diſtant the parts are the weaker are their powers.

This is, perhaps, better illuſtrated by diſeaſe than by any actions in health; for in health we have no comparative trials, as no two parts of the machine, at unequal diſtances from the heart, can be thrown into equal action, and therefore no concluſions can be drawn. I may juſt obſerve, that all the vital parts are near the heart.

In diſeaſes we ſee mortification, ariſing from debility, taking place in the extremities oftener than in other parts, more eſpecially if the perſon is tall; the heart not propelling the blood to theſe diſtant parts with equal force. In ſuch a ſtate of conſtitution, thoſe who labour under a hemiplegia, are often found to die at laſt, from mortification taking place in the extremities of the paralytic ſide. In ſome of thoſe caſes the arteries give way, and allow of extravaſation of the blood, and therefore we may reaſonably ſuppoſe, that they are proportionally weak in health. We alſo find, that ſuch extravaſation commonly begins in the extremities. This principle is not only evident in theſe two diſeaſes, but alſo in every diſeaſe that can affect an animal body. It appears in the readineſs with which diſeaſes come on, and proceed in parts diſtant from the ſource of the circulation, and alſo in the ſteps towards a cure.

Parts

Parts differ not only in their powers, in proportion as they are nearer or further from the heart, but likewise according to their peculiar structures, whereby they vary as much in the progress of diseased actions as in the operations of health.

An animal body is composed of a variety of substances, as muscle, tendon, cellular membrane, ligament, bone, nerve, &c.; we have therefore an opportunity of observing the comparative progress of diseases in them, and their comparative powers of performing a cure; and we find that they differ very much from one another in those respects. How far these differences take place in all diseases I have not been able to determine; but should suppose, that in specific diseases as scrofula and cancer, there is in general no difference in the mode of action in any of the structures,* these diseases producing the same specific effects in all the parts that are capable of being affected by them; but in diseases arising from accident, a great difference in the degrees of action takes place; the parts from such a cause being allowed to act according to their natures, which holds good also in the venereal disease. This difference appears to be chiefly in the degrees of strength and weakness in resisting diseased action. The less the natural powers of action are in any particular structure of parts, the less they are able to resist disease; therefore bone tendon ligament and cellular membrane go through their diseased actions more slowly than muscle or skin; and this principle is applicable to the venereal disease.

IV. OF PARTS SUSCEPTIBLE OF PARTICULAR DISEASES.

There are some parts much more susceptible of specific diseases than others. Poisons take their different seats in the body as if allotted for them. Thus we have the skin attacked with what are vulgarly called scorbutic eruptions, and many other diseases; it is also the seat of the small-pox

* Here it is to be understood, that we do not include those parts which have a greater tendency to specific diseases than what many others have, as the lymphatics to the scrofula, the breast to the cancer.

and the meaſles; the throat is the ſeat of action in the hydrophobia and the hooping-cough. The ſcrofula attacks the abſorbent ſyſtem, eſpecially the glands. The breaſts, teſticles, and the conglomerate glands are the ſeat of cancer. The ſkin throat and noſe are more readily affected by the *lues venerea* than the bones and perioſteum, which, on the other hand, ſuffer ſooner than many other parts, particularly the vital parts, which perhaps are not at all ſuſceptible of this diſeaſe.

V. OF INFLAMMATION.

I conſider common inflammation to be an increaſed action of the ſmaller veſſels of a part joined with a peculiar mode of action, by which they are enabled to produce the following effects; to unite parts of the body to each other; to form pus; and to remove parts of the ſolids. Theſe effects are not produced by a ſimple increaſe of action or enlargement of the veſſels, but by a peculiar action, which is at preſent perhaps not underſtood.

Theſe three effects of inflammation I have called, diſtinct ſpecies of inflammation. That which unites parts I have called, the *adheſive inflammation*; that which forms pus, *the ſuppurative inflammation*; and that which removes parts, the *ulcerative inflammation*.

In the adheſive inflammation the arteries throw out coagulable lymph which becomes the bond of union; this however is not ſimply extravaſated but has undergone ſome change before it leaves the arteries, ſince in inflamed veins it is found lying coagulated upon the internal ſurface of the veſſel, which could not have happened if ſimply extravaſated. In the ſuppurative inflammation a ſtill greater change is produced upon the blood before it is thrown out by the arteries, whereby it is formed into pus; which change is probably ſimilar to ſecretion. In the ulcerative inflammation the action of the arteries does not remove the parts; that office is performed by the abſorbent veſſels which are brought into action.

In the two firſt ſpecies of inflammation there muſt be a change in the diſpoſition and mode of action of the arteries; for the ſuppurative cannot be conſidered as ſimply an increaſe of the action of the adheſive, as its effects

are

are totally different; but in the third ſpecies there is probably no change of action in the arteries from that of the ſecond, the action only of the abſorbients being ſuperadded, by which ſolid parts and of courſe the arteries themſelves are removed.

VI. OF MORTIFICATION.

MORTIFICATIONS are of two kinds, one preceded by inflammation, the other not; but as the caſes of mortifications, which will be mentioned in this work, are all of the firſt kind, I ſhall confine my obſervations to that ſpecies.

I conſider inflammation as an increaſed action of that power which a part is naturally in poſſeſſion of; this increaſed action in healthy inflammations at leaſt is probably attended with an increaſe of power: but in inflammations which terminate in mortification there is no increaſe of power; on the contrary there is a diminution of power, which joined to an increaſed action becomes the cauſe of mortification, by deſtroying the balance which ought to ſubſiſt between the power and action of every part.

If this account of mortifications be juſt, we ſhall find it no difficult matter to eſtabliſh a rational practice; but before we attempt this, let us juſt take a view of the treatment hitherto recommended, and ſee how far it agrees with our theory.

It is plain from the common practice that the weakneſs has been attended to, but it is as plain that the increaſed action has been overlooked; and therefore the whole aim has been to increaſe the action with a view to remove the weakneſs. The Peruvian bark, confectio cardiaca ſerpentaria, &c. have been given in as large quantities as the caſe appeared to require, or the conſtitution could bear; by which means an artificial or temporary appearance of ſtrength has been produced, while it was only an increaſed action. The cordials and wine, upon the principle on which they have been given, are rationally adminiſtered; but there are ſtrong reaſons for not recommending them, ariſing from the general effect which all cordials have of increaſing the action without giving real ſtrength; and the powers of the body are afterwards ſunk proportionally as they have been raiſed, by which nothing can be gained but

but a great deal may be loſt; for in all caſes if the powers are allowed to ſink below a certain point they are irrecoverable.

The local treatment has been as abſurd as the conſtitutional; ſcarifications have been made down to the living parts, that ſtimulating and antiſeptic medicines might be applied to them, as turpentines, the warmer balſams, and ſometimes the eſſential oils; warm fomentations have been alſo applied as congenial to life, but warmth always increaſes action, and ſtimulants are improper where the actions are already too violent.

Upon the principles here laid down, the bark is the only medicine that can be depended upon, as it increaſes the powers and leſſens the action. Upon many occaſions opium will be of ſingular ſervice by leſſening the action, although it does not give real ſtrength; I have ſeen good effects from it both when given internally in large doſes, and when applied to the part. Keeping the parts cool is proper, and all the applications ſhould be cold. The above practice is to be kept in view in mortifications that happen in the venereal diſeaſe.

PART

PART I.

CHAPTER I.

OF THE VENEREAL POISON.

THE Venereal Disease arises from a poison, which as it is produced by disease, and is capable of again producing a similar disease, I call a morbid poison to distinguish it from the other poisons, animal, vegetable, and mineral.

The morbid poisons are many, and they have different powers of contamination. Those which infect the body, either locally or constitutionally, but not in both ways, I call *simple*. Those which are capable of affecting the body, both locally and constitutionally, I call *compound*. The venereal poison when applied to the human body, possesses a power of propagating or multiplying itself; and as it is also capable of acting both locally and constitutionally, it is a compound morbid poison. Like all such poisons, it may be communicated to others in all the various ways in which it can be received, producing the same disease in some one of its forms.

I. OF THE FIRST ORIGIN OF THE POISON.

THOUGH the first appearance of this poison is certainly within the period of modern history, yet the precise time and manner of its origin has hitherto escaped our observation; and we are still in doubt, whether it arose in Europe, or was imported from America. I shall not attempt to discuss this question, and those who wish to examine at length the facts, authorities and arguments brought in favour of the latter opinion, may consult Astruc; and for the former a ſhort treatiſe* publiſhed in one thouſand ſeven hundred and fifty-one, without a name. The author of this treatiſe appears to have conſidered the ſubject very fully, and as far as reaſoning goes on a ſubject of this kind, proves that the diſeaſe was not brought from the Weſt-Indies: not contented with this, he goes on to account for its firſt riſe in Europe; but in this he is not equally ſucceſsful. The ſubject is a difficult one; and the want of a ſufficient number of facts leaves too much room for conjecture.

We ſhall not therefore enter further into this queſtion, nor is it material to know at what period and in what country this diſeaſe aroſe; but we may in general affirm, that as animals are not naturally formed with diſeaſe, nor ſo as to run ſpontaneouſly into diſeaſed actions; but with a ſuſceptibility of ſuch impreſſions as produce diſeaſed actions, diſeaſes muſt always ariſe from impreſſions made upon the body: and as man is probably ſuſceptible of more impreſſions that become the immediate cauſe of diſeaſe than any other animal, and is beſides the only animal which can be ſaid to form artificial impreſſions upon himſelf, he is ſubject to the greateſt variety of diſeaſes. In one of thoſe ſelf-formed ſituations therefore the impreſſion moſt probably was given which produced the venereal diſeaſe.

II. BEGAN IN THE HUMAN RACE, AND IN THE PARTS OF GENERATION.

In whatever manner it aroſe, it certainly began in the human race; as we know no other animal that is capable of being infected with this poiſon. It is probable too, that the parts of generation were the firſt affected: for if it had taken place in any other part of the body it might probably never have gone farther than the perſon in whom it firſt aroſe; and therefore never have been known; but being ſeated in the parts of generation, where the only natural connection takes place between one human being and another, except the mother and child, it was in the moſt favourable ſituation for being propagated:

* Intitled, "A Diſſertation on the Origin of the Venereal Diſeaſe; proving that it was not brought from America, but began in Europe from an epidemical Diſtemper; tranſlated from the original Manuſcript of an eminent Phyſician. London, printed for Robert Griffiths, 1751."

and

and as we shall find hereafter in the history of the disease itself, that no constitutional effect of this poison can be communicated to others, we are led of necessity to conclude that its first effects were local.

III. OF THE NATURE OF THE POISON.

We know nothing of the poison itself, but only its effects on the human body. It is commonly in the form of pus, or united with pus, or some such secretion, and produces a similar matter in others, which shows that it is most generally, although not necessarily, a consequence of inflammation. It produces or excites therefore in most cases an inflammation in the parts contaminated; besides which inflammation, the parts so contaminated have a peculiar mode of action superadded, different from all other actions attending inflammation; and it is this specific mode of action which produces the specific quality in the matter. It is not necessary that inflammation should be present to keep up this peculiar mode of action, because the poison continues to be formed long after all signs of inflammation have ceased. This appears from the following facts: men having only what is called a gleet or healing chancre, give the disease to sound women: and many venereal gonorrhœas happen without any visible signs of inflammation.

In women the inflammation is frequently very slight, and often there is not the least sign of it; for they have been known to infect men though they themselves have had no symptoms of inflammation, or of the disease in any form. Therefore the inflammation and suppuration, when present, are only attendants on the peculiar mode of action; the degree in which they take place depending more on the nature of the constitution than on that of the poison.

The formation of matter also, though a very general, is not a constant attendant on this disease; for we sometimes find inflammation produced by the venereal poison which does not terminate in suppuration; such inflammation I suspect to be of the erysipelatous kind. It is the matter produced, whether with or without inflammation, which alone contains the poison; for without the formation of matter, no venereal poison can exist. Therefore a person

person having the venereal irritation in any form not attended with a discharge, cannot communicate the disease to another. To communicate the disease therefore it is necessary that the venereal action should first take place, that matter should be formed in consequence of that action, and that the matter should be applied to a sound person or part.

That the venereal disease is to be propagated only by matter is proved every day by a thousand instances. Married men contract the disease, and not suspecting that they have caught it, cohabit with their wives, even for weeks. Upon discovering symptoms of the disease they of course desist; yet in all my practice I never once found that the complaint was communicated under such circumstances, except where they had not been very attentive to the symptoms, and therefore continued the connection after the discharge had appeared. I have gone so far as to allow husbands to cohabit with their wives in order to save appearances, and always with safety. I could carry this still farther, and even allow a man who has a gonorrhœa to have connection with a sound woman, if he took great care to clear all the parts of any matter, by first syringing the urethra, making water, and washing the glans.

The matter which is impregnated with this poison, when it comes in contact with a living part, irritates that part, and inflammation is the common consequence. It must be applied either in a fluid state, or rendered fluid by the juices of the part to which it is applied. There is no instance where it has given the infection in the form of vapor, as is the case in many other poisons.

IV. OF THE GREATER OR LESS ACRIMONY OF THE POISON.

VENEREAL matter must in all cases be the same; one quantity of matter cannot have a greater degree of poisonous quality than another, and if there is any difference it is only in its being more or less diluted, which produces no difference in its effects. One can conceive however, that it may be so far diluted as not to have the power of irritation. Thus any fluid taken into the mouth, capable of stimulating the nerves to taste, may be so diluted as not to be tasted. But if the poison can irritate the part to which it is applied to action, it it is all that is required; the action will be the ſame whether from a large or ſmall quantity, from a ſtrong or a weak ſolution.

We find from experience, that there is no difference in the kind of matter; and no variation can ariſe in the diſeaſe from the matter's being of different degrees of ſtrength; for it appears that the ſame matter affects very differently different people. Two men having been connected with one woman, and both catching the diſeaſe, one of them ſhall have a violent gonorrhœa or chancre, while the other ſhall have merely a ſlight gonorrhœa. I have known one man give the diſeaſe to different women, and ſome of the women have had it very ſeverely, while in others it has been very ſlight. The ſame reaſoning holds good with regard to chancres. The variations of the ſymptoms in different perſons depend upon the conſtitution and habit of the patient at the time. What happens in the inoculation of the ſmallpox ſtrengthens this opinion. Let the ſymptoms of the patient from whom the matter is taken be good or bad, let it be from one who has had a great many puſtules, or from one who has had but few; let it be from the confluent or diſtinct kind, applied in a large quantity or a ſmall one, it produces always the ſame effect. This could only be known by the great numbers that have been inoculated under all theſe different circumſtances.

V. OF THE POISON BEING THE SAME IN GONORRHŒA AND IN CHANCRE.

It has been ſuppoſed by many that the gonorrhœa and the chancre ariſe from two diſtinct poiſons; and their opinion ſeems to have ſome foundation, when we conſider only the different appearances of the two diſeaſes, and the different methods of cure; which in judging of the nature of many diſeaſes is too often all we have to go by. Yet if we take up this queſtion upon other grounds, and alſo have recourſe to experiments, the reſult of which we can abſolutely depend upon, we ſhall find this notion to be erroneous.

If we attend to the manner in which the venereal poiſon was communicated to the inhabitants of the iſlands in the South Seas, there are many circumſtances which tend to throw light upon the preſent queſtion. It has been ſuppoſed, as no mention is made of a gonorrhœa at Otaheite, that it muſt have been the chancre that was firſt introduced into that iſland; and that of courſe nothing but a chancre could be propagated there; for as no gonorrhœa had been communicated no ſuch diſeaſe could take place. But if we were to reaſon upon all the probable circumſtances attending the voyages to that part of the world, we ſhould conclude the contrary; for it was almoſt impoſſible to carry a chancre ſo long a voyage without it's deſtroying the penis; while we know from experience, that a gonorrhœa may continue for a great length of time. It is mentioned in Cook's voyage, that the people of Otaheite, who had this diſeaſe, went into the country and got cured; but when it turned into a pox it was then incurable: this ſhows that the diſeaſe which they had muſt have been a gonorrhœa, for we know that it is only a gonorrhœa that can be cured by ſimple means; and further, if it had been a chancre, and they had been acquainted with the means of curing it, they could alſo have cured the *lues venerea*.

Wallis left Plymouth in Auguſt 1766, and arrived at Otaheite in July 1767, eleven months after his embarkation; and if none of his men had the diſeaſe when he failed, there was hardly a poſſibility of their contracting it any where afterwards in the voyage; this appears to be too long for a gonorrhœa to laſt. But let us ſuppoſe even that Wallis carried it thither in his ſhip, and that one or two of his crew had it; as he ſtaid there five weeks, it was very poſſible, even very probable, that ſuch perſon or perſons might have communicated it ſo quickly as to have become the cauſe of contamination of the whole crew of his ſhip; but as this did not happen, it is a preſumptive proof that Wallis did not carry it thither.

Bougainville left France in December 1766, but he touched at ſeveral places where ſome of his people might have got the diſeaſe; the laſt of which was Rio de la Plata, which he left in November 1767, and arrived at Otaheite in April 1768, five months after. This interval of time agrees better with the uſual continuance of the diſeaſe than the length of Wallis's voyage, and therefore from this circumſtance it becomes more probable that Bougainville carried it thither. Beſides, it is likely that he could guard his people leſs againſt the diſeaſe than Wallis, for Wallis could have his choice of men at his firſt ſetting out,

out, which was all that was necessary to prevent his carrying the disease with him, for he ran no risk of contracting it afterwards: but although Bougainville had the same advantage at first, yet he had it not afterwards, for his men were in the way of infection in several places, and he had no opportunity of changing them, and probably no great chance of having them cured. The circumstance of the disease being found by Bougainville at Otaheite soon after his arrival, is a kind of proof that he carried it thither himself; for I observed before, that if Wallis had carried it by one man only, this man could in a very few days have so far propagated it, as to have spread it through the whole ship's crew; and as Bougainville arrived at the island ten months after Wallis, there was a sufficient time for the inhabitants of the whole island to have been infected, and the ravages of the disease must have been evident to them immediately upon their arrival. Bougainville remained only nine days at the island of Otaheite, and observed nothing of the disease till some weeks after his departure, when it was found that several of the crew were infected, which most probably must have happened in consequence of the poison being carried there by some of his own people. It is also mentioned by Cook, that the Otaheiteans ascribed the introduction of the disease to Bougainville; and we can hardly suppose that they would be so complaisant to our countrymen as to accuse Bougainville, when they must have known whether the disease was imported by Wallis or not, especially as they had no reason to be partial in favour of the people who accompanied the latter. But as we find in Cook's last voyage, that the disease in every form is now there, and as we have no new intelligence of a gonorrhœa being since introduced, we must suppose that every form of the disease has been propagated from one root, which most probably was a gonorrhœa.

If any doubt still remain with respect to the two diseases being of the same nature, it will be removed by considering that the matter produced in both is of the same kind, and has the same properties; the proofs of which are, that the matter of a gonorrhœa will produce either a gonorrhœa, a chancre, or the *lues venerea*; and the matter of a chancre will also produce either a gonorrhœa, a chancre, or the *lues venerea*.

The following case is an instance of a gonorrhœa producing a *lues venerea*. A gentleman twice contracted a gonorrhœa, of which he was cured both

times

times without mercury. About two months after each he had ſymptoms of the *lues venerea*; thoſe in conſequence of the firſt infection were ulcers in the throat, which were removed by the external application of mercury; the ſymptoms in conſequence of the ſecond were blotches on the ſkin, for which alſo he uſed the mercurial ointment, and was cured. We have too many examples of chancres producing the *lues venerea*.

Since it ſhould appear from the above, that the gonorrhœa and chancre are the effects of the ſame poiſon, it may be worthy of inquiry, to what circumſtances two ſuch different forms of the diſeaſe are owing.

To account for theſe two very different effects of the ſame poiſon, it is only neceſſary to obſerve the difference in the mode of action of the parts affected when irritated, let the irritation be what it may. The gonorrhœa always proceeds from a ſecreting ſurface,* and the chancre is formed on a non-ſecreting ſurface; and in this laſt the part to which the poiſon is applied muſt become a ſecreting ſurface before matter can be produced. All ſecreting ſurfaces in the body being probably ſimilar, one mode of application only is neceſſary to produce this diſeaſe in them all, which is by the poiſonous matter ſimply coming in contact with them. But to produce the chancre, the venereal matter may be applied in three different ways; the firſt and moſt certain is by a wound, into which it may be introduced; the ſecond is by applying the matter to a ſurface with a cuticle, and the thinner that is it allows the matter to come more readily to the cutis; and the third is by applying the matter to a common ſore already formed.

The poiſon then being the ſame in both caſes, why do they not always happen together in the ſame perſon? for one would naturally ſuppoſe, that the gonorrhœa when it had taken place could not fail to become the cauſe of a chancre, and that this when it happened firſt would produce a gonorrhœa. Although it does not often happen ſo, yet it ſometimes does, at

* By *ſecreting ſurfaces* I mean all the paſſages for extraneous matter, including alſo the ducts of glands, ſuch as the mouth, noſe, eyes, anus, and urethra; and by *non-ſecreting ſurfaces*, the external ſkin in general. To which I may add a third kind of ſurface leading from the one to the other, as the glans penis, prolabium of the mouth, the inſide of the lips, the pudendum; which ſurfaces partaking of the properties of each, but in a leſs degree, are capable of being affected in both ways, ſometimes by being excited to ſecretion, and at other times to ulceration.

least

least there is great reason to believe so. I have seen cases where a gonorrhœa came on, and in a few days after in some, in others as many weeks, a chancre has appeared: and I have also seen cases where a chancre has come first, and in the course of it's cure a running and pain in making water have succeeded. It may be supposed that the two diseases arose from the original infection, and only appeared at different times; and their not occurring oftener together would almost induce us to believe it was so, since the matter is the same in both, and therefore capable of producing either the one or the other.

I suspect that the presence of one irritation in these parts becomes in general a preventive of the other. I have already observed, that the two parts sympathise in their diseases; and it is possible that, that very sympathy may prevent the appearance of the real disease; for if an action has already taken place which is not venereal, it is impossible that another should take place till that ceases, and it is probable that this sympathy will not cease while the cause exciting it exists; and therefore when both happen in the same person at the same time, I suspect that either the urethra never had sympathised with the chancre, or if it did at first that the sympathy had ceased, and then the venereal matter might stimulate the parts to action.

VII. OF THE CAUSE OF THE POISONOUS QUALITY—FERMENTATION—ACTION.

As the consideration of this point, and the being able to account for it, will throw some light upon the disease, and cure, I may be allowed to dwell a little upon it. It has been supposed by some, that the poisonous quality of the matter arises from a fermentation taking place in it as soon as it is formed. But whether this poisonous quality arises from that cause; or whether the animal body has a power of producing matter according to the irritation given, whereby the living powers whenever irritated in a particular manner produce such an action in the parts as to generate a matter similar in quality to that which excited the action, is what I am now to consider.

In the examination of this fubject I fhall confine myfelf to the gonorrhœa. In fupport of either of the two opinions, it muft be fuppofed that the venereal matter has by its fpecific properties, a power of irritation beyond common matter. I have already obferved, that it has the power of exciting inflammation even on the common fkin, and of forming a chancre, which power is not poffeffed by common matter. In the firft opinion it muft be fuppofed, that there is no fpecific inflammation or fuppuration produced by the application of the venereal matter, but only a common inflammation and fuppuration, and that the matter capable of producing thefe effects acts as a ferment upon the new formed matter, rendering it venereal as foon, or nearly as foon asi t is formed; and as there is a fucceffion of fecretions, there immediately follows a fucceffion of fermentations. Now, let us fee how far this idea agrees with all the variety of phænomena attending the difeafe. Firft, it may be afked, what becomes of this ferment in many cafes where the fuppuration does not come on for fome weeks after the irritation and inflammation have taken place? In fuch cafes we can hardly fuppofe the original venereal matter to remain, and to act as a ferment. Secondly, when there is a ceffation of the difcharge and no matter formed, which fometimes happens for a confiderable time, and yet all the fymptoms recur, what is it that produces this fermentation a fecond time? Nothing can, but a new application of frefh venereal matter. When, for example, the irritation is tranflated to the tefticle and the difcharge is totally ftopped, as often happens, what becomes of the virus; and how is a new virus formed when the irritation falls back upon the urethra? Thirdly, if the poifonous quality were produced by fermentation taking place in the matter already formed, it would not be an eafy matter to account for the fymptoms ever ceafing; for according to my idea of a ferment, it would never ceafe to act if new matter were continually added; nor could any thing poffibly check it but a fubftance immediately applied to the part, which could ftop or prevent the fermentation taking place in the new matter. But as the venereal inflammation in this fpecies of the difeafe is not kept up beyond a certain time, the production of the poifon cannot depend on fermentation. Fourthly, if it depended on a fermentation taking place in the fecreted matter all venereal cafes would be alike, nor would one be worfe than another, except from a greater or fmaller number of fermenting

ing places. Upon this ſuppoſition alſo all caſes would be equally eaſy of cure, for the fermentation would be equally ſtrong in a ſlight caſe as in a bad one; it can only be fermentation in the matter after it has left the veſſels; and the matter of every ſore or ſecreting ſurface would become venereal by applying venereal matter to it; which does not happen.

When the venereal matter has been applied to a ſore, ſo as to irritate, it produces a venereal irritation and inflammation. But even this does not always take place, for the common matter from the ſore may remove the venereal matter applied before it can affect the ſore, ſo as to produce the venereal inflammation and ſuppuration there. This experiment I have made ſeveral times, and never could produce the venereal inflammation but once. But if the venereal matter were capable of acting as a ferment, then it would in all caſes produce venereal matter, without altering the nature of the ſore.

The effects produced by the venereal poiſon appear to me to ariſe from it's peculiar, or ſpecific irritation, joined with the ſuſceptibility of the living principle to be irritated by ſuch a cauſe, and the parts ſo irritated acting accordingly. I ſhall therefore conſider it as a poiſon, which by irritating the living parts in a manner peculiar to itſelf, produces an inflammation peculiar to that irritation, from which a matter is produced peculiar to the inflammation. Let us conſider how far this opinion agrees with the various phænomena attending the diſeaſe.

Firſt, the venereal matter having a greater power of irritating than common matter, approaches nearer to the idea of irritation than of fermentation. Secondly, it's producing a ſpecific diſeaſe with ſpecific ſymptoms and appearances, ſhows that it has a ſpecific power of irritation, the living powers neceſſarily acting according to that irritation. Thirdly, the inflammation having it's ſtated time of appearing and terminating, is agreeable to the laws of the animal œconomy in moſt caſes, as it is a circumſtance that takes place in other diſeaſes that have a criſis; and when the diſeaſe is longer of duration in ſome than in others, it is becauſe they are much more ſuſceptible of this kind of irritation, and there may be perhaps other concurrent circumſtances. Fourthly, the venereal inflammation being confined to a ſpecific diſtance, is more agreeable to the idea of a ſpecific irritation, than that of a fermentation. Fifthly, we have a further proof of this opinion

opinion, from the appearance of the diſeaſe being tranſlated from one part of the body to another, as in the caſe of the ſwelled teſticle, in which the diſcharge is often ſtopped or otherwiſe affected. Sixthly, the diſcharge often ſtops from the conſtitution being attacked by a fever, and returns after ſome days or weeks, or not at all, according to the continuance of the fever: now we can plainly ſee why the fever ſhould put a ſtop to the diſcharge, as the diſpoſition produced by it in a part is very different from that diſpoſition which formed the matter; and we can plainly ſee why the ſame diſpoſition to form matter ſhould often return; but how that return ſhould be venereal, upon the principles of fermentation, we do not ſee. Seventhly, the produ-tion by art of an irritation of another kind, which is not ſpecific, removes the ſpecific irritation; now an irritation of another kind cannot prevent the fermentation from going on, but may deſtroy the venereal irritation. Eighthly, the circumſtance of particular parts of our body being much more readily irritated than others by the venereal poiſon, when in the conſtitution, ſhows that it ariſes from an irritation, and that of a particular kind. Ninthly, ſome animals are not ſuſceptible of the venereal irritation; for repeated trials have ſhewn that it is impoſſible to give it to a dog, a bitch, or an aſs*. It is much eaſier to ſuppoſe, that a dog or an aſs is not ſuſceptible of many irritations of which the human body is, which we find to be the caſe in all other ſpecific diſeaſes, and moſt poiſons, than that matter of the human body is ſuſceptible of a change, of which that of the dog or aſs is not.

This argument is ſtill further ſupported by comparing the venereal poiſon with other morbid poiſons. The animal poiſon, productive of the hydro-phobia, ſeems to be owing to a particular irritation affecting certain parts, which ſhews, that if the body or any part of the body is irritated, it takes on a diſpoſition to act in a peculiar manner, and that this mode of action is capa-ble of ſecreting ſuch juices as will throw another animal into the ſame action. In the hydrophobia the throat and its glands are particularly affected; and

* I have repeatedly ſoaked lint in matter from a gonorrhœa, chancre, and bubo, and introduced it into the vagina of bitches, without producing any effect. I have alſo introduced it into the vagina of aſſes, without any effect. I have introduced it under the prepuce of dogs, without any effect. I have alſo made inciſions and introduced it under the ſkin, and it has only produced a common ſore. I have made the ſame experiments upon aſſes, with the ſame reſult.

how

how the saliva should become of such a nature from the same kind of matter being either carried into the constitution, or perhaps only by the general sympathy of the constitution with a local affection, and more particularly with the parts about the throat, is not easily to be accounted for, without supposing either that the absorbed poison circulating can produce a specific constitutional action capable of affecting the throat and glands there, just as the poison of the small pox affects the skin, or that the circulating poison has power to affect or irritate the glands of the mouth only, or that those parts only are capable of immediately sympathysing with the part irritated, as the muscles of the lower jaw are when they produce the locked jaw.

If this theory is just, it accounts for epidemical diseases arising from seasons, air, &c. irritating in such a manner, as to produce a fever, the effluvia of which shall irritate in the same manner; for it is not in the least material how the original irritation arises, it is only necessary that the animal should act according to the stimulus given by that irritation.

CHAPTER II.

THE MODE OF VENEREAL INFECTION.

EVERY infectious diſeaſe has its peculiar manner of being caught, and among mankind there is generally ſomething peculiar in the way of life, or ſome attending circumſtance which expoſes them at one time or other to contract ſuch diſeaſes, and which if avoided would prevent their propagation. The itch for inſtance is generally caught by a ſpecies of civility, the ſhaking of hands, therefore the hand is moſt commonly the firſt part affected. And as the venereal poiſon is generally caught by the connection between the ſexes, the parts of generation commonly firſt ſuffer; from this circumſtance people do not ſuſpect this diſeaſe when the ſymptoms are any where elſe, while they always ſuſpect it in every complaint of thoſe parts.

In the lower claſs of people, one as naturally thinks of the itch when there is an eruption between the fingers, as we do in young men of the venereal diſeaſe from the genitals being affected; but as every ſecreting ſurface whether cuticular or non-cuticular, as was explained before, is liable to be infected by the venereal poiſon when it is applied to them, it is poſſible for many other parts beſides the genitals to receive this diſeaſe, therefore it appears in the anus, mouth, noſe, eyes, ears, and, as has been ſaid, in the nipples of women from giving ſuck to children who have it in their mouths; which children have been infected in the birth from the parts of the mother being diſeaſed.

CHAPTER III.

OF THE DIFFERENT FORMS OF THE DISEASE.

THE venereal poiſon is capable of affecting the human body in two different ways; locally, that is, in thoſe parts only to which it is firſt applied; and conſtitutionally, that is, in conſequence of the abſorption of the venereal pus which affects parts while diffuſed in the circulation.

Between the firſt and ſecond kind, or the local and conſtitutional*, certain intermediate complaints take place in the progreſs of abſorption; theſe are inflammations and ſuppurations forming what are called buboes, in which the matter is of the ſame nature with that of the original diſeaſe.

When the matter has got into the conſtitution, and is circulating with the blood, it there irritates to action. There are produced from that irritation many local diſeaſes, as blotches on the ſkin, ulcers in the tonſils, thickening of the perioſteum and bones.

The local or firſt kind is what I have called *immediate*, ariſing immediately upon the application of venereal pus. Of this kind there are two ſorts ſeemingly very different from one another. In the firſt there is a formation of matter without a breach in the ſolids, called a gonorrhœa. In the ſecond there is a breach in the ſolids, called a chancre. Neither of theſe two ways in which the diſeaſe ſhews itſelf is owing to any thing peculiar in the kind of poiſon applied, but to the difference in the parts contaminated.

The readineſs with which the parts run into violent action, in this ſpecies of inflammation, is greater or leſs according to the nature of the parts affected; which perhaps does not ariſe from any ſpecific difference in the parts, but is according to the common principle of ſenſibility and irritability; for we find that the vagina is not ſo much diſpoſed to inflammation in this diſeaſe, as the

* I have called this form of the diſeaſe, conſtitutional; yet it is not ſtrictly ſo, for every complaint in conſequence of it is truly local, and is produced by the ſimple application of the poiſon to the parts.

urethra

urethra is in the ſame ſex, becauſe it is not ſo ſenſible. However it is poſſible there may be ſome ſpecific diſpoſition to irritation and inflammation in the urethra in man; and what would incline me to think ſo is, that this canal is perhaps oftener out of order than any other, producing a great variety of ſymptoms.

I. VARIETIES IN DIFFERENT CONSTITUTIONS.

THIS diſeaſe when it appears in the form either of a gonorrhœa or a chancre differs very much in the violence of its ſymptoms in different people. In ſome it is extremely mild, in others extremely violent. When mild, it is generally ſimple in its ſymptoms, having but few and thoſe of no great extent, being much confined to the ſpecific diſtance; but when violent, it becomes more complicated in its ſymptoms, having a greater variety, and extending itſelf beyond the ſpecific diſtance. This does not ariſe from any variety in the ſpecific virtue of the poiſon, but from a difference in the diſpoſition and mode of action of the body, or parts of the body; ſome being hardly ſuſceptible of this or any irritation, others being very ſuſceptible of it, and of every other irritation, ſo as readily to run into violent action.

The venereal irritation however does not always follow theſe rules; for I have known young men, in whom a ſore from common accident healed up readily, yet the irritation attending a gonorrhœa would be violent, and a chancre would inflame and ſpread with great rapidity, and even mortify. On the other hand I have known young men in whom a ſore from common violence has been healed with great difficulty, yet when they had contracted a gonorrhœa or chancre, the diſeaſe has been mild and eaſily curable.

In particular people it is either mild or ſevere for the moſt part, uniformly. In the firſt ſtated diſpoſitions it is not invariably ſo, but then I believe there is ſome indiſpoſition at the time. I have known ſeveral gentlemen who had their gonorrhœas ſo ſlight in common, that they frequently cured themſelves; but it has ſo happened, that a gonorrhœa has been remarkably ſevere, which baffling all their ſkill they have applied for aſſiſtance, but then they were ſoon attacked with the ſymptoms of a fever, and when the fever has gone off the ſymptoms

ſymptoms of the gonorrhœa immediately became mild. I may now alſo obſerve, that when the diſeaſe is in the form of a *lues venerea*, different conſtitutions are differently affected, in ſome it's progreſs is very rapid, in others it is very ſlow.

CHAPTER IV.

OF THE LUES VENEREA BEING THE CAUSE OF OTHER DISEASES.

EVERY animal may be ſaid to have natural tendencies to diſeaſed actions, which may be conſidered as prediſpoſing cauſes, and theſe may be called into action whenever the immediate cauſe takes place, which may be ſuch as to have no connection with theſe tendencies, and cannot therefore be conſidered as the cauſe of the diſeaſe. One diſeaſe ſhall excite another, and therefore is ſuppoſed to be the ſole cauſe of it, as ſlight fevers, or colds, ſmall pox, and meaſles, become frequently the immediate cauſe of ſcrofula, and certain derangements of the natural actions of the body often bring on the gout, agues, and other diſeaſes; but theſe diſeaſes will be always more or leſs according to the conſtitution and parts; and the conſtitutions will differ according to circumſtances, which may be numerous; two of theſe however will be local ſituation, and age.

In this country the tendency to ſcrofula ariſes from the climate, which is in many a prediſpoſing cauſe, and only requires ſome derangement to become an immediate cauſe and produce the whole diſeaſe.

The venereal diſeaſe alſo becomes often the immediate cauſe of other diſorders, by calling forth latent tendencies to action. This does not happen from its being venereal, but from it's having deſtroyed the natural actions, ſo that the moment the venereal action and diſpoſition is terminated, the other takes place; and I have ſeen in many caſes the tendency ſo very ſtrong, that it has taken place before the venereal has been intirely ſubdued; for by purſuing the mercurial courſe the ſymptoms have grown worſe; but by taking up the new diſpoſition, and rendering it leſs active than the venereal, the venereal has come into action anew; and theſe effects have taken place alternately ſeveral times. In ſuch caſes it is a lucky circumſtance when the two modes of treatment can be united; but where they

act

act in opposition it is very unfortunate. If the venereal disease attacks the lungs, although that disposition may be corrected, consumption may ensue; and in like manner where the bones are affected, or the nose, scrofulous swellings or fistula lacrymalis may be the consequence, though the disease may have been cured.

Many of the diseases arising from this cause appear to be peculiar to such causes, and seem to be formed out of the constitution, the disease, and method of cure; therefore it is difficult to say of what nature such a disease may be; but it will in general have a particular tendency from the constitution; and if we are acquainted with the general tendency of a constitution we are to suspect that as the strongest cause, and that the disease will partake more of it than of the other. In this country these complaints have most commonly a scrofulous tendency, and are often truly scrofulous, the disease partaking more of that tendency than any other.

Parts have also their peculiar tendencies to diseases, which are stronger than those of the constitution at large, and when injured they will of course fall into the diseased action arising from such tendencies, therefore when parts have had their natural actions destroyed by a venereal irritation, those tendencies will be brought into action; and therefore the diseases arising from the tendencies of such parts are to be kept in view. They will be assisted likewise by local situation and age.

In particular countries, and in young people, the tendency to scrofula will be predominant; therefore buboes in them will more readily become scrofulous. In old people they may form cancers; and when in parts of the body which have a greater tendency to cancer, that disease will more readily take place.

The want of knowledge and attention to this subject has been the cause of many mistakes, for whenever such effects have been produced in consequence of the venereal disease it has immediately been blamed, and not only as a cause, but it has been supposed to be the disease itself. This is an inference natural enough for those who cannot see that a variety of causes are capable of producing one effect, or in other words, that where the predisposing cause is the same, a variety of immediate causes may produce the same action. It shews great

great ignorance however to suppose the venereal disease can be both the predisposing and immediate cause.

When the venereal disease attacks the urethra, it often becomes itself the predisposing cause of abscesses, and many other complaints; when it attacks the outside of the penis, forming chancres, they often ulcerate so deep as to communicate with the urethra, producing fistula in the urethra, and often continued phymoses.

In describing diseases which like the venereal disease admit of a great variety of symptoms, we should keep a middle line, first giving the most common symptoms of the disease in each form, then the varieties which most commonly occur, and last of all the most uncommon; but it will be impossible to take notice of every possible variety, therefore when a variety occurs not mentioned, it is not to be supposed that the author is leading his readers astray, or is unacquainted with the disease at large; for if his general principles are just, they will help to explain most of the singularities of the disease.

PART

PART II.

CHAPTER I.

OF GONORRHOEA.

WHEN an irritating matter of any kind is applied to a secreting surface, it increases that secretion, and changes it from it's natural state (whatever that be) to some other, which in the present disease is a pus.

When this takes place in the urethra it is called a gonorrhoea; and as it arises from the matter being applied to a non-cuticular surface, which naturally secretes some fluid, it is of no consequence in what part of the body this surface is; for if in the anus it will produce a similar discharge there, and a similar effect on the inside of the mouth, nose, eyes, and ears. It is conceived by some, that gonorrhoeas may take place without the above-mentioned immediate cause; that is, that they may arise from the constitution; if so, they must be similar to what is supposed to be a venereal ophthalmia. But from the analogy of other venereal affections proceeding from the constitution, I very much suspect the existence of either the one or the other: for when the poison is thrown upon the mouth, throat, or nose, it produces ulcers, and not an increased secretion like a gonorrhoea. But we never find an ulcer on the inside of the eye-lids in those ophthalmias; and gonorrhoeas in the urethra are too frequent to proceed from such a cause.

Till about the year 1753 it was generally supposed, that the matter from the urethra in a gonorrhoea arose from an ulcer or ulcers in that passage; but from observation it was then proved that this was not the case.

It may not be improper to give here a short history of the discovery of matter being formed by inflammation without ulceration. In the winter

1749, a child was brought into the room used for diſſection, in Covent Garden, on opening of whoſe thorax a large quantity of pus was found looſe in the cavity, with the ſurface of the lungs and the pleura furred over with a more ſolid ſubſtance ſimilar to coagulable lymph. On removing this from thoſe ſurfaces they were found intire. This appearance being new to Dr. Hunter, he ſent to Mr. Samuel Sharp, deſiring his attendance, and to him it alſo appeared new. Mr. Sharp afterwards in the year 1750, publiſhed his Critical Enquiry, in which he introduced this fact, " That matter may be formed without a breach of ſubſtance;" not mentioning whence he had derived this notion. It was ever after taught by Dr. Hunter in his lectures; we however find writers adopting it without quoting either Mr. Sharp or Dr. Hunter. So much being known, I was anxious to examine whether the matter in a gonorrhœa was formed in the ſame way. In the ſpring of 1753 there was an execution of eight men, two of whom I knew had at that time very ſevere gonorrhœas. Their bodies being procured for this particular purpoſe, we were very accurate in our examination, but found no ulceration, the two urethras appeared merely a little blood-ſhot, eſpecially near the glans. This being another new fact aſcertained, it could not eſcape Mr. Gataker, ever attentive to his emolument, who was then attending Dr. Hunter's lectures, and alſo practiſing diſſection under me. He publiſhed, ſoon after in 1754, a treatiſe on this diſeaſe, and explained fully, that the matter in a gonorrhœa did not ariſe from an ulcer, without mentioning how he acquired this knowledge; and it has ever ſince been adopted in publications on this ſubject. Since the period mentioned above, I have conſtantly paid particular attention to this circumſtance, and have opened the urethra of many who at the time of their death had a gonorrhœa, yet have never found a ſore in any; but always obſerved that the urethra near the glans was more blood-ſhot than uſual, and that the lacunæ were often filled with matter. I have indeed ſeen an inſtance of a ſore a little within the urethra; but this ſore was not produced by any ulceration of the ſurface, but from an inflammation taking place probably in one of the glands, which produced an abſceſs in the part, and that abſceſs opened its way into the urethra. The very ſame ſore opened a way through externally at the frænum, ſo that there was a new paſſage

ſor

the urine. Indeed the method of curing a gonorrhœa might have shown that it could not depend upon a venereal ulcer; for there is hardly an instance of a venereal ulcer being cured but by mercury, except by eschar-otics. We know however that most gonorrhœas are curable without mercury; and what is still more, without any medical assistance, which I believe is never the case with a chancre. This fact of there being no ulcers was first taught publicly by Dr. Hunter at his lectures in the year 1750, but he did not attempt to account for it.

I. OF THE TIME BETWEEN THE APPLICATION AND EFFECT.

In most diseases there is a certain time between the application of the cause, and the appearance of the effect. In the venereal disease this time is found to vary considerably, owing probably to the state of the constitution when the infection was received. Each form of the disease also varies in this respect; the gonorrhœa and chancre being earlier in their appearance after contamination than the *lues venerea*, and of the two former the gonorrhœa appearing sooner than the chancre. In the gonorrhœa the times of appearance are very different; I have had reason to believe that in some the poison has taken effect in a few hours, while in others it has been six weeks; and I have had examples of it in all the intermediate periods; so far however as we can rely upon the veracity of our patients, and farther evidence we cannot have, six, eight, ten, or twelve days would appear to be the most common period, though it is capable of affecting some people much sooner, and others much later. I was informed by a married gentleman who came from the country and left his wife behind him, that in a frolick he went to a bagnio and had connection with a woman of the town; the next morning he left her, and he had no sooner got to his lodging than he felt a moisture of the part, and upon inspection he found a beginning gonorrhœa, which proved a very troublesome one. I was told by another gentleman, that he had been with a woman over night, and in the morning the gonorrhœa appeared; the same happened to him twice. I was informed by a third gentleman, that the dis-

charge

charge appeared in ſix-and-thirty hours after the application of the poiſon. In the above-mentioned patients the infection muſt have ariſen from the poiſon applied at thoſe ſtated times, as none of them had an opportunity of receiving the infection for many weeks before.

Theſe aſſertions from men of veracity, and where there could be no temptation to deceive, not even an imaginary one, are ſufficient evidences. On the other hand, upon equally good authority, I have been informed that ſix weeks after the application had paſſed, before any ſymptom appeared. The patient had ſtrange and uncommon complaints preceding the running, ſuch as an unuſual ſenſation in the parts, with moſt of the other ſymptoms of gonorrhœa except the diſcharge. He had the ſame complaint about twelve months afterwards, and then it was four weeks from the application of the poiſon before it appeared, giving for ſome part of that time the former diſagreeable ſenſations; but from his late experience he ſuſpected what was coming. From this I am inclined to believe that it ſeldom or never lies perfectly quiet ſo long, and that the inflammatory ſtate may take place for ſome conſiderable time before the ſuppurative; and in theſe caſes there is leſs diſpoſition for a cure, as the very diſpoſition which forms a running is in general a ſalutary one, and is an intermediate ſtep between the diſeaſe, which is the inflammation, and the cure; for in the time of ſuppuration a change has taken place in the veſſels producing the formation of matter. If this change ſhould never take place it is not certain what would be the conſequence; whether the inflammation would go off without ſuppuration, as in many common inflammations, I have not been able to determine, but ſhould ſuſpect that it would continue much longer than uſual, becauſe the parts have not compleated their actions; and I alſo ſuſpect that ſuch caſes always ariſe from ſome peculiarity of conſtitution.

II. OF THE DIFFICULTY OF DISTINGUISHING THE VIRULENT FROM THE SIMPLE GONORRHŒA.

THE ſurface of the urethra is ſubject to inflammation and ſuppuration from various other cauſes beſides the venereal poiſon; and ſometimes diſcharges happen ſpontaneouſly when no immediate cauſe can be aſſigned; ſuch may be

called

called ſimple gonorrhœas, and have nothing of the venereal infection in them; though thoſe that have been formerly ſubject to virulent gonorrhœas are moſt liable to them. It is given as a diſtinguiſhing mark between the ſimple and the virulent gonorrhœa, that the ſimple comes on immediately after copulation, and is at once violent; whereas the virulent comes on ſome days after, and gradually. But the ſimple is not in all caſes a conſequence of a man's having had connection with women, it does not always come on at once, nor is it always free from pain. On the other hand we ſee many venereal gonorrhœas that begin without any appearance of inflammation; and I have been very much at a loſs to determine whether they were venereal or not; for there are a certain claſs of ſymptoms common to almoſt all diſeaſes of the urethra, from which it is difficult to diſtinguiſh the few that ariſe ſolely from the ſpecific affection. I have known the urethra ſympathiſe with the cutting of a tooth[a] producing all the ſymptoms of a gonorrhœa, and this happened ſeveral times in the ſame patient. The urethra is known to be ſometimes the ſeat of the gout.[b] I have known it the ſeat of the rheumatiſm. The urethra of thoſe who have had venereal complaints is more apt to exhibit ſymptoms ſimilar to gonorrhœa, than it is of thoſe who have never had any ſuch complaint; and it is generally in conſequence of the parts having been hurt by that diſeaſe that the ſimple gonorrhœa comes on; which perhaps is alſo a reaſon why they are in ſome meaſure ſimilar. In this complaint a diſcharge and even pain attacks the urethra, and ſtrange ſenſations are every now and then felt in theſe parts, which is either a return of the ſymptoms of the venereal diſeaſe without virus, may ariſe as it were ſpontaneouſly, or may be a conſequence of ſome other diſeaſe. When it is in conſequence of ſome former venereal gonorrhœa it is ſeldom conſtant, and may be called a temporary gleet, ceaſing for a time and then returning; but in ſuch caſes the parts ſeldom ſwell; the glans does not change to the ripe cherry colour, nor does it ſweat a kind of matter. Such a complaint, as a diſcharge without virus is known to exiſt by its coming on when there has been no late connection with women, and likewiſe by its coming on of its own accord where there had never been any former venereal complaint, nor any chance of infection.

[a] Nat. Hiſt. of Teeth, pt. II. p. 126. [b] Eſſays and Obſ. Phyſ. and Liter. of Edin. v. III. p. 425.

From its commonly going off soon, both in those who have had connection with women, and in those who have not, it becomes very difficult in many cases to determine whether it is venereal, for it is often thought venereal when it really is not so; and on the other hand it may be supposed to be only a return of the gleet, when it is truly venereal; but perhaps this is not so material a circumstance as might at first be supposed. These diseases may be considered only as an inconvenience intailed on those who have had the venereal gonorrhœa; no certain cure for them is known; they are similar to the fluor albus in women.

III. OF THE COMMON FINAL INTENTION OF SUPPURATION NOT ANSWERING IN THE PRESENT DISEASE.

When a secreting surface has once received the inflammatory action, it's secretions are increased, and visibly altered; also when the irritation has produced inflammation and an ulcer in the solid parts, a secretion of matter takes place, the intention of which in both seems to be to wash away the irritating matter; so that irritations are endeavouring to produce their own destruction, like a mote in the eye which by increasing the secretion of tears is itself washed away. But in inflammations arising from specific or morbid poisons this effect cannot be produced; for although the first irritating matter be washed away, yet the new matter formed has the same quality with the original; and therefore upon the same principle, it would produce a perpetual succession of irritations, and of course secretions, even if there were no other cause for the continuance than it's own matter. But the venereal inflammation is not kept up by the pus which is formed; but like many other specific diseases, by the specific quality of the inflammation itself. This inflammation however it would appear can only last a limited time; the symptoms peculiar to it vanishing of themselves by the parts becoming less and less susceptible of irritation. This circumstance is not peculiar to this particular form of the venereal disease; it is perhaps common to almost every disease that can affect the human body. From hence it will appear, that the consequent

consequent venereal matter has no power of continuing the original irritation, and indeed if this were not the case there would be no end to the disease.

As the living principle in many diseases is not capable of continuing the same action, it also loses this power in the present, when the disease is in the form of a gonorrhœa, and the effect is at last stopped, the irritation ceasing gradually. This cessation will vary according to circumstances; for if the irritated parts are in a state very susceptible of such irritations, in all probability their actions will be more violent and continued longer; but in all cases the difference must arise from the difference in the constitution, and not from any difference in the poison itself.

The circumstance of the disease ceasing spontaneously, only happens when it attacks a secreting surface, and when a secretion of pus is produced; for when it attacks a non-secreting surface, and produces it's effects there, that is an ulcer; the parts so affected are capable of continuing the disease, or this mode of action, for ever, as will be taken notice of when we shall hereafter consider chancre. But this difference between spontaneous and non-spontaneous cure, seems to depend more on the difference in the two modes of action, than on the difference in the two surfaces; for when the disease produces an ulcer on a secreting surface, which it often does from the constitution, as on the tonsils, it has no disposition to cure of itself; nor in the urethra, in a recent case, if ulcers are formed there, would they heal more readily than when formed any where else.

The common practice proves these facts; we every day see gonorrhœas cured by the most ignorant; but in chancre, or the *lues venerea*, more skill is necessary: the reason is obvious, gonorrhœa cures itself, whilst the other forms of the disease require the assistance of art.

It sometimes happens that the parts which become irritated first, get well, while another part of the same surface receives the irritation, which continues the disease, as happens when it shifts from the glans to the urethra.

From this circumstance of all gonorrhœas ceasing without medical help, I should doubt very much the possibility of a person getting a fresh gonorrhœa while he has that disease; or of his increasing the same by the application of fresh matter of it's own kind; and this observation holds in all the forms of the disease; for it has been proved that the application of the matter

matter from a gonorrhœa to a buboe does not in the leaſt retard the cure of that buboe; nor does the matter of a chancre applied to a buboe, nor the matter of a buboe applied to a chancre, produce any bad effect; though if venereal matter is applied to a common ſore it will often produce the venereal irritation. By all which I am led to believe that the venereal matter formed in a gonorrhœa does not aſſiſt in keeping up that gonorrhœa; for it is only an application of matter whoſe poiſon and effects are exactly ſimilar to the effects upon the ſolids already produced; and that nothing could increaſe or continue the effect but ſomething that is capable of increaſing the diſpoſition of the parts themſelves for ſuch inflammation, or making them more ſuſceptible of it. We find beſides, that a gonorrhœa may be cured while there is a chancre, and vice verſa: now if freſh venereal matter was capable of keeping up the diſeaſe, no gonorrhœa could ever get well, while there is this ſupply of venereal matter.* From all this it is reaſonable to ſuppoſe that ſuch a ſurface of an animal body is not capable of being irritated by it's own matter; nor is it capable of being irritated beyond a certain time; and therefore if freſh venereal matter were continued to be applied to the urethra of a man who had a gonorrhœa, that it would juſt go off as ſoon as if no ſuch application had been made, and get as ſoon well as if great pains had been taken to waſh it's own matter away. The ſame reaſoning holds good in chancres.

I carry this idea ſtill further, and aſſert that the parts become leſs ſuſceptible of the venereal irritation; and that not only a gonorrhœa could not be continued by the application of either it's own or freſh matter; but that a man could not get a freſh gonorrhœa nor a chancre if he applied freſh

* When treating of pus, in my lectures, I obſerved that I was inclined to believe that no matter, of whatever kind, can produce any effect upon the part that formed it: nor do I believe that the matter of any ſore, let it be what it will, ever does or can do any hurt to that ſore; for the parts which formed the matter are of the ſame nature, and cannot be irritated by that which they produced, except extraneous matter is joined with it. The gland which forms the poiſon of the viper, and the duct which conveys it to the tooth, are not irritated by the poiſon: and it would appear from Abbé Fontana's experiments, that the viper cannot be affected by it's own poiſon, Vide Traité ſur le Venin de la Vipere, par M. F. Fontana, vol. 1. page 22. If what I have now advanced is true, wiping, or waſhing away matter under the idea of keeping the parts clean, is in every caſe abſurd.

venereal

venereal matter to the parts when the cure is nearly completed, and continued the application ever after, or at least at such intervals as were within the effect of habit. For I can conceive that in time the parts may become so habituated to this application as to be insensible of it; for by a pretty constant application the parts would never be allowed to forget this irritation, or rather never become unaccustomed to it; and therefore this supply of fresh matter could not affect the parts so as to renew the disease till they first recovered their original and natural state, and then they would be capable of being affected again.

This opinion is not derived from theory only, but is deduced from experience and observation; for we find that a man shall immediately after having a gonorrhœa have frequent connections with women of the town, and that for years, without catching the disease; yet a fresh man shall contract it immediately from the very same woman; and if the first mentioned man was to be out of the habit of this irritation for some time, he then would be as ready to catch it as the other. Where this habit is not so strong as to prevent altogether the parts from being affected, yet it will do it in part; and it is a strong proof of this, that most people have their first gonorrhœa the worst, and the succeeding ones generally become milder and milder till the danger of infection almost vanishes.

The following facts seem to explain this: A married man who had connection only with his wife for several years, afterwards slept with a woman with whom he had formerly cohabited, but not for some time, she gave him a severe gonorrhœa, and declared that she knew nothing of it. He put himself and her under my care; and while they were going on with their cures they still continued to have connection with each other, which I readily allowed. He got well, and it was supposed she got well also; the intercourse was continued between them for many months after, without any mischief received on his side, or any suspicion of remaining disease on hers.

At last this connection was broken off, and she formed another attachment: she no sooner formed this new attachment than she gave her new lover a gonorrhœa; she now flew to me for a cure, and declared that she had no connection but with these two gentlemen; and therefore that the present disease must be the same for which I had attended her formerly. Her second lover was not a patient of mine; but I gave her medicines which she very much neglected taking. Her lover continued his connection, as the first had done, for several months after he had got well, without any further infection from her; but unfortunately her first lover returned about a twelvemonth after, and thinking himself secure, as she lived in peace with the present, had connection with her again, and but once, the consequence however was, a gonorrhœa.

Had the woman the gonorrhœa all this time? And what was the reason of these gentlemen not catching the disease, except after the acquaintance had been interrupted for some time; was it the effect of habit by which the parts lost their susceptibility of that irritation?

The case of a young woman from the Magdalen hospital is a striking proof of this, as far as circumstances can prove a fact. She was received into that house, and continued the usual time, which is two years. The moment she came out she was picked up by one who was in waiting for her with a post-chaise to carry her off immediately; she gave him a gonorrhœa.

This opinion of parts being so habituated to this irritation as hardly to be affected by it, is strengthened by observing, that in the gonorrhœa the violent symptoms shall often cease, and the disease shall still continue, spinning itself out to an amazing length, with no other symptoms than a discharge, yet that discharge shall be venereal; this I have frequently seen: and the following is an abstract of a singular case of this kind.

A gentleman had connection with a woman of the town, and received a venereal gonorrhœa in the beginning of April 1780. He, at first, could hardly believe it to be venereal, as he had kept the woman in the country, where she had scarcely ever been out of his sight; but the violent pain in making water, great running, chordee, and swelled testicle, convinced him that it was venereal. When the cure was going on tolerably well, and he had got the better of one swelled testicle, the other began to swell; however, all the symptoms gradually disappeared, except the chordee, hardness of the epididymis, and a small gleet which was slimy. On the 12th of June he went into the country; while in the country the chordee went off, and

and the hardneſs of the epididymis entirely diſappeared, but ſtill a ſlimy gleet remained, although but trifling.

September the firſt, he married a young lady, and endeavouring to enter the vagina, he found great difficulty, which brought on a return of the chordee, and an increaſed diſcharge. On the 10th, ſhe began to complain of heat, and pain, and of a difficulty and frequency in making water, and when ſhe made water there was forced out ſome matter; ſhe had alſo a dull heavy pain, and a ſenſe of weight at the bottom of her belly, and round her hips, with great ſoreneſs of the parts when ſhe ſat; theſe ſymptoms had been preceded by an itching about the orifice of the vagina.

By taking a mercurial pill, and rubbing the parts with mercurial ointment, in about eight days the violence of the ſymptoms abated; they were now allowed to cohabit, but whenever they came together, the pain which ſhe ſuffered was exceſſive. The parts were waſhed with a ſolution of corroſive ſublimate and ſugar of lead, and anointed with mercurial ointment, which applications being continued for ſome time, the ſoreneſs went off. He was treated medically, and afterwards all was well.

Here was a venereal gonorrhœa contracted about the beginning of April; all the ſymptoms had diſappeared by the firſt of June, and there only remained ſome of the conſequences, ſuch as chordee, hardneſs of the epididymis, and a diſcharge of a little ſlimy mucus, which could only be obſerved in the morning. In a ſhort time the chordee and hardneſs in the epididymis had intirely gone off, and merely the ſmall diſcharge of mucus which appeared only in the morning remained; yet three months after he communicated the diſeaſe to his wife.

I was conſulted in the following caſe by the ſurgeon who attended: July 13th, 1783, a perſon had connection with a woman of the town: the 30th, that is ſeventeen days after, a gonorrhœa came on, which was violent. He took mercurial pills and gentle purges; in twelve days the violent ſymptoms abated, and about the 4th of September the diſcharge was ſtopped. The 9th it began to appear again, but only laſted a few days; and would come and go in this way ſome times every two days; often ſix or ſeven days. On the 28th of September he had connection with his wife, while he had a ſmall diſcharge. The 9th of October he had connection again, and three days after ſhe complained

plained of heat in making water, with a discharge and other symptoms of gonorrhœa which were violent. About the latter end of October her complaints were almost removed; some only of the symptoms appearing and disappearing till January 1784, when he had connection with her to try whether she could give it him, viz. three months after the second connection, and in fourteen days after this he had all the symptoms of a gonorrhœa. April 29th he was not perfectly well, having a discharge with a pain in the perinæum, and she also had a discharge. If this last attack in January 1784, in him was a gonorrhœa, then of course she must have had it; and also of course he must have lost his in the intermediate time, between the 9th of October 1783, and January 1784; for if he had had it also then, it could not have produced any effect upon him.

It was impossible to say whether they had now the infection or not, for any trials upon themselves would prove but little, except one of them only had it so as to infect the other; but if both had it no alteration could take place in either; as it could not be ascertained whether they had the disease or not, and as there were suspicious symptoms in both, when joined with all the circumstances, the attending surgeon and I thought it most prudent to treat them as if actually affected with a gonorrhœa.

If it is true, as is asserted in the voyage round the world, that the venereal disease was carried to Otaheite, it shews that it can be long retained after all ideas of it's existence have ceased; and when it is retained for such a length of time it is most probably in the form of gonorrhœa.*

In like manner, a venereal buboe, if it could be kept a considerable time between the point of suppuration and resolution, would become indolent from habit, continue in that point of suspension, and remain perhaps almost incurable; such I think I have seen.

IV. OF THE VENEREAL GONORRHŒA.

In treating of the seat, extent, and symptoms of gonorrhœa, I shall begin with such particulars as are constant or most frequent, and take them as much

* Vide page 14.

as

as poſſible in the order they become leſs ſo; for there is conſiderable variety in different gonorrhœas.

V. OF THE SEAT OF THE DISEASE IN BOTH SEXES.

The ſeat of this diſeaſe in both ſexes is commonly the parts of generation: in men it is generally the urethra, though it ſometimes takes place on the inſide of the prepuce and ſurface of the glans: in women it is the vagina, urethra, labia, clitoris, or nymphæ.

The diſeaſe has it's ſeat in theſe parts from the manner in which it is caught; but if we were to conſider the ſurface of contact ſimply in men, we ſhould naturally ſuppoſe that the glans penis, or the orifice of the urethra would be the firſt, or indeed the only parts affected; yet moſt commonly they are not; for though there are caſes where the glans is affected, and where the diſeaſe goes no further, I believe it ſeldom attacks the orifice of the urethra, without paſſing ſome way along that canal. How far it ever can be ſaid to affect the prepuce only I am not quite certain, although I believe it ſometimes happens; for I have ſeen inflammation there, as well with as without a diſcharge from the urethra, which appeared to me to be venereal. I have ſeen in ſuch caſes the inflammation extending into the looſe cellular membrane of the prepuce and producing a phymoſis; and this inflammation I ſuſpect to be of the eryſipelatous kind.

When the diſeaſe attacks the glans, and other external parts as the prepuce, it is principally about the root of that body, and the beginning of the prepuce, the parts where the cuticle is thinneſt, and of courſe where the poiſon gets moſt readily to the cutis; but ſometimes it extends over all the glans and alſo the whole external ſurface of the prepuce. It produces there a ſoreneſs or tenderneſs, with a ſecretion of thinniſh matter, commonly without either excoriation or ulceration. I am not certain however, that it does not ſometimes excoriate thoſe parts, for I once ſaw a caſe where almoſt the whole cuticle came off the glans, and the patient aſſured me that it was venereal, for he had been picked up by a woman in the ſtreets a few nights before; he never had had any ſuch complaint from connection with women before that time. Perhaps the disease begins oftener on those parts than is commonly imagined, but the circumstance of their being little susceptible of this kind of irritation, from their having a cuticle, may be the reason why it does not produce a lasting effect, and is often so slight as not to be observed. When the glans or prepuce, or both, take on the venereal inflammation, it often rests there and goes no further, not being attended with a discharge of matter, nor with pain in the urethra, as the following case shews.

A young gentleman from Ireland, slept with a woman at Bristol, and a fortnight after he had intercourse in London with the maid of the house, which last happened to be on a Monday, and on the Tuesday, or the day following; he observed a running from the end of his penis when covered with the prepuce; on the Saturday following he applied to me; on examination I found that the running came from the inside of the prepuce near to the glans, and the *corona glandis*, as also that part of the prepuce behind it, appeared to be in a tender and excoriated state, and covered with matter. He told me he had once had a gonorrhœa before; and upon being asked if it was in the same place, he said it was; not being certain how far this might be venereal, I made the following inquiry; whether he had been subject to such excoriations before he had visited women? and his answer was, that he never had; and that he had not this complaint always after coition, but only twice, as has been above-mentioned, which being uncommon, made him suppose the effect to be venereal.

I suspect that when the prepuce swells in a gonorrhœa of the urethra, producing a phymosis, which is often the case, it arises from the same disease having taken place on it's inside, and that not being sufficient to produce ulceration it goes no further; and that this inflammation is of the erysipelatous kind; a circumstance very necessary to be known in the cure.

The urethra is the part in which this form of the venereal disease is most frequent; and although the inflammation attending the disease in this part has many of the common symptoms of inflammation, yet it can hardly be called such, when moderate; at least it does not constantly produce all the effects of common inflammation, though there is a tendency towards it. The parts seldom have all the characteristic symptoms; for there is no throbbing sensation; there is but little pain, except from the irritation of the urine and distention

diſtention of the parts; the inflammation ſeldom extends deeper than the ſurface, and we have therefore rarely any tumefaction or thickening of the parts. It would rather appear an error loci on the ſurface of the urethra like a blood-ſhot eye.

The ſecretion of pus with ſo little inflammation, is perhaps owing to theſe parts being naturally in a ſtate of ſecretion; therefore the tranſition from an healthy to a diſeaſed ſecretion is more eaſily produced. It ſometimes happens however, that the parts do inflame conſiderably, and the inflammation goes deep into the cellular or rather reticular membrane of the *corpus ſpongioſum urethræ*, eſpecially near the glans. Sometimes it extends further along the *corpus ſpongioſum urethræ*, producing tumefaction, that is, an extravaſation of the coagulable lymph, which is the common cauſe of chordee. It may be obſerved in general, that in moſt caſes when ſuppuration is produced, there is a decreaſe of inflammation. The inflammation in the reticular membrane of the ſurrounding parts would appear not to be always confined to the adheſive ſtage, for in thoſe parts we have ſometimes ſuppurations, eſpecially in the perinæum, which ſuppurations I ſuſpect to be in the glands, as will be taken notice of hereafter.

The gonorrhœa does not always attack urethras otherwiſe ſound, nor does it always attack urethras whoſe relative parts are always ſound. Thus we have people contracting this diſeaſe while they are affected with ſtrictures, ſwelled proſtate gland, as alſo diſeaſed teſticles, or ſuch teſticles as very readily run into diſeaſe; by which the diſeaſe becomes more complicated and requires more attention in the method of cure. Sometimes the diſeaſes are relieved by the gonorrhœa, at other times increaſed.

VI. OF THE MOST COMMON SYMPTOMS, AND THE ORDER OF THEIR APPEARANCE.

ALTHOUGH the irritation muſt always begin firſt, yet it is not certain which of the ſymptoms in conſequence of that irritation will firſt appear; for any one may appear ſingly without the others, though this is rarely the caſe. The firſt ſymptom, when carefully attended to, is generally an itching at the orifice of the urethra; ſometimes extending over the whole glans,* a little fulneſs of the lips of the urethra; the effects of inflammation is next obſervable, and ſoon after a running appears; the itching changes into pain, more particularly at the time of making water; there is often no pain till ſome time after the appearance of the diſcharge, and other ſymptoms; and in many gonorrhœas there is hardly any pain at all, even when the diſcharge is very conſiderable; at other times the pain, or rather a great degree of ſoreneſs will come on long before any diſcharge appears.

There is generally at this time a greater fulneſs in the penis, and more eſpecially in the glans, although it is not near ſo full as when erected, being rather in a ſtate of half erection. Beſides this fulneſs, the glans has a kind of tranſparency, eſpecially near the beginning of the urethra, where the ſkin is diſtended, being ſmooth and red, reſembling a ripe cherry; this is owing to the reticular membrane being loaded with a quantity of extravaſated ſerum, and the veſſels being filled with blood. Near the beginning of the urethra there is in many caſes an evident excoriation, which is marked by the termination of the cuticle all round; the ſurface of the glans alſo is often in an half excoriated ſtate, which gives it a degree of tenderneſs, and there ouſes out from it a kind of matter, as has been before obſerved. The canal of the urethra becomes narrower than uſual, which is known by the ſtream of the urine being ſmaller than common; this proceeds from the fulneſs of the penis in general, and from the internal membrane of the urethra being ſwollen by the inflammation, and alſo from it's being in a ſpaſmodic ſtate.

Beſides theſe changes, the *fear* the patient is in when he is making water aſſiſts in diminiſhing the ſtream of urine. The ſtream, as it flows from the urethra is generally much ſcattered and broken the moment it leaves the paſſage, which is owing to the internal canal having become irregular, and is not peculiar to a venereal gonorrhœa, but common to every diſeaſe of the urethra that alters the exact and natural figure of the canal, even although the irregularity is very far back, as we find in many diſeaſed proſtate glands.

* Theſe ſymptoms are moſt carefully obſerved by thoſe who are under apprehenſions of having the diſeaſe, and therefore are attentive to every little ſenſation about thoſe parts.

There

There is frequently a bleeding from the urethra, which I ſuppoſe ariſes from the diſtention of the veſſels, more eſpecially when there is a chordee, or a tendency to one.

There are often ſmall ſwellings obſervable along the lower ſurface of the penis in the courſe of the urethra. Theſe I ſuſpect are the glands of the urethra ſo enlarged as to be plainly felt on the outſide. They inflame ſo much in ſome caſes as to ſuppurate; and according to the laws of ulceration, the matter is brought to the ſkin, forming one, two, or more abſceſſes along the under ſurface of the urethra, and ſome of theſe breaking internally form what are called internal ulcers. I have obſerved in ſeveral caſes a tumor on the under ſide of the penis where the urethra is, which would ſwell at times very conſiderably, even to the ſize of a ſmall flattened nut, inflame, and then a guſh of matter flowing from the urethra, it would almoſt immediately ſubſide. The diſcharge has continued for ſome time, gradually diminiſhing till it has intirely gone off and the tumor has been almoſt wholly reduced; yet ſome months after it has ſwelled in the ſame manner again, and terminated in the ſame way. How far theſe tumors, and the matter they diſcharge, are really venereal when they appear firſt, may be doubtful; and it is difficult to determine this, from the patients in general having recourſe to medicine immediately; but in their ſubſequent attacks they are certainly not venereal, for they cure themſelves.

I have ſuſpected theſe tumors to be the ducts, or lacunæ of the glands of the urethra diſtended with their mucus from the mouth of the duct being cloſed, in a manner ſimilar to what happens to the duct leading from the lachrymal ſack to the noſe; and in conſequence of the diſtention of the ducts or lacunæ, inflammation and ſuppuration come on, and ulceration takes place, which opens a way into the urethra; but this opening ſoon cloſes up and occaſions a return. Cowper's glands have been ſuſpected to inflame, and hardneſs and ſwelling have been felt externally very much in their ſituation, which coming to ſuppuration have produced conſiderable abſceſſes in the perinæum. Theſe tumors break either internally or externally, and ſometimes in both ways, making a new paſſage for the urine, called fiſtulæ in perinæo.

A ſoreneſs is often felt by the patient all along the under ſide of the penis, owing to the inflamed ſtate of the urethra. This ſoreneſs often extends as far as the anus, and gives great pain, principally in erections; yet it is different from a chordee, the penis remaining ſtraight.

With moſt gonorrhœas there is a frequency in the erections, ariſing from the irritation at the time, which often approach to a priapiſm, eſpecially when there is the above-mentioned ſoreneſs, or when there is a chordee. Thoſe erections take place independent of the mind: they have been called involuntary; but all erections are involuntary. No man can will an erection.

Priapiſms often threaten mortification in men; and I have ſeen an inſtance of it in a dog. The erection never ſubſided, and the penis could not be covered by the prepuce, from the ſwelling of the bulb. The penis mortified and dropped off; and as a dog has a bone in the penis, this was denuded, and an exfoliation took place. As opium is of great ſervice in priapiſm, there is reaſon to ſuppoſe the complaint is of a ſpaſmodic nature.

VII. OF THE DISCHARGE.

The natural ſlimy diſcharge from the glands of the urethra is firſt changed from a fine tranſparent ropy ſecretion to a watery, whitiſh fluid; and the natural exhaling fluid of the urethra, which is intended for moiſtning that ſurface, and which appears to be of the ſame kind with that which lubricates cavities in general, becomes leſs tranſparent; and both theſe ſecretions becoming gradually thicker, aſſume more and more the qualities of common pus. In ſome caſes of gonorrhœa, the glands that produce the ſlime which is ſecreted in conſequence of laſcivious ideas, are certainly not affected; for I have ſeen caſes, when after the paſſages had been cleared of the venereal matter by making water, the pure ſlime has flowed out of the end of the penis, on theſe ideas taking place. When this matter is more in quantity than what lubricates the urethra, it is forced

forced out at the orifice by the periſtaltic action of that canal, and appears externally.[*]

The matter of gonorrhœa often changes its colour and conſiſtence, which is owing to the diſpoſition of the parts which form it; ſometimes from a white to a yellow, and often to a greeniſh colour. Theſe changes depend on the increaſe or decreaſe of the inflammation, and not on the poiſonous quality of the matter itſelf; for any irritation on theſe parts, equal to that produced in a gonorrhœa, will produce the ſame appearances; and the changes in the colour of the matter are chiefly obſervable after it has been diſcharged upon a cloth, and become dry. The appearance upon the cloth is of various hues; in the middle the matter is thicker or more in quantity, and it is therefore generally of a deeper colour; the circumference is paler, becauſe the watery or ſerous part of the matter has ſpread further, and at the outer edge of all it is darkeſt; this laſt appearance is owing to it's being only water with a little ſlime, in which ſome of the tinge is ſuſpended, which when dry gives a tranſparency to the part, that takes off from the white colour of the linen. It is very probable there is a ſmall extravaſation of red blood in all the caſes where the matter deviates from the common colour, and to this the different tinges ſeem to be owing. As this matter ariſes from a ſpecific inflammation, it has a greater tendency to putrefaction than common matter from a healthy ſore, and has often a ſmell ſeemingly peculiar to itſelf.

As it would appear that there is hardly a ſufficient ſurface of the urethra inflamed to give the quantity of matter that is often produced, eſpecially when we conſider that the inflammation does in common go no further than two or three inches from the external orifice, it is natural to ſuppoſe that the diſcharge is produced from other parts, the office of which it is to form mucus for natural purpoſes, and are therefore more capable of producing a great quantity upon ſlight irritations, which hardly riſe to inflammation. Theſe parts I have obſerved, are the glands of the urethra. In many caſes

[*] That the urethra has conſiderable powers of action, is evident in a vaſt number of inſtances, and that action is principally from behind forwards. We find that a bougie may be worked out by the action of the urethra. This action I believe is often inverted, as in ſpaſmodic ſtranguries.

where

where the glands have not been after death ſo much ſwelled as to be felt externally; and where I have had an opportunity of examining the urethra of thoſe who have had this complaint upon them, I have always been able to diſcover, that the ducts or lacunæ leading from them were loaded with matter, and were more viſible than in their natural ſtate; I have obſerved too, that the formation of the matter is not confined to theſe glands intirely, for the inner ſurface of the urethra is commonly in ſuch a ſtate as not to be able to ſuffer the urine to paſs without giving conſiderable pain, and therefore moſt probably this internal membrane is alſo affected in ſuch a manner as to ſecrete a matter.

This diſcharge in common caſes would ſeem not to ariſe much further back in the urethra than where the pain is felt, although it is commonly believed that it comes from the whole of the canal, and even from Cowper's and the proſtate glands, not excepting what are called the veſiculæ ſeminales.* But the truth of this I very much doubt. My reaſons for ſuppoſing that it comes only from the ſurface where the pain is, are the following. If the matter aroſe from the whole ſurface of the urethra, and from the glands near the bladder, we ſhould certainly have many other ſymptoms which we have not; for inſtance, if all the parts of the urethra beyond the bulb, or even in the bulb, were affected ſo as to ſecrete matter, that matter would be gradually ſqueezed into the bulb as the ſemen is, and from thence it would be thrown out by jerks; for we know that nothing can be in the bulbous part of the urethra, without ſtimulating it to action, eſpecially when in a ſtate of irritation and inflammation; in ſuch a ſtate we find that even a drop of urine is not allowed to reſt there; and alſo if an injection of warm water only is thrown into the urethra as far as the bulb, the *muſculi acceleratores* are uneaſy till they act, and throw it out. Hence it is natural to ſuppoſe that, if the membranous and bulbous part of the urethra, with the veſiculæ ſeminales, proſtate and Cowper's glands, aſſiſted in forming the matter, whenever it collected in the bulb it would probably be immediately

* Thoſe bags are certainly not reſervoirs for the ſemen. The difference between their contents and the ſemen gave me the firſt ſuſpicion of this; and from ſeveral experiments on the human body, as alſo a comparative view of them in other animals, I have been able to prove that they are not.

thrown

thrown forwards by the muſcles above-mentioned, and we ſhould be ſenſible of it every moment of the day. But ſuch ſymptoms ſeldom happen, ſometimes indeed a ſpaſmodic contraction of theſe muſcles takes place, which may probably ariſe from this cauſe, though it is more frequently felt immediately after making water.

When the inflammation is violent, it often happens that ſome of the veſſels of the urethra burſt, and a diſcharge of blood enſues, which is in greater quantity at the cloſe of making water; this however takes place at other times, and generally gives temporary eaſe: ſometimes this blood is in ſmall quantity, and only gives the matter a tinge, as I obſerved when treating of the colour of the diſcharge. The erections of the penis often ſtretch the part ſo much as to become a cauſe of an extravaſation of blood; his extravaſation generally increaſes the ſoreneſs at the time of making water, and in ſuch a ſtate of parts the urethra is uſually ſore when preſſed, yet the bleeding diminiſhes the inflammation, and often gives eaſe.

VIII. OF THE CHORDEE.

THE chordee appears to be *inflammatory* in ſome caſes, and *ſpaſmodic* in others; we ſhall treat firſt of the inflammatory.

When the inflammation is not confined merely to the ſurface of the urethra and it's glands, but goes deeper and affects the reticular membrane, it produces in it an extravaſation of coagulable lymph, as in the adheſive inflammation, which uniting the cells together, deſtroys the power of diſtention of the *corpus ſpongioſum urethræ*, and makes it unequal in this reſpect to the *corpora cavernoſa penis*, and therefore a curvature on that ſide takes place in the time of erection, which is called a chordee. The curvature is generally in the lower part of the penis, ariſing from the cells of the corpus cavernoſum penis of that ſide, having their ſides united by adheſions, ſometimes as it were ſpontaneouſly, at other times in conſequence of the inflammation attending bad chancres. Beſides this effect of inflammation, when the chordee is violent the inner membrane is I ſuppoſe ſo much upon the ſtretch, as to be in ſome degree torn, which frequently cauſes a profuſe bleeding from the urethra that often relieves, and even sometimes cures. As chordee arises from a greater degree of inflammation than common, it is an effect which may and often does remain after all infection is gone, being merely a consequence of the adhesive inflammation.

The spasmodic chordee arises from spasm, at least it cannot proceed from the same cause with the other, if my idea of that complaint be well founded. The spasmodic comes and goes, but at no stated times; at one time there will be an erection entirely free from it, at another it will be severely felt, and this will often happen at short intervals.

IX. OF THE MANNER IN WHICH THE INFLAMMATION ATTACKS THE URETHRA.

In what manner the disease extends itself to the urethra, is a question not yet absolutely determined; I suspect that it is communicated, or creeps along from the glans to the urethra, or at least from the beginning or lips of the urethra to it's inner surface; because it is impossible to conceive, that any of the venereal matter from the woman can get into the canal in the time of coition, although this is commonly believed and asserted; it is impossible at least that it can get so far as the common seat of the disease, or into those parts of the urethra where it very often exists, that is, through the whole length of the canal. The following case amounts almost to a proof of this opinion.

A gentleman, on whose veracity I have an entire confidence, when in Germany, where he had not lain with a woman for many weeks, was in a necessary-house and sat there some time; upon arising he found something that seemed to give the glans penis a little sharp pull, and he found a small bit of the plaister of the necessary-house sticking to it. He paid no further attention to it at that time than merely to remove what stuck to his penis; but five or six days after, he observed the symptoms of a clap, which proved a pretty severe one. The only way of accounting for this is, that some person who had a clap had been there before him, and had left some venereal matter

matter upon this place, and that the penis had remained in contact with it a sufficient time for the matter to dry.

When the disease attacks the urethra it seldom extends further than an inch and an half, or two inches at most, within the orifice, which distance appears to be truly specific, and what I have called the specific extent of the inflammation.*

As the cause of a gonorrhœa is commonly an inflammation, it is accompanied with pain and the formation of matter; in such a state neither the sensations of the patient, nor the actions of the parts themselves are confined to the real seat of the disease. In consequence of the neighbouring parts sympathising, a variety of symptoms are produced, many of which do not exceed what might arise from an irritable state; an uneasiness partaking of soreness and pain, and a kind of weariness, is every where felt about the pelvis: the scrotum, testicles, perinæum, anus and hips, become disagreeably sensible to the patient; and the testicles often require being suspended; and so irritable are they indeed in such cases, that the least accident or even exercise which would have no such effect at another time, will make them swell. The glands of the groin are often affected sympathetically, and will even swell a little, but do not come to suppuration: when they inflame from the absorption of matter they in general suppurate. I have seen cases where the irritation has extended so far as to affect with real pain the thighs, the buttocks, and the abdominal muscles, so that the patient has been obliged to lie quiet in an horizontal position; the pain has at times been so considerable as to make him cry out, and the parts have been very sore to the touch; they have even swelled, but the swelling has not been of the inflammatory kind; for though there was a visible fulness, yet the parts were rather soft. I knew one gentleman who never had a gonorrhœa, but that he was immediately seized universally with rheumatic pains, and this had happened several times. The blood at such times is generally free

* It is to be here remarked, that specific diseases, among which I shall reckon such as arise from morbid poisons, have their specific distance or extent as one of their properties; but this can only take place where the constitution is not susceptible of erysipelas, or any other uncommon mode of action; for where there is an erysipelatous disposition no bounds are set to the inflammation.

from

from the inflammatory appearance, and therefore we may suppose that the constitution is but little affected.

When the gonorrhœa (exclusive of the affections arising from sympathy) is not more violent than I have described, it may be called *common* or *simple venereal* gonorrhœa; but if the patient is very susceptible of such irritation, or of any other mode of action which may accompany the venereal, then the symptoms are in proportion more violent. In such circumstances we sometimes find the irritation and inflammation exceed the specific distance, and extend through the whole of the urethra. There is often also a considerable degree of pain in the perinæum, and a frequent, though not a constant, symptom is a spasmodic contraction of the acceleratores urinæ, which is always attended with contractions of the erectores muscles. Whether these spasms arise from a secretion of matter, which being collected in the bulbous part of the urethra produces uneasiness, and excites contractions in order to its own expulsion, like the last drops of urine, I have not been able to determine. I have seen such spasms in the time of making water, from the urine irritating the parts in it's passage through the urethra, and throwing the *musculi acceleratores* into contractions, so that the water came by jerks. This kind of inflammation sometimes is considerable, goes deep into the cellular membrane, and produces tumefaction without any other effect. In other cases it goes on to suppuration, often becoming one of the causes of fistulæ in perinæo. I have sometimes, as I have already observed, suspected Cowper's glands to be the seat of such suppurations; for I have observed externally, circumscribed swellings in the situation of those glands. The small glands likewise of the bulbous part of the urethra may be affected in a similar manner; and the irritation is often extended even to the bladder itself.

When the bladder is affected it becomes more susceptible of every kind of irritation, so that very disagreeable symptoms are often produced; it will not allow of the usual distention, and therefore the patient cannot retain his water the ordinary time, and the moment the desire of making water takes place, he is obliged instantly to make it with violent pain in the bladder, and still more in the glans penis, exactly similar to what happens in a fit of the stone. If the bladder be not allowed to discharge it's contents immediately, the pain becomes almost intolerable; and even when the water is evacuated

evacuated there remains for some time a considerable pain, both in the bladder and glans; because the very action of the muscular coat of the bladder becomes a cause of pain by it's own contraction.

The ureters, and even the kidnies sometimes sympathise, when the bladder is either very much inflamed, or under a considerable degree of irritation; however this but rarely happens; and if it should take place with any degree of violence, I should suppose that the stomach would also become affected, and of course the whole constitution. I have even reason to suspect that the irritation may be communicated to the peritonæum by means of the vas deferens; the following case appears to have been an instance of this. A gentleman had a gonorrhœa which was treated in the antiphlogistic way; the discharge in some degree stopped, a tension came upon the lower part of the belly on the right side just above Poupart's ligament, but rather nearer to the ilium; there was hardness and soreness to the touch, this soreness spread over the whole belly, producing rigors every third day, with a low pulse, which to me indicated a peritonæal inflammation, arising, in my opinion, from the vas deferens of that side being affected in it's course through the belly and pelvis.

When the inflammation, or perhaps only the irritation, runs along the whole surface of the urethra, attacks the bladder, and even extends to the ureters and the kidnies so as to cause a disagreeable sensation in all these parts, the disease is generally very violent, and I suspect is something of the erisypelatous kind; at least it shows an irritable sympathising habit.

This disease sometimes produces very uncommon symptoms: A gentleman had a gonorrhœa, and when the inflammatory symptoms were abating the urethra lost both the involuntary and voluntary powers of retaining the urine: his water came away involuntarily, nor could he stop it: I advised him to do nothing, and to wait for some time, as probably the method of cure might be more disagreeable than the disease itself, although it was very troublesome to him when in company. The complaint gradually lessened, and in time went entirely off. If I had recommended any medicine it would have been the tincture of cantharides.

X. OF THE SWELLED TESTICLE.

A very common symptom attending gonorrhœa is a swelling of the testicle. This I believe like the affection of the bladder, and many of the symptoms mentioned before, is only sympathetical, and not to be reckoned venereal, because the same symptoms follow every kind of irritation on the urethra, whether produced by strictures, injections, or bougies. It may be observed here, that those symptoms are not similar to the actions arising from the application of the true venereal matter, whether by absorption or otherwise; for they seldom or ever suppurate, and when suppuration happens the matter produced is not venereal.

The testicles seem as it were in many cases rather to be acting for the urethra, than for themselves, thus the swelling and inflammation appears suddenly, and as suddenly disappears, or in a few minutes goes from one testicle to the other; the affection depending upon the state of the urethra, and not at all upon the part itself. A part however of the testicle, the epididymis, assumes all the characters of inflammation, remaining swelled even for a considerable time after the inflammation has subsided.

The first appearance of swelling in the testicle is generally a soft pulpy fulness of the body of the testicle, which is tender to the touch; this increases to a hard swelling, accompanied with considerable pain. The hardest part is generally the epididymis, and principally that portion of it which is at the lower end of the testicle, as may be distinctly felt; the hardness and swelling however often run the whole length of that body, and form a knob at the upper part. The spermatic chord is likewise often affected, and more especially the vas deferens, which is thickened, and sore to the touch. The veins of the testicle sometimes become varicose. I have seen such a state of veins accompany a swelling of the testicle in two instances. A pain in the small of the back generally attends inflammations of the testicles of all kinds, with a sense of weakness of the loins and pelvis. The bowels generally sympathise with most complaints of the testicle, in some by cholicky pains, in others by an uncommon sensation both in the stomach and intestines: sickness is a common symptom, and even vomiting; the powers

of

of digestion by this means are impaired, and a disposition for the accumulation of air takes place which is often very troublesome. Here we have from the testicles a chain of sympathies, as we had in consequence of the irritation running along the whole urinary passages; first the testicle is affected from the urethra, then the spermatic chord, the loins, intestines, stomach, and from thence in some measure the whole body.

In a case of swelled testicle I have known the buttocks swell, but the swelling was not of the inflammatory kind, and in making water pain was felt there. Whether this symptom arose from the swelling of the testicle, or from the same common cause, that is the gonorrhœa, is not easily determined; although the latter supposition is the most probable.

It has been asserted, but without proof, that in cases of swelled testicles in consequence of a gonorrhœa, it is not the testicle that swells, but the epididymis. The truth is, it is both the one and the other. Any man that is accustomed to distinguish between a swelling of the whole testicle, and that of the epididymis only, will immediately be sensible, that in the *hernia humoralis* the whole testicle is swelled; the testicle assumes the same shape that it does from other causes, where we know from being obliged to remove it, that the whole has swelled. The pain is in every part of the testicle. I have seen such swellings suppurate on the fore part, and have known several instances of adhesions between the tunica albuginea and vaginalis from such causes: this has only been discovered after death, or in the operation for a partial hydrocele; such changes could not have taken place if the body of the testicle had not been in a state of inflammation. This inflammation of the testicle most probably arises from it's sympathising with the urethra, and in many cases it would appear to arise from what is understood by a translation of the irritation from the urethra to the testicle: thus a swelling of the testicle coming on shall remove the pain in making water, and suspend the discharge; which shall not return till the swelling of the testicle begin to subside; or the irritation in the urethra first ceasing shall produce a swelling of the testicle, which shall continue till the pain and discharge return; thus rendering it doubtful, which is cause and which is effect. I have nevertheless known cases where the testicle has swelled, and yet the discharge become more violent; nay I have seen instances where a swelling has come on after the

the difcharge had ceafed, yet the difcharge has returned with violence, and remained as long as the fwelling of the tefticle. Sometimes the epididymis only is affected, fometimes the vas deferens, and at other times only the fpermatic chord, producing varicofe veins; no reafon can be affigned why one of thefe parts is affected more than another, and indeed the immediate caufe in all is yet unknown. For although an action in the urethra is the remote caufe, yet it is ftill impoffible to fay whether it be the ceffation of that action that is the caufe of the fwelling in the tefticle, or the fwelling in the tefticle the caufe of the ceffation. It is defcribed as arifing from an irritation taking place in the mouths of the vafa deferentia, were this the caufe it ought in general to affect both tefticles at the fame time; but I have feen this complaint happen as often where the inflammation went no further back in the urethra than about an inch and a half, or two inches, as where it has extended further; and the fwelling fhifting fuddenly from one tefticle to the other, fhews it to arife from fome other principle in the animal œconomy.

A ftrangury often attends fuch cafes of fympathy, and more frequently when the running ftops, than when that difcharge is continued along with the fwelling of the tefticle; indeed any fudden ftopping of the difcharge gives a tendency to a ftrangury.

As fingular a circumftance as any refpecting the fwelling of the tefticle is, that it does not always come on when the inflammation in the urethra is at the height: I think it oftener happens when the irritation in the urethra is going off, and fometimes even after it has entirely ceafed, and when the patient conceives himfelf to be quite well.

I may be allowed to remark, that fwellings in the tefticle in confequence of venereal irritation in the urethra, fubject it to a fufpicion that every fwelling of this part is venereal: but from what I have faid of it's nature when it arifes from a venereal caufe, which was that it is owing to fympathy only, and from what I fhall now fay, that it is never affected with the venereal difeafe either local or conftitutional, as far as my obfervation goes, we muft infer that fuch fufpicions are always ill-founded; this perhaps is an inference to which few will fubfcribe.

I have known the gout produce a fwelling in the tefticle of the inflammatory kind, and therefore fimilar to the fympathetic fwelling from a venereal

caufe,

caufe, having many of it's characters. Injuries done to the tefticle produce fwellings, but they are different from thofe above-mentioned, being more permanent, having the difeafe or caufe in the part itfelf. Cancers and the fcrofula produce fwellings of the tefticle, but thefe are generally flow in their progrefs, and not at all fimilar to thofe arifing from an irritation in the urethra.

XI. OF THE SWELLINGS OF THE GLANDS FROM SYMPATHY.

SINCE our knowledge of the manner in which fubftances get into the circulation, and our having learned that many fubftances efpecially poifons, in their courfe to the circulation, irritate the abforbent glands to inflammation and tumefaction, we might naturally fuppofe fuch fwellings, accompanying complaints in the urethra attended with a difcharge, to be owing to the abforption of that matter, and therefore if it be a venereal difcharge, that they muft alfo be venereal. But we muft not be too hafty in drawing this conclufion; for we know that the glands will fometimes fwell from an irritation at the origin of the lymphatics, where no abforption could poffibly have taken place. They often fwell and become painful upon the commencement of inflammation, before any fuppuration has taken place, and fubfide upon the coming on of fuppuration; becaufe when the fuppuration begins, the inflammation abates. I have known a prick in the finger with a clean fewing needle, produce a red ftreak all up the fore-arm, pain along the infide of the biceps mufcle, a fwelling of the lymphatic gland above the inner condyle of the humerus, and alfo of the glands of the arm-pit, immediately followed by ficknefs and a rigor, all of which however foon went off. As it would therefore appear, that the abforbent fyftem is capable of being affected as well by irritation, as by the abforption of matter, in all difeafes of this fyftem arifing from local injuries attended with matter, one muft always have thefe two caufes in view, and endeavour if poffible to diftinguifh from which the prefent affection proceeds. For in thofe arifing from an irritated furface in confequence of poifon, efpecially the venereal, it is of confiderable confequence to be able to ſay from which of the two it ariſes; ſince it ſometimes happens, although but ſeldom, that the glands of the groin are affected in a common gonorrhœa with the appearance of beginning buboes, but which I ſuſpect to be ſimilar to the ſwelling of the teſticle, that is, merely ſympathetic; the pain they give is but very trifling, when compared to that of true venereal ſwellings ariſing from the abſorption of matter; and they ſeldom ſuppurate; however there are ſwellings of theſe glands from actual abſorption of matter in gonorrhœa, and which conſequently are truly venereal; and as it is poſſible to have ſuch they are always to be ſuſpected. As they have ſometimes ariſen upon a ceſſation of the irritation in the urethra, ſimilar to the ſwelling of the teſticle, it has been ſuppoſed that the matter was driven as it were into them by unſkilful treatment. From our knowledge of the abſorbing ſyſtem, we know that the matter can go that way; but we alſo know that we have no method of driving it that way; and if we had, there is no reaſon why more ſhould not be formed in the urethra; this therefore does not account for the ceſſation of ſecretion of matter in that part.

It is difficult to ſay, what is the nature of thoſe ſympathetic diſeaſes. They are not venereal, for they ſubſide by the common treatment of inflammation without the uſe of mercury; and I have known an inſtance of a ſwelled teſticle from a venereal gonorrhœa, that ſuppurated, and was treated by my advice as a common ſuppuration, and healed without a grain of mercury being given. Neither can they be called truly inflammatory, having rarely any of the true characters of inflammation, ſuch as thickening of the parts, ſymptomatic fever, or ſizy blood, except in ſwellings of the teſticle and glands. The ſwelling of the teſticle has ſeveral peculiarities attending it; it is often very quick in its increaſe, and not being of the true inflammatory diſpoſition, it requires leſs time for the removal of the inflammation; but even where it appears to have more of the true inflammatory action, we find that the removal of the inflammation and tumefaction take place more rapidly than when proceeding from other cauſes. A ſwelled teſticle in conſequence of the radical cure in the hydrocele does not ſubſide after inflammation is gone, in as many weeks; as the ſwelled teſticle in conſequence of its ſympathy with other parts, does in days; and probably the reaſon of this is, that it ariſes from ſympathy; for an inflammation ariſing from real diſeaſe

in

in a part, or from an external injury, as in the hydrocele, must always last either till the disease be removed, or the injury repaired; but that from sympathy will vary as the cause varies, which may happen very quickly; for we find a testicle swell in a few minutes, and in as little time subside; and also the swelling move suddenly from one testicle to the other. These sympathies are often peculiar to constitutions, and even to temporary constitutions, in so much as to be in some degree epidemic; for there is often such an influence in the atmosphere as predisposes the body to this kind of irritation; and bodies so predisposed require only the immediate cause to produce the effect.

XII. OF THE DISEASES OF THE LYMPHATICS IN A GONORRHŒA.

Another symptom which sometimes takes place in gonorrhœa, is a hard chord leading from the prepuce, along the back of the penis, and often directing its course to one of the groins, and affecting the glands; there is most commonly a swelling in the prepuce at the part where the chord takes it's rise. This happens sometimes when there is an excoriation, and discharge from the prepuce or glans, which may be called a venereal gonorrhœa of these parts. Both the swelling in the groin, and the hard chord, we have reason to suppose arise from the absorption of pus, and therefore are the first steps towards a lues venerea; but as that form of the disease seldom happens from a gonorrhœa, I shall not take any further notice of it in this place; however, I may remark, that from this observation of the lues venerea being seldom produced from a gonorrhœa, it would appear that a whole surface, or one only inflamed, does not readily admit of the absorption of the venereal poison; and therefore although the venereal matter lies for many weeks in the passage, and over the whole glans, it seldom happens that any absorption takes place. I have seen a case where blood has been discharged from the urethra, and the above symptoms have come on, and I at first suspected that the absorption had taken place where the vessel gave way; but as this symptom rarely happens, even where there has

has been a confiderable difcharge of blood, I am inclined to think that wounds are alfo bad abforbing furfaces, efpecially when I confider that few morbid poifons are abforbed from wounds.

XIII. SHORT RECAPITULATION OF THE VARIETIES IN THE SYMPTOMS.

FROM what has been advanced above, it muft appear that the variety of fymptoms in gonorrhœa, and their difference in different cafes, are almoft endlefs. I fhall now recapitulate a few of the moft material or common varieties. The difcharge often appears without any pain, and the coming on of the pain is not at any ftated time after the appearance of the difcharge. There is often no pain at all, although the difcharge be confiderable in quantity, and of a bad appearance; the pain often goes off, while the difcharge continues, and will fometimes return again. An itching in fome cafes is felt for a confiderable time, which fometimes is fucceeded by pain; though in many cafes it continues to the end of the difeafe: on the other hand, the pain is often troublefome, and confiderable even when the difcharge is trifling or none at all. In general the inflammation in the urethra does not extend beyond an inch or two from the orifice; fometimes it runs all along the urethra to the bladder, and even to the kidnies, and in fome cafes fpreads into the fubftance of the urethra, producing a chordee. The glands of the urethra inflame, and often fuppurate; and I fufpect that Cowper's glands fometimes do the fame. The neighbouring parts fympathife, as the glands of the groin, the tefticle, the loins, and pubes, with the upper parts of the thighs and abdominal mufcles. Sometimes the difeafe appears foon after the application of the poifon, as in a few hours, at other times not till after fix weeks. It is often not poffible to determine whether it is venereal, or only an accidental difcharge arifing from fome unknown caufe.

It may not be improper to mention here, that I have feen a chancre on the prepuce produce a pain in the urethra in making water; which moft probably depended upon a fympathy fimilar to that by which the application of venereal matter to the glans produces a difcharge from the urethra, as was obferved above.

above. If the application of venereal matter to the glans can produce a discharge from the urethra, it is possible that any acrid matter, though not venereal may have a similar effect. The discharge from the vagina in cases of what is called fluor albus is sometimes extremely irritating, in so much as to excoriate the labiæ and thighs; and the following history shews that it may sometimes produce effects similar to venereal matter.

Mr. and Mrs. ——— have been married these twenty years and upwards; she has for many years past been at times troubled with the *fluor albus*. When he has connection with her at such times, it generally, although not always, produces an excoriation of the glans and prepuce, and a considerable discharge from the urethra, attended with a slight pain. These symptoms commonly take a considerable time to go off, whether treated as a gonorrhœa or as a weakness. Is this a new poison? And does it go no further because the connection takes place only between two? What would be the consequence, if she were to have connection with other men, and these with other women? Such cases, as far as I have seen have only been in form of a gonorrhœa, they have not produced sores in the parts; nor as far as I know do they ever produce constitutional diseases.

CHAPTER II.

OF THE GONORRHOEA IN WOMEN.

THE venereal diſeaſe in the form of gonorrhœa in women, is not ſo complicated as in men; the parts affected are more ſimple, and fewer in number. But it is not ſo eaſily known in them as it is in men, becauſe the parts commonly affected in women are very ſubject to a diſeaſe reſembling the gonorrhœa, called *fluor albus*; and the diſtinguiſhing marks, if there are any, have not yet been completely aſcertained. A diſcharge ſimply from theſe parts in women, is leſs a proof of the exiſtence of the venereal infection than even a diſcharge without pain in men; therefore in general little or no attention is paid to it by the patient herſelf, and we often find the venereal virus formed in thoſe parts without any increaſe of the natural diſcharge. The kind of matter gives us no aſſiſtance in diſtinguiſhing the two diſeaſes; for it often happens that the diſcharge in the fluor albus puts on all the appearances of the venereal matter; and an increaſe of the diſcharge is no better mark by which we can diſtinguiſh the one from the other. Pain or any peculiarity in the ſenſations of the parts, is not a neceſſary attendant upon this complaint in women, therefore not to be looked for as a diſtinguiſhing ſymptom.

The appearances of the parts often give us but little information, for I have frequently examined the parts of thoſe who confeſſed all the ſymptoms; ſuch as increaſe of diſcharge, pain in making water, ſoreneſs in walking, or when they were touched, yet I could ſee no difference between theſe and ſound parts. I know of no other way of judging in caſes where there are no ſymptoms ſenſible to the perſon herſelf, or where the patient has a mind to deny having any uncommon ſymptoms, but from the circumſtances preceding the diſcharge; ſuch as her having been connected with men ſuppoſed to be unſound, or her being able to give it to others; which laſt circumſtance being derived from the teſtimony of another perſon, is not always to be truſted

to,

for very obvious reaſons. Thus a woman may have this ſpecies of the venereal diſeaſe without knowing it herſelf, or without the ſurgeon being able to diſcover it, even on inſpection. It may appear very ſtrange, that a diſeaſe which is ſo violent and well marked in men ſhould be ſo obſcure in women: but when we conſider that this poiſon generally produces ſymptoms according to the nature of the parts affected by it; it becomes an eaſy matter to account in ſome meaſure for this difference.

When we attend to the manner in which this diſeaſe is contracted by women, it is evident that it muſt principally attack the vagina, a part that is not endowed with much ſenſation, or action of any kind. While it is confined to the vagina it may be compared to the ſame diſeaſe on the glans penis in men. In many caſes however it extends much further, and becomes the cauſe of diſagreeable feelings, producing a conſiderable ſoreneſs in all the parts formed for ſenſation, ſuch as the inſide of the labia, nymphæ, clitoris, carunculæ myrtiformes, the orifice of the meatus urinarius, and often affecting that canal in its whole length. Thoſe parts are ſo ſore in ſome caſes, as not to bear being touched; the perſon can hardly walk; the urine gives pain in it's paſſage through the urethra, and when it waſhes the abovementioned parts, which can hardly be avoided; ſuch ſymptoms are not much encreaſed at one time more than another, excepting at the time of making water, and then principally in thoſe who have the urethra affected; for as theſe parts are leſs expoſed to circumſtances of change, the increaſed irritation ariſing from ſuch change of parts muſt neceſſarily in this ſex be leſs; but in men the urethra, which is the part moſt commonly affected, has great ſenſibility, is capable of violent inflammation, is often diſtended with a ſtimulating fluid, and the body of the penis, urethra, and glans, ſtretching the paſſage with erections, always produce an increaſe of the ſymptoms, eſpecially of the pain.

But as this diſeaſe frequently attacks parts more ſenſible than the vagina, and which are more ſuſceptible of inflammation, as has been obſerved, under ſuch circumſtances women have nearly the ſame ſymptoms as men; a fulneſs about the parts, almoſt like an inflamed tonſil, a diſcharge from the urethra, violent pain in making water, and great uneaſineſs in ſitting from preſſure on thoſe parts.

The

The bladder ſometimes ſympathiſes, producing the ſame ſymptoms as in men, and it is probable that the irritation may be communicated even to the kidnies. It has been aſſerted that the ovaria are ſometimes affected in a ſimilar manner to the teſticles in men: I have never ſeen a caſe of this kind, and I ſhould very much doubt it's exiſtence; for we have no inſtance in other diſeaſes of the ovaria ſympathiſing with thoſe parts, or at leaſt producing ſuch ſymptoms as would enable us to determine that they did. That there are however uncommon ſymptoms every now and then taking place, would appear from the following caſe.

A lady had all the ſymptoms of a venereal gonorrhœa, ſuch as a diſcharge, pain and frequency in making water, or rather a continued inclination to void it, and a heavineſs approaching to pain about the hips and loins. The uncommon ſymptom in this caſe, was great flatulence in the ſtomach and bowels; this laſt ſymptom was moſt probably a ſympathy with the uterus: there may poſſibly be ſympathies therefore with the ovaria.

The inflammation frequently goes deeper than the ſurface of the parts; often running along the ducts of the glands, and affecting the glands themſelves ſo as to produce hard ſwellings under the ſurface on the inſide of the labia, which ſometimes ſuppurate, forming ſmall abſceſſes, opening near the orifice of the vagina. Theſe are ſimilar to the inflammations and ſuppurations of the glands of the urethra in men. The different ſurface or parts which the diſeaſe attacks, make no diſtinction in the diſeaſe itſelf: it is immaterial whether it is a large or ſmall ſurface, it only ſhows that in one caſe the parts are more ſuſceptible of this irritation than in another, yet it may make the method of cure more complicated.

It ſometimes happens, that the venereal matter from the vagina runs down the perinæum to the anus, producing a gonorrhœa or chancres there.

How far the gonorrhœa in women is capable of wearing itſelf out, as in men, I cannot abſolutely determine; but am much inclined to believe that it would; for I have known many women who have got rid of a violent gonorrhœa without uſing any means to cure it; and indeed the great variety of methods of cure made uſe of in ſuch caſes, all of which cannot poſſibly do good, though the patients get well, ſeems to confirm this opinion. One circumſtance which appears as curious as any, is the ſeeming continuance of of the diſeaſe in the vagina for years; at leaſt we have reaſon to believe this, as far as the teſtimony of the patient can be relied on; and this long continuance of it, without being cured, or tiring itſelf out as it does in men, is probably owing to it's being leſs violent in the vagina.

I. OF THE PROOFS OF A WOMAN HAVING THIS COMPLAINT.

It may be aſked, what proof there is of a woman having a gonorrhœa when ſhe is not ſenſible of having any one ſymptom of the diſeaſe, and none appears to the ſurgeon on examination? In ſuch a caſe the only thing we can depend upon is, the teſtimony of thoſe whom we look upon as men of veracity: ſuch men aſſert that they have been infected by a woman in the ſituation above-deſcribed, although they have had no connection for ſome months with any other woman. From this evidence it is reaſonable to ſuppoſe that the diſeaſe has been caught from ſuch women; and it would ſeem to put it beyond a doubt, when the ſame woman gives the diſeaſe in this way to more than one man. The caſe of the woman giving the diſeaſe to two men alternately at an interval of twelve months each time,[a] which gives a ſpace of at leaſt two years for the continuance of the diſeaſe, proves that it's communication is almoſt the only criterion of it's preſence. The caſe too of the young woman at the Magdalen hoſpital,[b] confirms the ſame opinion. Yet all this does not amount to an abſolute proof, for a ſound woman may have had connection with a man who had a gonorrhœa, or a man with chancres, and ſoon after, that is perhaps within forty-eight hours, ſhe may have admitted the embraces of a ſound man; in ſuch a caſe it is very poſſible that he may receive the infection from that matter which was lodged in the vagina by the unſound man, and yet the woman may not catch the diſeaſe; for the matter may be waſhed away before it irritates the vagina, and this woman may be ſuſpected of having a gonorrhœa, and apparently with great juſtice. A repetition of

[a] See page 37. [b] See page 38.

these circumstances may be the cause of many women appearing to have the disease for years, without really having it. Again, I have seen a buboe come on when the patient knew nothing of the complaint till that appeared, which one would think is an absolute proof that there may be a gonorrhœa without the patient knowing; but even this is not altogether without fallacy, for there may have been an absorption of venereal matter deposited in the vagina by some infected man, which did not produce any irritation there.

CHAPTER III.

OF THE EFFECTS OF THE GONORRHOEA ON THE CONSTITUTION IN BOTH SEXES.

THE diſeaſe I have been deſcribing both in men and women, is local, and generally confined to the part affected, yet it ſometimes happens that the whole conſtitution is more or leſs affected by it. Thus we find before there is any appearance of matter from the parts, that ſome patients complain of ſlight rigors: theſe are moſt conſiderable when the ſuppuration is late in taking place. A remarkable inſtance of this happened in a gentleman who had the infection twice*, the firſt time he aſſured me that it was ſix weeks between the time it was poſſible for him to have contracted the diſeaſe, and it's appearance; and that for a conſiderable part of that time he had often been indiſpoſed with ſlight rigors, attended with a little fever and reſtleſſneſs, for which he could aſſign no cauſe; nor was he relieved by the uſual remedies preſcribed in ſuch caſes. A violent gonorrhœa came on, and theſe ſymptoms went off, which appeared to me to explain the caſe. The ſecond time it was a month from the time of infection before the gonorrhœa appeared, and for ſome weeks of that time he was ſubject to a ſimilar indiſpoſition, which went off as before when the running came on. Here it would appear that we have ſomething of a ſuppurative fever, which perhaps often happens in this diſeaſe; but the inflammation being ſmall and the fever therefore inconſiderable, it is commonly little noticed by the patient. The above gentleman not ſuſpecting any ſuch complaint in the firſt attack, had connection with his wife as uſual, and was afraid when the diſeaſe appeared that he might have given it to her; but ſhe never complained, which is a ſtrong circumſtance in confirmation of the principle laid down above, that it cannot be communicated but by matter.

* The caſe is mentioned before, page 39.

Theſe

Theſe conſtitutional ſympathies from local ſpecific diſeaſes, are the ſame from whatever cauſe they proceed; they are the ſympathetic effects of irritation or of violence, and it is probable that all remote ſympathies are, at leaſt in this reſpect ſimilar; for if they were ſimilar to their cauſe, it is moſt probable that they would produce in the conſtitution the ſame kind of diſeaſe which gave riſe to them.

CHAPTER

CHAPTER IV.

OF THE CURE OF GONORRHOEA.

FROM the idea which I have endeavoured to give of the venereal disease in general, showing that whatever form it appears in, it always arises from the same cause, we should be induced to suppose that since we have a specific for some of the forms of the disease, this specific should be a certain cure for every one; and therefore that it would be no difficult task to cure the disease when in the form of inflammation and suppuration upon the secreting surfaces of any of the ducts or outlets of the body; but from experience we find the gonorrhoea the most variable in it's symptoms while under a cure; and the most uncertain in the cure, of any of the forms of this disease; many cases terminating in a week, while others continue for months though under the same treatment.

The only thing necessary to be done for the cure is, to destroy the disposition and specific mode of action in the solids of the parts, and as that is changed the poisonous quality of the matter produced will also be destroyed; this is the cu e of the disease, but not always of it's consequences.

I have already observed, that this form of the disease was not capable of being continued beyond a certain time in any constitution; and that in cases where it was violent, or lasted very long, it was owing to the parts being very susceptible of such irritation, and readily going on with it. As we have no specific medicine for gonorrhoea, it is fortunate that time alone will effect a cure: it is therefore very reasonable to suppose, that every such inflammation gets well of itself; yet although this appears to be nearly the truth, it is worthy of consideration, whether medicine can be of any service in this form of the disease. I am inclined to believe it is very seldom of any kind of use, perhaps not once in ten cases; but even this would be of some consequence, if we could distinguish the cases where it is of service, from those where it is not. Upon this idea of every gonorrhoea curing itself,

I gave certain patients pills of bread which were taken with great regularity. The patients always got well, but ſome of them I believe not ſo ſoon as they would have done had the artificial methods of cure been employed.

The methods of cure hitherto recommended, and ſtill practiſed by different people of the profeſſion, are of two kinds, conſiſting either of internal remedies, or local applications; but in whichever of theſe two ways this diſeaſe is to be treated, we are always to pay more attention to the nature of the conſtitution, or to any attending diſeaſe in the parts themſelves, or parts connected with them, than the diſeaſe itſelf.

The nature of the conſtitution is principally to be learnt from the local effects; for the local effects of this poiſon are ſo different in different people as to require a treatment ſuited to each variety; but this has been too little attended to, from every one endeavouring to attack the immediate ſymptoms, as if they had a ſpecific for gonorrhœa.

Whether the cure be attempted conſtitutionally, locally, or in both ways, nearly the ſame principles are to be adhered to, except when evacuations are made uſe of, for we cannot evacuate locally.

The firſt thing to be conſidered is, the inflammation itſelf, whether violent or mild, whether common or irritable; yet even where this is aſcertained, we have not in all caſes the cure in our power; for I have already obſerved, that ſome people are very ſuſceptible of this irritation, who are as it were inſenſible to others; and on the contrary, many are eaſily affected by common inflammation, who are inſenſible to this. Theſe laſt are rather uncommon diſpoſitions, and the cure being always eaſy they demand little attention. When the ſymptoms are violent, but of the common inflammatory kind, which is to be collected from the attending circumſtances, particularly the extent of the inflammation not exceeding the ſpecific diſtance, the local mode of cure may be either irritating or ſoothing, till the original violence is over. Irritation in the preſent caſe may be attended with leſs danger than in the irritable inflammation*, and may alter the ſpecific action; but

* It is very difficult to give clear ideas of diſtinctions in diſeaſe, when they are not marked by ſomething permanent as to time, ſpace, &c. I have uſed the term *irritable inflammation*, becauſe I think this kind of inflammation takes place more in weak irritable habits than in others: it appears

but to produce this effect it must be greater than the irritation from the original injury. The parts would afterwards recover of themselves, as from any other common inflammation. After all however, I believe the soothing plan is the best at the beginning. If the inflammation be great, and of the irritable kind, no violence is to be used in the cure, for it will only increase the symptoms, unless we knew that the great degree of inflammation arose entirely from a susceptibility of this irritation, and that there was no general irritability in the constitution, which seldom can be ascertained. In cases where the symptoms run high, nothing should be done that may tend to stop the discharge, either by internal or external means, for by this nothing would be gained; as merely stopping the discharge does not put an end to the inflammation. The constitution is to be altered if possible, by remedies adapted to each disposition, with a view to alter the actions of the parts arising from such dispositions, and reduce the disease to it's simple form. If the constitution cannot be altered, nothing is to be done but to allow the parts to tire themselves out by a continuance of the same action.

When the inflammation has considerably abated, the disease only now remaining in a mild form, it may be attacked either by internal remedies, or local applications. If it be attacked locally, violence is still to be avoided; because it may bring back the irritation. At this period gentle astringents may be applied with a prospect of success; or if the disease has begun mildly, and there are no signs of an inflammatory disposition, either of the common or the irritable kind; in order to get rid of the specific mode of action quickly, an irritating injection may be used, which will increase the symptoms for a time, but when it is left off they will often abate, or wholly disappear. In such a state of parts, astringents may be used; for the only thing to be done, is to procure a cessation of the discharge, which is now the principal symptom.

appears to be guided by no law that I am acquainted with. It may be called an ill-formed inflammation, as not going through the usual process to a natural termination, but continuing with little variation; and if such inflammation took place in the cellular membrane, it would rather produce an oedematous swelling than such as arises from the extravasation of coagulable lymph, which takes place in what I would call the true or healthy inflammation.

In

In thoſe caſes where the itching, pain, and other uncommon ſenſations begin and go on long before the diſcharge appears, I ſhould be inclined to recommend the quieting or ſoothing plan inſtead of the irritating, with a view to bring on the diſcharge, as that effect is a ſtep towards a reſolution of the irritation; but how far it would really be the proper plan I cannot abſolutely ſay, not having had experience enough in ſuch caſes. One thing however I think I may aſſert from reaſoning, that to uſe aſtringents would be bad practice, as they would rather tend to prevent the diſcharge from taking place, which might prolong the inflammation and protract the cure. In caſes of ſtricture, or in caſes of diſeaſed teſticles, I believe aſtringents ſhould not be uſed, for we find in either caſe, while the diſcharge laſts, both complaints are relieved; therefore it ſhould be left to itſelf more than when all the parts are otherwiſe ſound. If we had a ſpecific for venereal gonorrhœa, the queſtion would be, would this ſpecific cure the irritation, before the full action ſhould have taken place?

I. OF THE DIFFERENT MODES OF PRACTICE—EVACUANTS—ASTRINGENTS.

THE remedies commonly recommended in gonorrhœa, are of two kinds, *internal and local*. The former may be divided into evacuants, and aſtringents.

The evacuants are principally of the purgative or diuretic kind, without being confined to any particular medicines of theſe claſſes, every practitioner ſuppoſing that he is in poſſeſſion of the beſt. Some uſe mercurial evacuants, while others carefully avoid mercury in every form. The neutral ſalts have been given from the idea of their being cooling. Some of the profeſſion have kept principally to diuretics, perhaps with two views, as evacuants acting upon the urinary paſſages mechanically to waſh off the venereal matter, or as ſpecifics for the latter purpoſe: nitre has been given with this view; beſides it has been ſuppoſed to leſſen inflammation; but it's powers in this way I very much doubt. Under theſe different modes of treatment the patients always get well, and the cures have been aſcribed by each to his own method of treatment.

Keeping

Keeping the body open in moſt caſes, even when the patient is otherways in health, muſt no doubt be proper; but what idea can we form of an irritation produced all along the inteſtinal canal, curing a ſpecific inflammation in the urethra; yet there are caſes where a briſk purge has been of ſervice, and even in ſome has performed a cure; but I ſuſpect that in ſuch caſes the diſeaſe was continued by habit only, and that this practice therefore would not have ſucceeded in the beginning of the ſame diſeaſe. A gentleman had a gonorrhœa, all the ſymptoms of which continued for two months, and by taking at once ten grains of calomel, which purged him moſt violently, he was almoſt immediately cured. The calomel could not have acted ſpecifically, but by a kind of derivation, that is, an irritation produced in one part, curing one that ſubſiſted in another; but even if it ſhould be granted, that in ſome conſtitutions purges have the power of making the ſolids leſs ſuſceptible of this irritation, it cannot be ſuppoſed they will have this effect in every caſe; in ſome conſtitutions they might debilitate, increaſe irritability, and of courſe increaſe the ſymptoms. Theſe contrary effects muſt take place in different conſtitutions in which a medicine has no ſpecific action. On the ſuppoſition of the cure being promoted by an evacuation from the blood, what ſervice can purging out ſome of the blood in form of a ſecretion from one part do, to an inflammation of another part? On ſuch a ſuppoſition, would not a ſweat, or an increaſe of ſaliva by chewing tobacco, or ſtimulating the noſe by ſnuff, all tend equally to cure a gonorrhœa? But humors having been conſidered as the univerſal cauſe of every diſeaſe, eſpecially thoſe in which pus was formed or a diſcharge produced, and purging having been ſuppoſed to be the cure for humors, purgatives were of courſe made uſe of in this diſeaſe; and as the patients always got well, the practice became generally eſtabliſhed.

Thoſe who recommended mercury in this form of the diſeaſe, did it moſt probably from the opinion that this medicine was a ſpecific for the venereal diſeaſe in all it's forms. On this ſuppoſition we can ſee ſome reaſon for their practice, as it would be abſorbed from the inteſtines, circulate through the inflamed veſſels of the urethra, and thereby deſtroy the venereal irritation. Here we can only ſuppoſe it to act by it's ſpecific virtue; but I doubt very much of mercury having any ſpecific virtue in this ſpecies of the diſeaſe, for I find that it is as ſoon curable without mercury as with it; and where it is only ufed as a purge, or purged off the next day, and therefore only allowed to act upon the bowels, I cannot conceive that it could have any more effect upon the venereal inflammation in the urethra, than an irritation in the bowels arifing from any other purgative. So little effect indeed has this medicine upon a gonorrhœa, that I have known a gonorrhœa take place while under a courfe of mercury fufficient for the cure of a chancre. Whether the gonorrhœa arofe from the fame infection that produced the chancre I cannot fay, nor can it be eafily determined in fuch cafes. Men have alfo been known to contract a gonorrhœa when loaded with mercury for the cure of a *lues venerea*, the gonorrhœa neverthelefs has been as difficult of cure as in ordinary cafes.

A gentleman put himfelf under my care on the 27th of June, for the cure of two chancres and a buboe. I difperfed the buboe, but as he difliked the unction, I was obliged to fubftitute *mercurius calcinatus* daily inftead of it, giving two grains in the evening and one in the morning. About the middle of July his mouth became fore, and the mercury was left off; we began it's ufe again in a week, and he appeared to be quite well of his venereal complaints. I however continued the ufe of mercury, keeping his mouth fore, and on the 16th of Auguft while in this ftate, he had connection with a woman, both on that and the following evening, and in five days after, a gonorrhœa appeared, and proved to be very violent.

The fame general obfervations may be made with refpect to diuretics.

It is poffible that fpecific medicines taken into the conftitution, (if we had fuch) and paffing off by urine, might act upon the urethra in their paffage through it. The balfams and turpentines pafs off in this way, and become fpecifics for many irritations in the urinary paffages; but how far medicines which have the power of affecting particular parts when found, or when under difeafes peculiar to thofe parts, have alfo the powers of affecting a fpecific irritation in thefe parts, I know not; but do not believe they have any confiderable powers in this way; it is poffible however, that they may remove any attending irritation, although not the fpecific one. Diuretics have neverthelefs their advantages, for if they produce a greater quantity of water, they do good; but I believe this had better be effected by fimple

water,

water, or water joined with ſuch things as will encourage the patient to drink a good deal, as tea, capillaire, orgeate, and the like.

Aſtringents although often given, yet have always been condemned by thoſe who have called themſelves the judicious and regular practitioners; becauſe, according to them, there is ſomething to be carried off, and if that is not carried off a lues venerea is to be the conſequence. This reaſoning is not juſt, and therefore the thing to be conſidered is, do they, or do they not aſſiſt us in the cure of the gonorrhœa. I believe they do not in any caſe leſſen the venereal inflammation; but certainly they often leſſen the diſcharge. As that effect however does not conſtitute a cure, it is not neceſſary to produce it.

I can conceive that a combination of aſtringents, eſpecially the ſpecific aſtringents of thoſe parts, as the balſams, with any other medicine which may be thought to be of ſervice, may help to leſſen the diſcharge in proportion as the inflammation abates; and this I have often ſeen, as will be explained more at length hereafter.

II. OF LOCAL APPLICATIONS—DIFFERENT KINDS OF INJECTIONS—IRRITATING—SEDATIVE—EMOLLIENT—ASTRINGENT.

LOCAL applications may be either internal to the urethra, external to the penis, or both; all of which will in many caſes be neceſſary. The internal, or thoſe applied to the urethra would ſeem the moſt likely to cure this ſpecies of diſeaſe, by coming immediately in contact with the diſeaſed parts; for if they have any power of action, whatever that be, it muſt be in oppoſition to the venereal irritation; therefore we might ſuppoſe that moſt irritations that are not venereal would tend to a cure; but certainly this is not univerſally the caſe. If on the contrary the applications are ſuch as quiet irritation, they muſt alſo be of ſervice.

Local applications to the urethra may be either in a ſolid or fluid form, each of which has it's advantages and diſadvantages. A fluid is only a temporary application, and that of very ſhort duration, and is ſimilar to the waſhing

washing of a sore, which is I believe in most cases unnecessary, for I imagine that matter, from any sore whatever, is always such as cannot stimulate that sore into any action; it can be of no consequence therefore whether the matter is allowed to lie upon it or not; but by removing it the medicines are allowed to come in contact with the inflamed surface. I apprehend it is only in this way the removal of it can be of service. The solid applications may remain a long time, and are similar to the dressings in the case of a wound. When the parts are not so much inflamed as to prevent their use, they would appear to have an advantage over the fluid applications by their continuance; but they in general irritate immediately, from their solidity alone. These applications must be in the form of a bougie; but I should be inclined to suppose, that the less use we make of bougies when these parts are in an inflamed state, the better; although I cannot say that I ever saw any bad effect from them in any case, when properly applied.

Fluid applications to the inside of the urethra are commonly called injections, and like the internal remedies, are without number; every one thinking, or wishing to make the world think, that his own is the best. But the great variety of injections, and every venereal inflammation getting well during their use, which was likewise observed to happen when internal medicines were given, are strong corroborating circumstances in favour of the opinion, that every such complaint will in time cure itself; I think however it appears from practice, that an injection will often have almost an immediate effect upon the symptoms, therefore they must have some powers; and yet the kind of injection which would have the greatest specific powers, I believe is not yet known: if an injection has no specific powers, it must be very uncertain in it's effects, and can only be of service as far as it may be adapted to a peculiarity of constitution or parts. As injections are only temporary applications, it becomes necessary to use them often, especially in cases where they are found to be of service; they should therefore be applied as often as convenient, perhaps every hour, or even oftener; but this must be regulated in some measure by the kind of injection; for if it be irritating it will not be proper to use it so often, as it may be productive of bad consequences.

Many

Many injections immediately, or at least soon after their application, remove the symptoms, and prevent the formation of matter, which has given rise to the notion of their shutting up the disease, and driving it into the constitution: but this supposed mode of producing a constitutional complaint, is the reverse of what really happens; for I have already endeavoured to prove, that matter is the only substance in which the poison is contained, and that the formation of the poison is inseparable from the formation of matter; therefore if we can prevent the one, the other cannot take place, and of course there can be no room for absorption, so that there can neither be any power of infecting the constitution in the same person, nor of communicating the infection to others.*

When the discharge is an effect of present inflammation it may be stopped by injections, though the inflammation still continue in some degree, and may afterwards be removed without the discharge ever reappearing. But I believe that by this practice little is gained, for the effect of the inflammation is not the disease which we wish to remove; however we find that the same method which stops the discharge, also removes the inflammation, although not always, and only I believe when the inflammation is slight.

I shall divide injections according to their particular effects upon the urethra into four kinds, the irritating, sedative, emollient, and astringent. The specific I believe is not yet discovered, although a mercurial injection in some form or other is by most people supposed to be possessed of such a power, and of course this mineral makes part of many of the injections now in use.

Irritating injections of whatever kind I suspect in this disease act upon the same principle, that is by producing an irritation of another kind, which ought to be greater than the venereal, by which means the venereal is destroyed and lost, and the disease is cured, although the pain and running may still be kept up by the injection, yet those effects will soon go off when the injection is laid aside, because they arise only from it's irritating qualities. In this way bougies, as well as many injections may be supposed to cure; and although they increase the symptoms for the time they never

* Vide page 12, what was said in the method of contracting the lues venerea.

can increaſe the diſeaſe itſelf, any more than the ſame injection which would produce the ſame ſymptoms if applied to the urethra of a ſound man can communicate the diſeaſe. Moſt of the irritating injections have an aſtringent effect, and prove ſimply aſtringent when mild, their irritating quality depending chiefly upon their ſtrength.

As irritating injections do not agree with all inflammations ariſing from the venereal poiſon,[a] it may be aſked in what caſes are the irritating injections to be uſed with advantage? This I have not been able to determine abſolutely; but I think irritating injections ſhould never be uſed where there is already much inflammation, eſpecially in conſtitutions which cannot bear a great deal of irritation, as a previous knowledge of the diſeaſe in the ſame perſon ſometimes teaches us; nor ſhould they be uſed where the irritation has ſpread beyond the ſpecific diſtance; nor where the teſticles are tender, nor where upon the diſcharge ſtopping quickly they have become ſore; nor where the perinæum is very ſuſceptible of inflammation, and eſpecially if it formerly has ſuppurated; nor where there is a tendency in the bladder to irritation, which is known from the patient having had for ſome time a frequency in making water. In ſuch caſes I have not ſucceeded with them; they not only do no good, but they often do harm; for I have ſeen them make the inflammation ſpread further in the urethra[b]; and I think I have had reaſon to ſuſpect that they have been the cauſe of abſceſſes *in perinæo*. But in caſes that are mild, and in conſtitutions that are not irritable, injections often ſucceed, and remove the diſeaſe almoſt immediately. The practice however ought to be attempted with caution, and not perhaps till milder methods have failed: two grains of corroſive ſublimate diſſolved in eight ounces of diſtilled water, or roſe-water, is nearly as good an injection as any of the kind. But an injection of only half this ſtrength may be uſed, where it is not intended to attempt a cure ſo quickly. If however the injection, even in that proportion, gives conſiderable pain in it's application, or if it occaſions a great increaſe of pain in making water, it ſhould be diluted.

[a] For I have already remarked, that the inflammation varies according to the conſtitution.

[b] It is however to be remarked, that this ſymptom is not always to be attributed to the injections, for it often happens when none have been uſed.

Sedative

Sedative injections will always be of service in cases where the inflammation is considerable, not by lessening the disease itself, but by lessening the diseased action, which always allows the natural actions of the part more readily to take place; they are likewise very useful in relieving the painful feelings of the patient. Perhaps the best sedative we have is opium, as well when given by the mouth or anus as when applied to the part affected in the form of an injection. But even opium will not agree, or act as a sedative in all constitutions or parts; on the contrary it often has opposite effects, producing great irritability. Lead may be reckoned a sedative, so far as it abates inflammation, while at the same time it may act as a gentle astringent. Fourteen grains of saccharum saturni, in eight ounces of rose-water, make a good sedative astringent injection.

The drinking freely of diluting liquors may perhaps be considered as having a sedative effect, as it in part removes some of the causes of irritation, rendering the urine less stimulating, either to the bladder when the irritation is there, or to the urethra in it's passage through it; and it is possible that diluting may lessen the susceptibility of irritation. The vegetable mucilages of certain seeds and plants, and the emollient gums are recommended; but I suspect that this practice is founded on a mechanical notion, and that none of them are of much service. I believe the advantage arises chiefly from the quantity of water that is drank, therefore if the water be joined with any thing, spirits excepted, that can induce the patient to drink freely, the purpose is fully answered. I have however been informed by some patients that they thought when the liquids they drank were impregnated with those substances, they had less uneasiness in making water.

Emollient injections are the properest applications where the inflammation is very great; they are most probably useful by first simply washing away the matter, and then leaving a soft application to the part; in which way I can conceive them to be of singular service, by lessening the irritating effects of the urine; and indeed practice proves this, for we often find that a solution of gum arabic, milk and water, or sweet oil, will lessen the pain and other symptoms, when the more active injections have done nothing, or to appearance have done harm.

It

It very often happens that the irritation is so great at the orifice of the urethra, that the point of the syringe, cannot be suffered to enter; when this is the case nothing should be done in the way of injection till the inflammation abate. Emollients may likewise be used externally in form of fomentation.

The astringent injections can only act by lessening the discharge, they can have no specific effect upon the inflammation; but as they must affect the actions of the living powers, it is possible they may alter the venereal disposition. They should only be used towards the latter end of the disease, when it has become mild, and the parts begin to itch. But this should be according to circumstances, and if the disease began mildly they may be used at the very beginning; for by gradually lessening the discharge without increasing the inflammation, we complete the cure, and prevent a continuation of the discharge, called a gleet. Injections of this kind very probably stimulate in such a way as to make the vessels of the part contract, and probably hinder the act of secretion; we can hardly suppose that they act chemically by coagulating the juices. They will have an irritating quality if used strong, which in some measure destroys their astringency, or rather makes the parts act contrary to what they would do from the application of a simple astringent; so that they often increase the discharge instead of lessening it, by which means the disease also may be cured, in the same way as by irritating injections, that is by altering the disposition of the inflammation. When more mild, they often stop the discharge, without however in all cases hastening the cure; for the inflammation may still continue even longer than it otherways would have done if the tendency to secretion had not been stopped; for I have already observed, that a surface that discharges has assumed the complete action of the disease, which is one step towards a cure or termination. However it sometimes happens, that an astringent injection will cure a slight irritation in a very few days. My experience has not taught me that one astringent is much better than another.

The astringent gums, as dragon's blood, the balsams, and the turpentines dissolved in water; the juices of many vegetables, as oak bark, Peruvian bark, tormentil root, and perhaps all the metallic salts, as green, blue, and white vitriols;

vitriols; the salts of mercury, and also alum; probably all act as far as we yet know much in the same way; although we may assert that they do not always act equally well in every gonorrhœa, for on our changing the injection a new one will sometimes succeed after several others have been tried in vain.

The external applications are generally poultices, and fomentations; but they can be of little service, except when the external parts, such as the prepuce, glans, and orifice of the urethra, are in some degree inflamed; the last indeed is almost always more or less affected.

When the glands of the urethra are swelled so as to be felt externally, the application of mercurial ointment to the part may be proper, but most probably this will be of more service after the inflammation has subsided. Indeed mercurial ointment is often applied to all the external surfaces of those parts when in a state of inflammation, with an emollient poultice over it; but I am not perfectly satisfied of the utility of this practice.

CHAPTER V.

OF THE CURE OF GONORRHOEA IN WOMEN.

IN women the cure of the gonorrhœa is nearly the ſame as in men; but the diſeaſe itſelf being milder, and the ſecondary ſymptoms leſs numerous in women, owing to there not being ſo many parts to be affected, and to theſe parts not being either of ſo great extent, or ſo liable to inflammation, the cure becomes more ſimple.

When the diſeaſe is in the vagina only, it is eaſily cured. Injections are the beſt means that can be uſed, and after injecting it may be proper to anoint the parts as far up as poſſible with mercurial ointment,[*] and alſo to waſh the external parts often with the injection.

If the inflammation has attacked the urethra, injections there cannot be ſo conveniently uſed, as it is almoſt impoſſible for the patient to throw an injection into that canal.

The injections recommended in the cure in men are equally ſerviceable here, but they may be made doubly ſtrong, as the parts are not nearly ſo irritable as the common ſeat of this diſeaſe in men.

If what I have ſaid of the diſeaſe in women be juſt, we muſt ſee that it will be a difficult thing to ſay, with any degree of certainty, when the patient is well; becauſe whenever the ſymptoms are gone, the ſurgeon and the patient will naturally ſuppoſe the cure to be complete; but a new trial of thoſe parts may prove the contrary; or in caſes where the diſeaſe has never affected the urethra, but only the vagina, and ſtill more where no ſymptoms have ever been obſerved, it will be more difficult to fix the date of the cure; but general experience muſt direct the practitioner.

[*] How far mercurial ointment aſſiſts in the cure I have not been able to determine; the practice rather ariſes more from a kind of practical analogy than real knowledge of it's uſe in ſuch caſes.

When

When the inflammation runs along the ducts of the glands, whether those of the mouth of the vagina, or urethra, or affects the glands themselves, the same method is to be followed; in particular the mercurial ointment is to be freely applied to the parts. If the inflammation on the mouths of the ducts is so great as to shut them up, the duct and glands will suppurate and form abscesses; in such cases it will be necessary to open them, or enlarge the opening already formed, and dress the abscess as a chancre or buboe.

In the case of a simple running the constitutional treatment will be taken notice of hereafter; but if any suppuration take place, the constitution is to be treated as in chancres or buboes; for most probably absorption will take place, and it's effects must be guarded against.

CHAPTER

CHAPTER VI.

OF THE TREATMENT OF THE CONSTITUTION IN THE CURE OF GONORRHOEA.

IN the cure of gonorrhœa, the conſtitution is in ſome caſes to be as much attended to as the parts affected, if not more; but in general this is not neceſſary. The knowledge of the conſtitution is to be obtained in a great meaſure from the local ſymptoms, and as far as the conſtitutional treatment can be made ſimilar to the local, they ſhould correſpond.

We find in many ſtrong plethoric conſtitutions, where both the powers and actions are great, that the ſymptoms are often violent. Theſe conſtitutions have generally a ſtrong tendency to fever of the inflammatory kind; and probably the moſt diſtinguiſhing mark of ſuch a conſtitution will be that of the ſymptoms not extending beyond the ſpecific diſtance. Many medicines which might be of ſervice in another conſtitution will often prove hurtful here, in ſo much as to increaſe the very ſymptoms they were meant to relieve. I have ſeen even opiate clyſters though they relieved at firſt, yet in the end produce or increaſe fever, and by that means increaſe all the ſymptoms. I have ſeen the balſam capivi given in ſuch caſes increaſe the inflammatory ſymptoms, probably by ſtopping the diſcharge in part, which appears to be ſalutary.

The treatment of ſuch a conſtitution when affected with this diſeaſe conſiſts chiefly in evacuations, the beſt of which are bleeding and gentle purging.

To live ſparingly, and above all to uſe little exerciſe, is neceſſary; for although ſuch a treatment does not leſſen the venereal irritation, yet it removes the violence of the inflammation, and allows the parts to relieve themſelves. In this kind of conſtitution therefore the diſeaſe is in the end ſooneſt cured, as there is not a diſpoſition to continue inflammation long.

In the weak and irritable conſtitution, the ſymptoms are frequently very violent, ariſing from great action in the parts, and often extend beyond the ſpecific diſtance; the inflammation running along the urethra, and even affecting the bladder. Inſtead of evacuation, which would rather aggravate the ſymptoms than relieve them, the conſtitution ſhould be ſtrengthened, which will make it leſs ſuſceptible of irritation in general.

I have ſeen patients whoſe conſtitutions were ſuch, that they were never ſure of twenty-four hours health, and were always expecting when well, to be ill ſoon, where the inflammation has been both conſiderable, and extenſive; I have ſeen evacuations tried, and the ſymptoms increaſed; but as ſoon as the bark was given freely, they have become almoſt immediately mild; and without uſing any other medicine the patients have got ſoon well. The medicine here acted upon the conſtitution, deſtroyed the irritability, gave the parts a true and healthy ſenſation of the venereal irritation, and brought the inflammation to that ſtate in which it ought to be in a healthy ſubject, whereby the conſtitution was enabled to cure itſelf.

So capricious ſometimes is this form of the diſeaſe in it's cure, that I have ſeen by an accidental fever coming on, the diſcharge ſtop, the pain in making water go off, and the gonorrhœa finally terminate with the fever.

In others I have ſeen all the ſymptoms of the gonorrhœa ſtop by the coming on of a fever, and return again when it went off. In ſome I have ſeen a gonorrhœa begin mildly, but a ſevere fever coming on, and continuing for ſeveral days, has greatly increaſed the ſymptoms, and on the fever going off, the gonorrhœa has alſo gone off. Although a fever does not always cure a gonorrhœa, yet as it may, nothing ſhould be done while the fever laſts; and if it continues after the fever is gone, it is then to be treated according to the ſymptoms.

Unfortunately there are caſes where no known method leſſens the ſymptoms; evacuations have produced no abatement, the ſtrengthening plan has been as unſucceſsful: ſedatives and emollients have procured no relief; and time alone has performed the cure. With ſuch the ſoothing plan I believe is the beſt, till we know more of the diſeaſe. Aſtringents ſhould not be uſed, their action upon the inflamed parts is uncertain, for they often do not leſſen the inflammation or the pain, although they may perhaps leſſen the diſcharge. The turpentines, eſpecially the balſam capivi, and Canada balſam, leſſen the diſpoſition of the parts to form matter, which effect has always a falutary appearance; but as they have not at the fame time the power of leffening the inflammation, they can be of little fervice.

Befides the various effects arifing from the difference of conftitution in the gonorrhœa, we find that it is confiderably affected by the way of life, during the inflammatory ftate, and alfo by other difeafes attacking the conftitution at the fame time. But this is common to all other difeafes; for whenever we have a local difeafe, in which light I have confidered a gonorrhœa, it is always affected by whatever affects the conftitution. Moft things that hurry, or increafe the circulation, aggravate the fymptoms, fuch as violent exercife, drinking too much of ftrong liquors, eating ftrong indigeftible food; fome kinds of which act fpecifically on thefe parts, and thereby increafe the fymptoms more than fimply heating the body, fuch as peppers or fpices of all kinds, and fpirits.

From what has been faid in general, it muft appear that a gonorrhœa is to be cured in the fame way as every other inflammation; and it muft alfo appear, that all the methods ufed are only to be confidered as correctors of of irritation in general, and of difordered circulation. In cafes that have begun mildly, where the inflammation has been but flight, or in thofe cafes where the violent fymptoms above taken notice of have fubfided, fuch medicines as have a tendency to leffen the difcharge may be given along with the local remedies before-mentioned. The turpentines I believe are the moft efficacious; cantharides; the falts of fome metals, fuch as of copper, zink, and lead, and alfo of fome earths, as alum, are ftrongly recommended as aftringents when given internally.

Whatever methods are ufed for the cure, either locally or conftitutionally, it is always neceffary to have in view the poffibility of fome of the matter being abforbed, and afterwards appearing in the form of a lues venerea; to prevent which I fhould be inclined to give fmall dofes of mercury internally. At what time this mercurial courfe fhould begin I am not certain, but if the obfervation be juft, that a difpofition once formed is not to be cured by mercury, but that mercury has the power of preventing a difpofition from forming, as was formerly explained, we fhould begin early and continue it to the end of the difeafe, till the formation of venereal matter ceafes, and even

for

for ſome time after. The mercurial ointment may be uſed where mercury diſagrees with the ſtomach and inteſtines, which is ſometimes the caſe.

This practice appears to be more neceſſary if the diſcharge has continued a conſiderable time, and eſpecially if the treatment has been ſimply by evacuants, for in the former there is a greater time for abſorption, and in the latter we may ſuppoſe a greater call for it, ſuch medicines having no effect in carrying off the virus.

The quantity of mercury neceſſary will be proportioned to the duration of the diſeaſe; a grain of mercurius calcinatus made into a pill, and taken every night, or one at night and another in the morning may be ſufficient.

The ſucceſs of this practice in any particular caſe can never be aſcertained, becauſe it is impoſſible to ſay when matter has been abſorbed, except in caſes of buboes; and where it is not known to be abſorbed, it is impoſſible to ſay that there would have been a lues venerea if mercury had not been given, as very few are infected from a gonorrhœa, although they have taken no mercury. It is however going upon the ſureſt grounds to give mercury, as we may reaſonably ſuppoſe it will often prevent a lues venerea, as it does when given during the cure of a chancre or buboe, where we know from experience that without it lues venerea would certainly take place.

CHAPTER

CHAPTER VII.

OF THE TREATMENT OF OCCASIONAL SYMPTOMS OF GONORRHOEA.

AS the following ſymptoms are only occaſional conſequences of venereal gonorrhœa, being the effects of an irritation on the urethra, and therefore not venereal, they are to be treated in the ſame manner as if they aroſe from any other cauſe.

I. OF THE BLEEDINGS FROM THE URETHRA.

I have already obſerved, that when the inflammation is violent, or ſpreads along the urethra, there is frequently a diſcharge of blood from the veſſels of that part. In ſuch bleedings I have ſeen the balſam capivi given internally of ſervice, and I ſhould ſuppoſe that all the turpentines would be equally uſeful. I cannot ſay that I have done any good by aſtringent injections; and in ſome caſes, I have even ſuſpected that they have been the cauſe of this complaint. They always go off in the uſual time of the cure of the gonorrhœa.

II. OF PREVENTING PAINFUL ERECTIONS.

OPIUM given internally appears to have great effects in preventing painful erections in many caſes; I have known twenty drops of tinctura thebaica taken at bed-time procure eaſe for a whole night; I think the cicuta has likewiſe ſome powers in this way.

III. OF

III. OF THE TREATMENT OF THE CHORDEE.

In the beginning of this complaint, bleeding from the arm is often of service, but it is of more immediate service to take away blood from the part itself by leeches; for we often find by a vessel giving way in the urethra, and a considerable hæmorrhage ensuing, that the patient is greatly relieved. Fomenting the penis by holding it over the steam of warm water will give ease, as will also poultices; and if camphire be added to the fomentation and poultice, it will in many cases assist in taking off the inflammation. Opium given internally is of singular service, and if joined with camphire the effect will be still greater; but opium in such cases acts rather by lessening the pain than by removing the inflammation, though by preventing erections it may be said to obviate the immediate cause of the complaint.

When the chordee continues after all other symptoms are gone, I believe that little or nothing in the way of evacuation is necessary, the inflammation being gone and a consequence of it only remaining, which will go off gradually by the absorption of the extravasated coagulable lymph; therefore bleeding in this case can be of no use. Rubbing the parts with mercurial ointment will promote the absorption of the extravasated coagulable lymph, for we find that mercury has considerable powers in exciting absorption; the friction also will be of use. In one case I thought I saw considerable benefit from giving the cicuta, after I had tried the common methods of cure. Electricity may be of service.

This symptom is often longer in going off than either the running or pain, but no bad consequences arise from it; it's declension is gradual and uniform, as happens with most consequences of inflammation.

In relieving the chordee, or the remains of it which appear to arise from spasm, I have known the bark of great service. Evacuations whether from the part, or from the constitution, generally do harm.

IV. OF THE TREATMENT OF THE SUPPURATION OF THE GLANDS OF THE URETHRA.

SUPPURATIONS in the glands of the urethra I suspect should be treated as chancres, therefore mercury ought to be given, as will be explained in speaking of that form of the disease.

Should a suppuration take place in Cowper's glands, it demands more attention; the abscess must be opened freely, and pretty early, as the matter if confined might make it's way either into the scrotum or urethra, which would be productive of bad consequences. Here also mercury I believe must be given, and perhaps as freely as in a buboe; in short, the treatment should be the same as in a venereal ulcer; and in this respect it will differ from the treatment of those abscesses which arise in consequence of stricture, to be taken notice of hereafter.

V. OF THE TREATMENT OF THE AFFECTION OF THE BLADDER.

WHEN the disease extends as far as the bladder I do not know a more troublesome complaint. It is however one of those complaints from which seldom or ever any bad consequences arise, and in general it will get well of itself; but I suspect that it sometimes lays the ground-work of future irritation in that viscus, which may prove very troublesome, and even dangerous; but this is only conjecture.

Opiate clysters, if nothing in the constitution forbids the use of them, procure considerable temporary relief. The warm bath is of service, altho' not always; and bleeding pretty freely, if the patient is of a full habit often gives great relief; leeches also applied to the perinæum have good effects; but in many constitutions bleeding will rather do harm; and I believe we should be cautious in making use of this evacuation, for I have already observed, that many of these cases are rather sympathetic than inflammatory.

tory. How far an opiate plaister applied to the region of the pubis would be of service I do not know. If applied to the small of the back, or origin of the nerves of the bladder, it might perhaps be of use; and probably a small blister on the perinæum would answer in such cases as well as it does in those irritations of the bladder which arise from other causes, as will be taken notice of hereafter. But in spite of every attempt, the affection of the bladder often continues for a considerable time, producing other sympathies in the neighbouring parts.

VI. OF THE TREATMENT OF THE SWELLED TESTICLE.

When the testicle sympathises either with the urethra or bladder, and inflames, I believe that rest is the best remedy; lying in an horizontal position is the easiest, as such a position of body is the best for a free circulation. If the patient cannot submit to an horizontal position, it is absolutely necessary to have the testicle well suspended; indeed the patient's feelings will make him fly to that expedient the moment he is acquainted with the ease it procures.

In this complaint perhaps there is no particular method of cure; it is to be treated as inflammation in general, by bleeding and purging, if the constitution requires them, fomentation and poultices. Bleeding with leeches I have often seen of service, although we cannot well account for this, as the vessels of the scrotum have but little connection with those of the testicle.

As I do not look upon the swelling of the testicle to be venereal, mercurials can be of no service in these cases when in a state of inflammation, but are useful when the inflammation is gone, and the induration only remains.

Vomits have been recommended in such cases, and are sometimes of service. I have known a vomit act like a charm, however this is not a constant effect. The effects of the vomit most probably arise from the sympathy between the stomach and the testicle. Opiates are of service, as they are in most irritations of those parts. When such swellings suppurate, which

which they seldom do, they require only to be treated as common suppurations, and mercury need not be given.

In the history of this disease I observed, and indeed it has been observed by most writers, that when a swelling came upon the testicle in consequence of a gonorrhœa, the running stopped; or when the running stopped, the testicle swelled; but which was the cause, or which was the effect, has not yet been ascertained. It has been also observed, that when the running returned, the testicle then showed the first symptoms of recovery, so that by the testicle losing it's sympathising action, the action was restored to the urethra; and here also it has not yet been ascertained, which is the cause, and which is the effect; but from a supposition that the stopping of the discharge in the urethra was the cause of the swelling, it has been attributed to the mode of treatment of that irritation, and by some to injections.

It has been advised by many, and some have attempted, to procure a return of the running; but the methods they used were hardly founded upon any sound principle. Mr. Bromfield appears to have been the first who recommended a treatment suitable to this theory, which was to irritate the urethra to suppuration again, by introducing bougies. I cannot say that I have seen that benefit that could have been wished, or that the first idea might make us expect, from this practice. Some have gone further, by recommending the introduction of venereal matter into the urethra; but this appears to be only conceit, and is founded upon a supposition that such diseases arise only from venereal irritations; but I have already observed that they are produced by others.

It is generally a long time before the swelling of the testicle intirely subsides, although it does so more quickly at first than swellings of this part arising from other causes; but when the inflammation is removed, and the swelling only remains, evacuations never are of service. Before it becomes less, it generally becomes softer, commonly on the anterior surface; and this goes on till the whole becomes perhaps softer than natural, and then it diminishes.

It is still much longer before the epididymis comes to its natural state, and indeed it is often years before it returns to it's natural size and softness, and sometimes it never does; however this is of no great consequence, as there

there is no inconvenience arifing from a continuance of the hardnefs fimply; though fometimes I am inclined to believe fuch tefticles are rendered totally ufelefs. I never had an opportunity of examining the tefticle of one that I knew to have this complaint; but I have examined tefticles where the epididymis had the fame external feel, and the canal of the vas deferens was obliterated; but this I rather fufpect is feldom the cafe, for there are people who have them both fwelled, and notwithftanding have evacuations of the femen as before.

It is in this ftage of the complaint that refolvents might be of fervice, fuch as mercurial friction joined with camphire. Fumigations with aromatic herbs, which may ftimulate the abforbents to action in order to take up the fuperfluous matter. Electricity has been in fome cafes of fingular fervice.

VI. OF THE DECREASE AND TERMINATION OF THE SYMPTOMS OF GONORRHŒA.

The decreafe of the difeafe is generally known by an abatement of fome or all of the above-mentioned fymptoms. The pain in the part becomes lefs, or terminates in an itching fimilar to the beginning of many gonorrhœas, and at laft entirely goes off; the fenfe of wearinefs about the loins, hips, tefticles, and fcrotum, is no longer felt, and the tranfparent cherry-like appearance of the glans penis gradually vanifhes; thefe are the beft figns of an abatement of the difeafed action.

The running becomes lefs, or if it does not diminifh becomes firft whiter, then of a paler colour, and gradually becomes more flimy and ropy in confiftence, which has always been confidered as the moft certain fign of an approaching cure; and at laft it entirely difappears. When the running becomes more flimy it is then changed from matter to the natural fluid which lubricates the paffage, and alfo to that fluid which appears to be preparatory to coition; but it is often very inconftant in it's appearances, arifing frequently from different modes of living, &c.

It very often happens that all the fymptoms fhall totally difappear, and the patients fhall think themfelves cured, and yet all the fymptoms fhall come upon them anew, but commonly milder, though in ſome caſes they are as violent, or even more violent than at firſt; and this takes place ſometimes at a conſiderable diſtance of time. I have known the ſymptoms return a month after every appearance of the diſeaſe had been removed; however in ſuch caſes they ſeldom laſt long. How far this ſecond attack is to be looked upon as truly venereal is not yet I believe aſcertained: nothing can prove it abſolutely but the circumſtance of giving it to a ſound perſon. What may be the caſe with thoſe in whom it has returned ſoon after the going off of the ſymptoms, I will not pretend to ſay; but I ſhould very much ſuſpect that where it has continued well for a month, a return would not be venereal; but this is only conjecture, and if we were to reaſon upon it, we might eaſily reaſon ourſelves into a belief that it was venereal; for if the parts can fall back again into one mode of action, that of inflammation and ſuppuration, there can be no reaſon why they ſhould not fall back again into the ſpecific mode of action; however as the common effect of irritation is ſuppuration, and as the ſpecific ſuppuration requires a peculiar irritation, it is eaſier to conceive that the parts ſhould fall into the common mode of action, than into both. It is poſſible however that in ſuch caſes it is only the venereal action that is ſuſpended, and thus becomes ſimilar to what happens between the contamination and complete appearance of the diſeaſe.

In women returns of the ſymptoms are more frequent than in men, particularly of the diſcharge; which being ſimilar to the fluor albus, and frequently taken for that diſeaſe, gives leſs ſuſpicion, although it is perhaps equally bad.

The diſtinction between a gonorrhœa and a gleet is not yet aſcertained, for the inflammation ſubſiding, the pain going off, and the matter altering, are no proofs that the poiſon is deſtroyed; for it is no more neceſſary there ſhould be a continuance of the inflammation to produce the ſpecific poiſon, than it is neceſſary for a continuance of the inflammation to produce the gleet, as will appear evident from two caſes before related.*

* Vide page 38 and 39.

The

The firſt of theſe caſes ſhows that the inflammation is not neceſſary to the exiſtence of the venereal poiſon; and on the contrary, the inflammation may exiſt after the matter diſcharged has ceaſed to be venereal; for I have known caſes where the inflammation and diſcharge have continued for twelve months, and with conſiderable violence; and there has been a connection with women without a ſuſpicion of giving them the diſeaſe; however this is not an abſolute proof that there is no virus in the diſcharge.

CHAPTER

CHAPTER VIII.

GENERAL OBSERVATIONS ON THE SYMPTOMS WHICH OFTEN REMAIN AFTER THE DISEASE IS SUBDUED.

IT often happens after the virus is deſtroyed, and the venereal inflammation removed, that ſome one, two, or more of the ſymptoms ſhall continue, and perhaps prove more obſtinate than the original diſeaſe itſelf; ſome of them ſhall continue through life, and even new ones ſhall ſometimes ariſe as ſoon as the firſt ſubſide. All theſe ſymptoms are commonly imputed by the patients themſelves, and what is ſtill worſe, either ignorantly or illiberally by ſome of the profeſſion, to the original diſeaſe having been ill treated, or as is vulgarly ſaid ill cured. But certainly ſo far as we are yet acquainted with the diſeaſe and method of cure, this is not true; for the methods of treatment, though numerous, may be ſaid to be very ſimilar, and we ſhall find theſe ſymptoms not to be conſequences of any one mode of treatment, but that they happen indiſcriminately after them all. Yet I can conceive that many conſtitutions, and particular parts, often require one mode of treatment in preference to another, and probably require modes that we are not yet acquainted with; but if theſe peculiarities of conſtitution or parts are not known, which muſt often be the caſe, the practitioner is not to be raſhly accuſed of ignorance.

In the introduction I obſerved, that the venereal diſeaſe is capable of calling into action ſuch ſuſceptibilities as are remarkably ſtrong, and peculiar to certain conſtitutions, and countries; and as the ſcrofula is predominant in this country, ſome of the effects of gonorrhœa may partake of a ſcrofulous nature.

The ſymptoms which continue after the virus is gone, do not owe their continuance to the ſpecific qualities of the virus, but to it's effects upon the parts, ſuch as inflammation and it's conſequences; for the ſame degree

of

of inflammation ariſing from any other cauſe would leave moſt of the ſame effects. But I ſuſpect that the continuance of the diſcharge called a gleet is an exception to this; for we find that it is often cured by the ſame mode of action which would produce the other ſymptoms, that is, inflammation; and we find in general that a diſcharge brought on by violence of no ſpecific kind, does not laſt longer than the violence, even although the cauſe has been continued for ſome time, as is often the caſe during the uſe of bougies.

The firſt of the continued ſymptoms may be reckoned the remains of the diſagreeable ſenſations excited by the original diſeaſe.

The ſecond, the diſcharge called a gleet.

The third, the chordee.

The fourth, the irritable ſtate of the bladder.

The fifth, the increaſe and hardneſs of the epididymis.

I. OF THE REMAINS OF THE DISAGREEABLE SENSATIONS EXCITED BY THE ORIGINAL DISEASE.

The ſtrange kind of ſenſations which continue in the urethra and glans, happen more frequently when the bladder has ſympathiſed with the urethra in the time of the diſeaſe; for then there is often the remains of the old ſhooting pains in the glans, or on it's ſurface, which take their riſe from the bladder. Theſe however commonly go off, ſeldom being the forerunners of any bad ſymptoms, and therefore are not to be conſidered as part of the diſeaſe but merely a conſequence, yet they are often very troubleſome, and teazing to the patient, keeping his mind always in doubt whether he is cured or not, which makes him frequently become the dupe of ignorant or deſigning men.

As theſe remaining ſenſations vary conſiderably in their nature perhaps no one method of treatment will always be proper. I have known a bougie introduced a few times take off entirely the diſagreeable ſenſation in the urethra, and I have known it do no good. Gentle irritating injections uſed occaſionally will often alleviate in ſome degree thoſe complaints. A grain of corroſive ſublimate to eight ounces of water makes a good injection for this purpoſe, but ſuch applications are in general no more than palliatives.

C c I have

I have known the uſe of hemlock relieve the ſymptoms very much, and in ſome caſes entirely cure them, while in many others it has not had the leaſt effect.

A bliſter applied to the perinæum will entirely cure ſome of the remaining ſymptoms, even when they extend towards the bladder, as will be explained hereafter; indeed it appears to have more effect than any other remedy. A bliſter to the ſmall of the back will alſo give relief, but not ſo effectually as when applied to the perinæum.

The following caſes are remarkable inſtances of this. A Portugueſe gentleman about twenty-five years of age had contracted a venereal gonorrhœa of which he was cured, but for two years after many of the ſymptoms ſtill continued, and even with conſiderable violence. The ſymptoms were the following; a frequency in making water, and when the inclination came on he could not retain it a moment; a ſtraining, and pain in the bladder after voiding it; a conſtant pain in the region of the bladder; a ſhooting pain in the urethra, which extended often to the anus; ſtrange ſenſations in the perinæum; a ſenſe of wearineſs in the teſticles; and if he at any time preſſed his thighs cloſe together, it brought on the pain or ſenſation in the perinæum. It was ſuppoſed at Liſbon that he had the ſtone, and he came over to London for a cure of that diſeaſe. He was examined, but no ſtone was found. He was ordered to waſh the external parts every morning with cold water, which he did for a fortnight, but found no benefit. I was conſulted, and informed of all the above-mentioned circumſtances. As a ſtaff had been paſſed, there could be no ſtricture; however I thought it was poſſible there might be a diſeaſed proſtate gland, and therefore examined him by the anus; but found that gland of it's natural ſize and firmneſs. As there was no viſible alteration of ſtructure any where to be found, I looked upon the diſeaſe as only a wrong action of the parts, and therefore ordered a bliſter to be applied to the perinæum, which relieved him almoſt immediately; it was only kept open for a few days, and the whole of the ſymptoms were entirely removed. He retained his water as uſual, all the ſtrange ſenſations went off, and the bliſtered part was allowed to heal. About a fortnight after, he got a freſh venereal gonorrhœa, which alarmed him very much, as he was afraid it might bring back all his former ſymptoms, which however did not return,

and

and he was soon cured of the gonorrhœa. He stayed in London some time after, without any relapse.

Another case, was that of a gentleman's servant in the country. He had, from a venereal cause, a disagreeable sensation whenever he made water, also a running, and some degree of chordee, and had laboured under these symptoms for a considerable time. He had undergone a course of mercury which lasted two months, on a supposition of the venereal virus not being destroyed, but without effect. He had after that been bled, used powders of gum arabic and tragacanth, and taken calomel in small doses, with no better success. He then had recourse to injections and bougies of all kinds, but without receiving any benefit from them. On the ground of the symptoms not being venereal, but only wrong actions of the parts, a blister was applied upon the perinæum, repeated and kept open six days, when the symptoms totally disappeared, and had not recurred a twelvemonth after.

This practice is not only of service where there has been a preceding gonorrhœa, but I have found it remove almost immediately common stranguries, where the turpentines and opium, both by the mouth and anus, had proved ineffectual, and when the catheter had been necessarily introduced twice a day to draw off the water. But of this more fully hereafter.

Electricity has been found to be of service in some cases, and therefore may be tried either in the first instance, or when other means have failed.

II. OF A GLEET.

Whatever method has been used in the cure of the venereal inflammation, whether injections, or internal medicines, mercurials, purgatives, or astringents, it often happens that the formation of pus shall continue, and prove more tedious and difficult of cure than the original disease. For as I have already observed, the venereal inflammation is of such a nature as to go off of itself, or to wear itself out; or, in other words, it is such an action of the living powers as can subsist only for a certain time. But this is not the case with a gleet, which seems to take it's rise from a habit of action which the parts have contracted, and as they have no disposition to lay

lay aside this action it of course is continued; for we find in those gonorrhœas which last long, or are tedious in their cure, that this habit is more rooted than in those which go off soon.

This disease however has not always the disposition to go on, for it often appears to stop of itself, even after every method has been ineffectually used. It is most probable that this arises from some accidental changes in the constitution, not at all depending upon the nature of the disease itself.

I have suspected that there was something of a scrofulous action in some gleets. We find frequently that a derangement of the natural actions of a part will be the cause of that part falling into some new diseased action, to which there may be a strong tendency in the constitution. We find that a cold falling on the eyes produces a scrofulous weakness in those parts, with a considerable discharge. There are often scrofulous swellings in the tonsils from the same cause.

This opinion of the nature of some gleets is strengthened by the methods of cure, for we find that the sea-bath cures more gleets than the common cold-bath, or any other mode of bathing. I have never yet tried the internal use of those medicines which are generally given in the scrofula; but I have found sea-water diluted, and used as an injection cure some gleets, though not always effectual.

A gleet is generally understood to arise from a weakness; this certainly gives us no idea of the disease, and indeed there is none which can be annexed to the expression. By mechanical weakness is understood the not being able to perform some action, or sustain some force; by animal weakness the same; but when the expression is applied to the animal's performing an uncommon, or an additional action, I do not perfectly understand it.

Upon this idea of weakness depended in a great measure the method of cure; but we shall find that the treatment founded on this idea is so far from answering in all cases, that it often does harm, and a contrary practice is successful.

A gleet differs from a gonorrhœa, first in this, that though a consequence of it, it is perfectly innocent with respect to infection. Secondly, when it is a true gleet it is generally different in some of the constituent parts of the discharge, which consists of globular bodies floating or wrapt in a slimy

mucus

mucus instead of a serum. But the urethra is so circumstanced as easily to fall back into the formation of pus, and this commonly happens upon the least increase of exercise, eating or drinking indigestible food, or any thing which increases the circulation or heats the patient. The virus however I believe does not return; but of this I am not certain, for there are cases that make it very doubtful, as was before observed.

I am inclined to suspect that a gleet arises from the surface of the urethra only, and not from the glands; for I have observed in several instances, that when the passage has just been cleared either by the discharge of urine, or by the use of an injection; a lascivious idea has caused the natural slime to flow very pure, which I do suppose would not have happened if the parts secreting the liquor had assisted in forming the gleet.

A gleet is supposed to be an attendant upon what we call a relaxed constitution; but I can hardly say that I have observed this to be the case; at least I have seen instances where I should have expected such a termination of a gonorrhœa if this had been a general cause, but did not find it so; and I have seen it in strong constitutions, at least in appearance, in every other respect. Gleets do not in all cases arise from preceding gonorrhœas, but sometimes from other diseases of the urethra. A stricture in the urethra is I believe almost always attended with a gleet: it sometimes arises also from a disease in the prostate gland.

When a gleet does not arise from any evident cause, nor can be supposed to be a return of a former gleet in consequence of a gonorrhœa, a stricture, or diseased prostate gland is to be suspected; and inquiry should be made into the circumstances of making water, whether the stream is smaller than common? whether there be any difficulty in voiding it? and whether the calls to make it are frequent? If there should be such symptoms, a bougie of a size rather less than the common, ought to be used, which will if there is a stricture stop when it reaches it; and if it passes on to the bladder with tolerable ease, the disease is probably in the prostate gland, which should be next examined. But more fully of both these complaints hereafter.

CHAPTER IX.

OF THE CURE OF GLEETS.

As this discharge has no specific quality, but depends upon the constitution of the patient, or nature of the parts themselves, there can be no certain or fixed method of cure; and as it is very difficult to find out the true nature of different constitutions, or of parts, it becomes equally difficult to prescribe with certainty the medicines which will best suit this disease; for so great is the variety in constitutions, that what in one case proves a cure, will in another aggravate the complaint.

The cure would appear to depend upon a change being produced in the action of the parts, and that change may be produced in a great many ways, in different constitutions, each having a mode of action peculiar to itself, which I believe cannot be at first known.

Whatever method of cure is followed, it will probably be a continuation of that which was put in practice towards the latter end of the cure of the gonorrhœa, and which was meant as a prevention of gleet. If such methods have not been already used, they may be tried now, and varied according to circumstances.

There are two ways of attempting the cure of this complaint, constitutional, or local.

I. OF THE CONSTITUTIONAL METHOD OF CURE.

Medicines, when taken into the constitution with a view to the cure of gleet, may be supposed to act in three ways, as specifics,* strengtheners, and astringents.

* It may be necessary to remark here, that by specific I do not mean a specific for the disease, but only such medicines as act specifically on those parts, as the turpentines, cantharides, &c.

The

The ſpecific power of internal medicines upon thoſe parts is not very great, however we find that ſome of them, ſuch as the balſams, turpentines, cantharides, &c. are of uſe, eſpecially in ſlight caſes. I think I have been able to aſcertain this fact, that when the balſams, turpentines, or cantharides, are of ſervice they are almoſt immediately ſo; therefore if upon trial they are not found to leſſen, or totally remove the gleet in five or ſix days, I have never continued them longer. And even where they have either leſſened or totally removed the gleet in that time it will often recur upon leaving them off, and therefore they ſhould be continued for ſome time after the ſymptoms have diſappeared. I have known caſes where the gleet has diſappeared immediately upon taking the balſam capivi, and recurred upon leaving it off; and I have alſo ſeen where that medicine has kept it off for more than a month, and yet it has recurred immediately upon laying it aſide, and ſtopped again as quickly, upon having recourſe to it. In ſuch caſes the other methods of cure ſhould be tried. The balſams may either be given alone, or mixed with other ſubſtances ſo as to make them leſs diſagreeable.

The general ſtrengtheners of the habit need only be given when the parts act merely as parts of that habit, and by diſpoſing the whole to act properly, theſe parts are alſo diſpoſed to act in the ſame way, ſuch are the cold-bath, ſea-bathing, the bark, ſteel, &c.

Aſtringents taken into the conſtitution have no great powers, and if they had, they might be very improper, as any thing that could act with powers in the conſtitution equal to what would be neceſſary here, might very much affect many natural operations in the animal economy. The aſtringent gums, and ſalt of ſteel, are commonly given.

II. OF THE LOCAL METHOD OF CURE.

THE ſecond mode of cure is by local applications; theſe may be divided into four, which are, ſpecifics, aſtringents, irritating medicines, and ſuch as act by derivation.

The

The ſpecifics applied locally, we may reaſonably ſuppoſe will have greater effects than when given internally; becauſe they may be applied ſtronger than can ſafely be thrown into the circulation; and I think I have had experience of this.

The aſtringents commonly uſed are, the decoction of the bark, white vitriol, alum, and preparations of lead. The aqua vitriolica cœrulea, of the London Diſpenſatory, diluted with eight times it's quantity of water, makes a very good aſtringent injection. The ſame obſervations that I made on the ſpecifics are applicable to the aſtringents; I believe that they act nearly in the ſame manner, and have the ſame effect. What their mode of action is I can hardly ſay.

When either of theſe methods have been uſed, and have had the deſired effect, they ſhould be continued for a conſiderable time after the ſymptoms have diſappeared, and the time muſt be in proportion to the duration of the complaint, or the frequency of it's returns. If it has been of long ſtanding we may be ſure that the diſpoſition for ſuch a complaint is ſtrong; and if it has returned frequently, upon the leaſt increaſe of circulation, we may expect the ſame thing to happen again; therefore to correct the bad habits it is neceſſary to continue the medicines for a conſiderable time.

Irritating applications are either injections or bougies, ſimple, or medicated with irritating medicines; violent exerciſe may be conſidered as having the ſame effect. Such applications ſhould never be uſed till the other methods have been fully tried and found unſucceſsful. They differ from the foregoing by producing at firſt a greater diſcharge than the one they are intended to cure; and the increaſed diſcharge may or may not continue as long as the application is uſed. It becomes therefore neceſſary to inquire how long they are to be uſed to produce a cure of the gleet. That time will generally be in proportion to the violence uſed, and the nature of the parts which form the matter; and according to the diſpoſition being ſtrong or weak joined to it's duration, and the greater or leſs irritability of the parts. If the parts are either weak or irritable, or both, an irritating injection ſhould not be uſed; if ſtrong, and not irritable, it may be uſed with ſafety. In this laſt caſe, if it is an injection that ſtimulates very conſiderably, perhaps uſing it twice, or thrice, may be ſufficient. I knew a gentleman who threw into the urethra,

for

for a gleet of two years ſtanding, Goulard's extract of lead undiluted, which produced a moſt violent inflammation, but when this inflammation went off, the gleet was cured. Two grains of corroſive ſublimate to eight ounces of water is a very good irritating injection.

If it is a gleet of old ſtanding it may require a week or more to remove it, even with an irritating injection; and if the injection is leſs irritating, ſo as to give but little pain and increaſe the diſcharge in a ſmall degree, it may require a fortnight. But one precaution is very neceſſary reſpecting the uſe of irritating injections; it ſhould be firſt known if poſſible, that they will do no harm. To know this may be difficult in many caſes, but the nature of the parts is to be aſcertained as nearly as poſſible, that is, whether they had ever been hurt before by ſuch treatment; whether they were ſo ſuſceptible of irritation, as that the irritation would run along the urethra and produce ſymptoms in the bladder; for in ſuch caſes I think irritating applications do not anſwer, but on the contrary, often produce worſe diſorders than thoſe they were meant to cure.

Bougies may be claſſed with the irritating applications, and in many caſes they act very violently as ſuch. They appear to be more efficacious than injections, but they require longer time to produce their full effect. A ſimple, or unmedicated bougie, is in general ſufficient for the cure of a gleet, and requires a month or ſix weeks application before the cure can be depended on. If they are made to ſtimulate otherwiſe than as extraneous bodies, then a ſhorter time will generally be ſufficient; probably the beſt mode of medicating them, would be by mixing a little turpentine, or a little camphire with the compoſition, ſo as to act ſpecifically on the parts; but great care ſhould be taken not to irritate too much.

The ſize of the bougie ſhould be ſmaller than the common, and need only be five or ſix inches long, as it ſeldom happens that a greater extent of the urethra has the diſpoſition for gleet; although no harm will ariſe from paſſing a bougie of the common length through the whole extent of the urethra.

In the cure of gleet attempted by means of the bougie, we have no certain rules to direct us when it ſhould be left off; as the diſcharge will often continue as long as the bougie is uſed. If upon leaving off the bougie after having uſed it for ſeveral weeks, the running ſtops, then we may hope there is a cure performed; but if it ſhould not be in the leaſt diminiſhed, it is more than probable that bougies will not effect a cure, and therefore it is hardly neceſſary to have recourſe to them again; yet if the gleet is in part diminiſhed, it will be right to begin again, and probably it may be proper to increaſe the irritating quality of the bougie to ſuit it to the diminiſhed irritability of the parts.

The fourth mode of cure is by ſympathy, or by producing an irritation in another part of the body, which ſhall deſtroy the mode of action in the urethra.

I knew a caſe of obſtinate gleet attended with very diſagreeable ſenſations in the urethra, eſpecially at the time of making water, removed entirely by two chancres appearing upon the glans. The gentleman had taken all the medicines commonly recommended, and had applied the bougie, without effect.

A gentleman informed me that he had cured two perſons of gleets, by applying a bliſter to the underſide of the urethra, and I have known ſeveral gleets of old ſtanding, after having baffled all common attempts, cured by electricity. All theſe different methods of cure alter the diſpoſition of the part.

In whatever way the cure is attempted, reſt or quietneſs in moſt caſes is of great conſequence; for as I have obſerved, exerciſe is often a cauſe, not only of it's continuance, but of it's increaſe and return. But this idea is not to be too rigidly adhered to, eſpecially in caſes which have been treated unſucceſſfully; as I have known ſome that have got immediately well by riding on horſeback after long diſuſe of that exerciſe.

Regularity and moderation in eating and drinking ſhould be particularly attended to, for irregularities of this kind either hinder the cure or bring on a return of the diſeaſe.

Connection with women often cauſes a return, or increaſe of gleet, and in ſuch caſes it gives ſuſpicion of a freſh infection; but I believe the difference between this, and a freſh infection is, that the return will follow the connection ſo cloſe, as to be almoſt immediate, and that circum-

ſtance

ſtance joined with the other ſymptoms will in general aſcertain the nature of the diſcharge.

III. OF GLEETS IN WOMEN.

This diſeaſe is more frequent in women than in men, at leaſt a diſcharge from the vagina is very common in them, which probably will be called a gleet, when following a venereal taint, although only the fluor albus.

The cure of the gleet in women is nearly the ſame as in men, except in the uſe of what I have called ſpecifics to the parts; for as the gleet in women is principally from the vagina, I believe that this part is not more affected by the turpentines than other parts are. Neither can we uſe the bougie in caſes of gleet in the vagina; and when the gleet is only from the urethra, I imagine it is hardly ever attended to in women.

IV. OF THE REMAINING CHORDEE.

This ſymptom I have already obſerved often remains after every mark of the true virus is removed, and may or may not be an attendant on any of the other continuing ſymptoms.

Rubbing the part externally with mercurial ointment may be of ſervice, and if joined with camphire, it's powers will be increaſed. I have known electricity cure a chordee of long ſtanding. If it is the ſpaſmodic chordee that remains, bark ſhould be given.

V. OF THE CONTINUANCE OF THE IRRITATION OF THE BLADDER.

The irritation of the bladder ſometimes continues after every other ſymptom is gone, and it may be an attendant upon all, or any of the other continuing ſymptoms; it ſeldom laſts with the ſame violence, although it is often very troubleſome. When this irritation is kept up with the ſame violence,

violence, the bladder itself may be suspected of being diseased; or it may arise from it's connection with other parts, such as the urethra, or prostate gland; for a stricture in the urethra coming on will continue it, and a disease in the prostate gland will do the same.

Neither of these diseases will probably follow the gonorrhœa so closely as to continue this irritation, though perhaps they may have been taking place prior to the gonorrhœa, and so contribute to it's increase, and continuance; which may probably be ascertained by a history of the patient preceding the present complaint; however before the bladder itself is attempted to be cured, a bougie should be passed, and if no stricture is found, then the prostate gland should be examined, as shall be described.

When the disease is in the bladder only, I think the pain is principally at the close of making water, and for a little while after. The cure of this symptom consists in opiate clysters, cicuta, bark, sea-bathing, and I should be inclined to recommend the application of a blister to the perinæum in men. How far opiate clysters can affect the bladder in women as they do in men, I am not certain.

VI. OF THE REMAINING HARDNESS OF THE EPIDIDYMIS.

This symptom I have observed remains long after every other symptom is removed, and may continue even for life, but seldom or ever any bad consequences happen from it, if the vas deferens is not rendered impervious; and not even then if it is only in one testicle, the other being equal to all the purposes of generation. As this is the case, we must at once see, that no certain method of resolution is yet known. Sitting over the steam of warm water with camphire, might be tried, especially in such cases as are not disposed to be permanent, and rubbing the scrotum with mercurial ointment joined with camphire. But in most cases this practice will prove too tedious, or rather too inefficacious to be long persisted in.

CHAPTER

PART III.

CHAPTER I.

OF DISEASES SUPPOSED TO ARISE IN CONSEQUENCE OF VENEREAL INFLAMMATION IN THE URETHRA OF MEN.

GONORRHŒA either produces, or is supposed to produce, many disorders besides those already mentioned, and which are totally different from the original disease. How far they do all or any of them arise in consequence of this disease, is not clear; but as they are diseases of the urethra and are both numerous and important, I mean to treat fully of them in this place. If any of these diseases arise from gonorrhœa, they are most probably not the consequences of any specific quality in the venereal poison, but are such as might be produced by any common inflammation in those parts, as was observed of the *continued symptoms*.

In this investigation we shall find some of the complaints arising out of each other, so that there is frequently a series of them. Thus a stricture of the urethra produces an irritable bladder, a frequent desire to make water, increased strength of the bladder, a dilatation of the urethra between the bladder and stricture, ulceration, fistulæ in perinæo, dilatation of the ureters and enlargement of the pelvis of the kidneys, besides other complaints that are sympathetic, such as swellings of the testicle, and of the glands in the groin.

I shall treat of the diseases of those parts in the order in which they most commonly arise. It may be observed that most of these diseases, especially the diminution of distensibility in the bladder, attack men advanced beyond middle age, although many if not all of them are at times found in younger men, and the circumſtance of their appearing at this period ariſes probably in ſome degree from a long habit of an unnatural mode of life producing many diſeaſes, ſuch as gout; for certainly ſuch complaints do not ſo frequently take place among the more uncivilized nations.

The moſt frequent diſeaſe in the urethra is an obſtruction to the paſſage of the urine; it happens both in young and old, although moſt frequently in the latter. Before I begin to treat of this ſubject, I ſhall for the better underſtanding of the whole, make ſome obſervations on the uſes of this paſſage in it's natural ſtate.

It may firſt be obſerved, that the urethra in man is employed for two purpoſes, and on this occaſion I may be allowed to make the following general remark, that nature has not been able to apply any one part to two purpoſes with advantage, as might be illuſtrated in many inſtances in different animals. The animals whoſe legs are adapted both for ſwimming, and walking, are not good at either, as ſeals, otters, ducks, and geeſe; the animals alſo whoſe legs are intended both for walking and flying, are but badly formed for either, as the bat; the ſame obſervations are applicable to fiſh, for the flying fiſh neither ſwims, nor flies well; and whenever parts intended for ſuch double functions are diſeaſed, both are performed imperfectly. This is immediately applicable to the urethra, for it is intended for two purpoſes, as a canal or paſſage, both for the urine, and the ſemen. The urine requires the ſimpleſt of all canals, and of no greater length than the diſtance from the bladder to the external ſurface, as we find the urethra in women, birds, the amphibia, and fiſh; but the paſſage for the ſemen in the quadruped required to be a complicated canal, and of a length capable of conveying the ſemen to the female, provided with many additional and neceſſary parts, as the *corpus ſpongioſum urethræ*, *muſculi acceleratores*, *Cowper's glands*, *proſtate gland*, and *veſiculæ ſeminales*. As all theſe parts are ſuperadded for the purpoſes of generation, and as the diſeaſes of this canal are principally ſeated in them, we muſt at once ſee how much the urinary organs muſt ſuffer from a connection with parts ſo numerous, and ſo liable to diſeaſe; and what adds to the evil is, that the actions of the urinary organs are conſtant, and abſolutely neceſſary for the well-being of the

the machine; whereas the evacuation of the ſemen takes place only during a certain portion of life, is then only occaſional, and never eſſentially neceſſary to the exiſtence of the individual. The force of this obſervation is at once ſeen by making the compariſon between the inconveniences that attend the expulſion of the urine in the male, and in the female.

The canal of the urethra is liable to ſuch diſeaſes as are capable of preventing in ſome degree the paſſage of the urine through it; and in ſome of theſe diſeaſes the paſſage at laſt becomes completely obſtructed. In all caſes there is a diminution of the ſize of the canal, but in different ways. There are five modes of obſtruction, four of which are diſeaſes of the paſſage itſelf, the fifth is a conſequence of the diſeaſes of other parts. Three of the former are a leſſening of the diameter of the paſſage; the fourth an excreſcence in the paſſage; the fifth ariſes from the ſides being compreſſed, which may be done either by exterior contiguous ſwellings, or by a ſwelling of the proſtate gland.*

I. OF STRICTURES.

The three firſt I ſhall now conſider, of which the firſt is the true permanent ſtricture ariſing from an alteration in the ſtructure of part of the urethra. The ſecond is a mixed caſe, compoſed of a permanent ſtricture and ſpaſm. The third is the true ſpaſmodic ſtricture. Moſt obſtructions to the paſſage of the urine, if not all, are attended with nearly the ſame ſymptoms, ſo that there are hardly ſufficient marks for diſtinguiſhing the different cauſes. Few take notice of the firſt ſymptoms of a ſtricture till they have either become violent, or have been the cauſe of other inconveniences: for inſtance, a patient ſhall have a conſiderable ſtricture without obſerving that he does not make water freely; he ſhall even have, in conſequence of a ſtricture, a tendency to inflammation, and ſuppuration in the perinæum, and not feel any obſtruction to the paſſage of his urine, nor ſuſpect that he has any other

* Many other kinds of obſtruction are deſcribed by authors, none of which I have ever ſeen; and as probably I have opened more urethras after death, where there was an obſtruction of the paſſage, than all the authors who have written on this ſubject, I am inclined to believe that they wrote from imagination only.

complaint

complaint but the inflammation in the perinæum. In all of these obstructions the stream of water becomes small, and that in proportion to the obstruction; but this symptom, though probably it is the first, is not always observed by the patient. In some the water is voided only in drops, and then it cannot escape notice; in others the stream of urine is forked, or scattered: under such circumstances the passage should be examined with a bougie; and if one of a common size passes with tolerable ease, the fifth cause of obstruction is to be suspected, which will most probably be found to be a swelled prostate gland; for any other cause that can produce a compression of the sides of the urethra, sufficient to obstruct the urine, will be known to the patient, such as a tumor forming any where along the canal, or an inflammation along it's sides; therefore if neither of these are known to exist, the prostate gland should be examined, as will be described hereafter.

The spasmodic obstruction will commonly explain itself when the symptoms are well investigated; for the obstruction arising from this cause will not be permanent. These obstructions, but more particularly that from a permanent stricture, is generally attended with a discharge of matter or a gleet. This is often considered by the patient as the whole disease, and he applies to the surgeon for the cure of a gleet. The surgeon often goes on attempting the cure of this disease; but not succeeding at last other symptoms are observed, and a stricture is suspected either by the surgeon or patient. In diseases of this passage, and also of the prostate gland and bladder, there is commonly an uneasiness about the perinæum, anus, and lower part of the abdomen, and the person can hardly cross his legs without pain.

CHAPTER

CHAPTER II.

OF THE PERMANENT STRICTURE.

IN the permanent ſtricture* the patient ſeldom complains till he can hardly get the water to paſs; and frequently has a conſiderable degree of ſtrangury, and even other ſymptoms that happen in ſtone and gravel, which are therefore too frequently ſuppoſed to be the cauſes of the complaint. The diſeaſe generally occupies no great length of the paſſage; at leaſt in moſt of the caſes that I have ſeen it extended no further in breadth than if the part had been ſurrounded with a piece of packthread; and in many it had a good deal of that appearance. I have however ſeen the urethra irregularly contracted for above an inch in length, owing to it's coats, or internal membrane, being irregularly thickened, and forming a winding canal.

A ſtricture does not ariſe in all caſes from an equal contraction of the urethra all round, but in ſome from a contraction of one ſide, which probably has given the idea of it's having ariſen from an ulcer on that ſide. This contraction of one ſide only, throws the paſſage to the oppoſite ſide, which often renders it difficult to paſs the bougie. The contracted part is whiter than any other part of the urethra, and is harder in it's conſiſtence. In ſome few caſes there are more ſtrictures than one. I have ſeen half a dozen in one urethra; ſome of which were more contracted than others; and indeed many urethras that have a ſtricture have ſmall tightneſſes in other parts of them; this we learn from ſucceſſive reſiſtance felt in paſſing the bougie.

Every part of the urethra is not equally ſubject to ſtrictures, for there appears to be one part which is much more liable to them than the whole of the urethra beſides, that is about the bulbous part. We find them how-

* Vide plate I, fig. 1.

ever ſometimes on this ſide of the bulb, but very ſeldom beyond it. I never ſaw a ſtricture in that part of the urethra which paſſes through the proſtate gland; and the bulb, beſides being the moſt frequent ſeat of this diſeaſe, has likewiſe the ſtrictures formed there of the worſt kind. They are generally ſlow in forming, it being often years from their being perceived before they become very troubleſome.

The ſame ſtricture is not at all times equally bad; for we find that in warm weather it is not nearly ſo troubleſome as in cold: theſe changes are often very quick, a cold day, even an hour of cold weather, ſhall produce a change in them; and the ſame ſtricture is almoſt always worſe in winter than in ſummer; however this obſervation is not free from exceptions, I know one caſe that was always worſe in the ſummer. There are other circumſtances beſides cold that make a ſtricture worſe; a gentleman who had an ague, always found the ſtricture increaſed during the fit; it is alſo increaſed by drinking, violent exerciſe, and by the retention of urine after an inclination to void it. This laſt cauſe is often ſo great as to produce a total ſtoppage for a time. It is ſometimes rendered much worſe by a ſmall calculus paſſing from the bladder, of the formation of which this ſtricture was probably the cauſe. The calculus not being able to paſs will produce a total ſtoppage of urine, the cauſe of which can hardly be known at the time; and if known it could not be remedied without an operation.*

It is impoſſible to ſay what is the cauſe of that alteration in the ſtructure of the urethra which diminiſhes the canal: it has been aſcribed to the effects of the venereal diſeaſe, and often to the method of cure; but I doubt very much if it commonly, or even ever, ariſes from theſe cauſes; yet as moſt men have had venereal complaints ſome time or other, it is natural to aſcribe the ſtricture to them; and therefore it may be very difficult to refute this opinion. Many reaſons however can be given why we ſhould ſuppoſe that it is not commonly a conſequence of a venereal inflammation. Strictures are common to moſt paſſages in the human body; they are often to be found in the œſophagus; in the inteſtines, eſpecially the rectum; in the anus; in the prepuce producing phymoſis; in the lachrymal duct pro-

* Vide plate IV.

ducing

ducing the disease called fistula lachrymalis, where no disease had previously existed. They sometimes happen in the urethra where no venereal complaint had ever been; I have seen an instance of this kind in a young man of nineteen who had had the complaint for eight years, and which therefore began when only eleven years of age. It was treated at first as stone, or gravel. He was of a scrofulous habit, the lips thick, the eyes sore, a thickened cornea of one eye, and of a weak habit. This stricture was in the usual place, about the membranous part of the urethra. I have seen an instance of a stricture in the urethra of a boy of four years, and a fistula in perinæo in consequence of it. They are as common to those who have had the gonorrhœa slight, as those who have it violently.

I knew a young gentleman who had a very bad stricture; he had had several gonorrhœas, but they were so slight that they seldom lasted a week; nor in any of them did the pain extend beyond the frænum, but the stricture was about the membranous part; cases of this kind occur every day. They are never found to come on during the venereal inflammation, nor for some time after the infection is gone. There have been thirty, and sometimes forty, years between the cure of a gonorrhœa and the beginning of a stricture, the health being all that time perfectly good. If they arose in consequence of the venereal inflammation we might expect to find them of some extent, because the venereal inflammation extends some way; and we should also expect to find them most frequent in that part of the urethra which is most commonly the seat of the venereal disease; but I remarked before, that they are not so frequent there as they are in other parts of the urethra.

It is supposed by many that strictures arise from the use of injections in the cure of gonorrhœa, but this opinion appears to be founded in prejudice; for I have seen as many strictures after gonorrhœas that have been cured without injections, as after those cured with them.

These modes of accounting for strictures give no explanation of those where there has been no previous gonorrhœa, or where the gonorrhœa has not been cured by injections; and indeed if we consider the mode of cure of strictures we must see that an injection is a mild application to the urethra, compared to a bougie; yet a bougie has never been supposed, or known to be the cause of a stricture. Further, some have injected by mistake very irritating

ting liquors, ſuch as the undiluted extract of lead, and cauſtic alkali, without giving the leaſt tendency towards a ſtricture, although they produced violent inflammation, and even ſloughing of the internal membrane of the urethra.

By many they have been ſuppoſed to have ariſen from the healing of ulcers in the urethra; but as I never ſaw an ulcer in theſe parts, except in conſequence of a ſtricture, and as I do not believe there ever is an ulcer in the caſe of a common gonorrhœa, I can hardly attribute them to that cauſe.

I. OF THE BOUGIE.

The bougie, with it's application, is perhaps one of the greateſt improvements in ſurgery which theſe laſt thirty or forty years have produced. When I compare the practice of the preſent day with what it was in the year 1750, it hardly appears to be the ſame diſeaſe we are treating. I remember about that time when I attended the firſt hoſpitals in this city, the common bougies were either a piece of lead* or a ſmall wax candle; and although the preſent bougie was known at that time, yet a due preference was not given, or it's particular merit underſtood, as we may ſee from the publications of that time.

Daran was the firſt who improved the bougie and brought it into general uſe. He wrote profeſſedly on the diſeaſes for which it is a cure, and alſo of the manner of preparing it; but he has introduced ſo much abſurdity in his deſcriptions of the diſeaſes, the modes of treatment, and of the powers and compoſition of his bougies, as to create diſguſt; yet this abſurdity has been much more effectual in introducing the bougie into univerſal uſe, than all the real knowledge of that time directed by good ſenſe could have been. Such extravagant recommendations of particular remedies are not at all times without their uſe. Inoculation would have ſtill been practiced with caution, if it had not been for the enthuſiaſm of the Suttons. Preparations of lead

* When lead was uſed in place of bougies, it has happened that a piece of the end has broken off in the bladder, which has been diſſolved by throwing quickſilver into that viſcus. I ſuſpected that quickſilver could not come in contact with lead while in water ſo as to diſſolve it, but upon making the experiment I found it did.

would

would not have been so univerſally applied if they had not been recommended by Goulard in the moſt extravagant terms; nor would the hemlock have come into ſuch general uſe if it's true merits only had been held forth. Improvements are often over rated, but they come to their true value at laſt: Sutton has told us, that the cold regimen in extreme is infinitely better than the old method; but from general practice we have learned that moderation is beſt, which is all we yet know.

When Daran publiſhed his obſervations on the bougie, every ſurgeon ſet to work to diſcover the compoſition, and each conceived that he had found it out from the bougies he had made producing the effects deſcribed by Daran. It never occurred to them that any extraneous body of the ſame ſhape and conſiſtence would do the ſame thing.

II. OF THE TREATMENT OF THE PERMANENT STRICTURE.

The cure of the permanent ſtricture is I believe to be accompliſhed only by local applications; mercury has been given upon the erroneous ſuppoſition of it's being venereal, but without ſucceſs. The cure is either a dilatation of the contracted part, or a deſtruction of it by ulceration, or eſcharotics. The dilatation is performed by the bougie, and is ſeldom or ever more than a temporary cure; for although the paſſage may be dilated ſufficiently for the urine to paſs, yet there is always the original tendency for contraction which generally recurs ſooner or later.* The ulcerative proceſs is alſo effected by a bougie, and the deſtruction by eſcharotics, is by means of cauſtics, as the lunar cauſtic. It often happens in ſtrictures that the paſſage is ſo diminiſhed

* In caſes of ſtricture when a patient applies for relief, it may often be proper to inquire into the hiſtory of the caſe, previous to the paſſing of a bougie; eſpecially to enquire if he ever uſed bougies before; if he has, then to enquire into the reſult; if they paſſed readily, or if they did not paſs the ſtricture at all: if the firſt, then nothing further need be aſked, but if the laſt then enquire if he or his ſurgeon obſerved that they were gaining ground with the bougie, viz. if the bougie went further in before they left them off than at firſt; if ſo, then to aſk him how far. If they have viſibly gained ground without getting through the ſtricture, I am afraid that the uſe of the bougie muſt not be purſued, becauſe it is moſt probable a new paſſage has been formed, which makes the paſſing of the bougie into the ſtricture impoſſible.

as hardly to allow any water to paſs, producing often a total ſtoppage; nor will a bougie immediately paſs, and if it can be made to paſs, yet no water follows it when withdrawn. In ſuch caſes therefore we muſt have recourſe to temporary relief; ſuch as the warm-bath, which counteracts the effects of cold, and quiets any ſpaſms that may have taken place in the parts, and clyſters alſo with opium, which have ſtill more effect. Producing an evacuation by ſtool, often leſſens the ſpaſm, for a ſpaſmodic ſuppreſſion of urine often ariſes from a conſtipation, even where there is no ſtricture.

Probably a bliſter to the perinæum will be of ſingular ſervice, if there be time for it's operation.

The cure by dilatation is I imagine principally mechanical when performed by bougies, whoſe powers are in general thoſe of a wedge; however their ultimate effect is not always ſo ſimple, as that of a wedge upon inanimate matter; for preſſure produces action of the animal powers, either to adapt the parts to their new poſition, or to recede by ulceration, which gives us two very different effects of a bougie, and of courſe two different intentions in applying them; one to produce dilatation the other ulceration, which laſt is not always ſo readily effected.

It generally happens, as has been already obſerved, that the diſeaſe has gone conſiderable lengths before application has been made for a cure, and therefore the ſtricture has become conſiderable, in ſo much that it is often with great difficulty that a ſmall bougie can be made to paſs. If the caſe is ſuch as will readily admit the end of a ſmall bougie to paſs, let it be ever ſo ſmall, the cure is then in our power; it often happens however, that the ſtricture is ſuch, as will reſiſt the paſſing of a ſmall bougie at firſt, and even after repeated trials. Yet it is neceſſary to perſevere with the ſmall bougie, for ſometimes it happens that the paſſage through the ſtricture is not in a line with the urethra itſelf, which of courſe obſtructs the bougie; ſuch ſtrictures I ſuſpect are not equally placed all round ſo as to throw the ſmall paſſage remaining into the centre of the canal.

In many caſes where the ſtricture is very conſiderable, we are often teazed with occaſional ſpaſms, which will either refuſe the bougie altogether, or only let a very ſmall one paſs; though at another time they will admit one larger: in ſuch caſes I have been able to get the point of the bougie ſometimes

to

to enter, by rubbing the perinæum externally with the finger of one hand while I pushed the bougie on with the other. This though it does not always succeed yet is worth trying. Whether it alters the position of the stricture so as to give entrance to the point of the bougie, or by sympathy removes the spasm I will not absolutely determine, but I believe it rather acts by sympathy.

In such cases of spasm in the stricture, I have often succeeded by letting the bougie remain a little while close to the stricture, and then pushing it on; this mode so often succeeds that it should always be attempted when the bougie does not pass, or only passes occasionally, which will be mentioned more fully when on the spasmodic stricture.

Dipping the glans penis into cold water might probably take off the spasm, as it does sometimes in common strangury, but this cannot be so easily done while a bougie is in the passage.

In cases of a permanent stricture, though the bougie does not at first pass, yet upon repeated trials it will every now and then find it's way, which helps to render a future trial more certain and easy. Yet it too often happens that the future success does not immediately depend upon passing the bougie once or twice, for it shall pass to-day and not to-morrow; and this uncertainty shall last for weeks, notwithstanding every trial we can make. I may however observe that in general it's introduction becomes gradually less difficult, and therefore in no case should we despair of success.

It is imagined by some that the best time for trial in these cases is just after making water, as the passage is supposed to be clear and more in a straight line; but this is not confirmed by practice.

It is not an easy matter in cases where the passage is very small, to tell whether the bougie has entered the stricture or not; for such slender bougies as must generally be used at first, bend so very easily that the introducer is apt to think it is passing while it is only bending. A surgeon however should generally first make himself acquainted with the situation of the stricture, by a common sized bougie, and when that is known he should try a smaller one, and when he comes to the stricture push gently, and for a little time only. If he has pressed so as make the bougie pass further into the penis, he will know how far it has entered the stricture by taking off the pressure from

from the bougie; for if it recoil he may be ſure that it has not paſſed, at leaſt has not paſſed far but only bent, for the natural elaſticity of the bougie and the direction of the paſſage having been altered by it will force it back again. But if it remain fixed and do not recoil, he may be ſure that it has entered the ſtricture; in uſing a very ſmall bougie however theſe obſervations do not ſo well apply, for it may be bending, or bent, without being perceptible. It often happens that a bougie will enter only a little way, perhaps not more than one-tenth of an inch, and then bend if the preſſure be continued. To know whether this be the caſe it is neceſſary to withdraw the bougie and examine it's end; if the end be blunted we may be ſure the bougie has not entered in the leaſt, but if it be flattened for an eighth or tenth of an inch, or grooved, or have it's outer waxy coat puſhed up for that length, or if there be a circular impreſſion made upon the bougie where the ſtricture is, or only a dent on one ſide, both of which laſt I ſuſpect ariſe from ſpaſm at the time, we may then be ſure that it has paſſed as far as theſe appearances extend. It becomes then neceſſary to introduce another exactly of the ſame ſize and in the ſame manner, and to let it remain as long as the patient can bear it, or convenience will allow; and by repeating this the ſtricture will be overcome. Sometimes we can judge of it's having entered the ſtricture, by pulling it gently out; for if it ſtick a little at the firſt pull we may be certain it has entered; but the appearance of the bougie itſelf will give the beſt information.* In ſuch caſes I have always directed my patient to preſerve the bougie for my inſpection, exactly in the ſame form it was when it was withdrawn; but when it paſſes with eaſe this nicety is not neceſſary.

* It may be remarked, that there are ſome lacunæ (Vide plate I, fig. 2.) near, and alſo a little way beyond the glans penis, which often ſtop the bougie, and give at firſt the idea of a ſtricture. I have known them taken for ſuch; and when the bougie ſtops ſo near to the glans this is to be ſuſpected, and therefore the direction of the point of the bougie ſhould be varied, bearing it againſt the under ſide of the urethra. When the bougie ſtops in one of thoſe lacunæ I think that the patient appears to have more pain than from a real ſtricture. The valvular part of the proſtate gland formed by diſeaſe (Vide plate V.) very often obſtructs the bougie and is taken for a ſtricture by thoſe who are not well acquainted with the different obſtructions in this canal; and by thoſe who are, it is a means of diſcovering diſeaſe in this part; and indeed in a natural ſtate of parts I think I can tell when I come to this part with a bougie.

The

The time that each bougie ſhould remain in the paſſage muſt be determined by the feelings of the patient, for it ſhould never give pain if poſſible. Going beyond this point is deſtroying the intention, increaſing the very ſymptoms that are meant to be relieved, and producing irritation, which for a time renders the further application of the bougie improper. While the bougie is paſſing, if the patient feel very acutely, it ſhould not be left in above five or ten minutes, or not ſo long if it give great pain; and each time of application ſhould be lengthened ſo gradually, as to be inſenſible to the feelings of the mind, and the irritability of the parts. I have known it days, nay in many patients weeks, before they could allow the bougie to remain in the paſſage five or ten minutes, and yet in time they have been able to bear it for hours, and at laſt without any difficulty. The beſt time to let them remain in the paſſage is when the patient has leaſt to do; or in the morning while he is in bed, provided he can paſs it himſelf.

The bougie ſhould be increaſed in ſize according to the facility with which the ſtricture dilates, and the eaſe with which the patient bears the dilatation. If the parts are very firm, or very irritable, the increaſe of the ſize of the bougie ſhould be ſlow, gradually ſtealing upon the parts, and allowing them to adapt their ſtructure to the increaſed ſize. But if the ſenſibility of the parts will allow, the increaſe of the ſize of the bougie may be ſomewhat quicker, though never more quick than the patient can bear with eaſe; the increaſe ſhould be continued till the largeſt ſized bougie paſſes freely; nor ſhould this be laid aſide till after three weeks, or a month, in order to habituate the dilated part to it's new poſition, or to take off the habit of contracting from the part as much as poſſible; but as was obſerved before, the permanency of this cure can ſeldom be depended upon.

Inſtead of proceeding with the caution recommended, it has been practiſed with ſucceſs for a time, to force a common ſized bougie through a ſtricture that only allowed a ſmall one to paſs. This I ſuppoſe either tore the ſtricture or weakened it by ſtretching it ſuddenly ſo as to render it unable to recover it's contractile power for a conſiderable time after. I have ſeen where this has produced good effects, and for a time removed the permanent ſtricture, and prevented ſpaſm from taking place. This is a practice however which I have never tried; always preferring the mild treatment where I could paſs a bougie.

I have known the paſſing of the bougie remove almoſt immediately a ſwelling of the teſticle which had ariſen from the ſtricture; therefore ſuch a ſymptom ſhould not prevent the uſe of the bougie.

In caſes of ſtrictures where the bougie is uſed, the patient is commonly in other reſpects well, and is with difficulty perſuaded to reſtrain from his common habits, often making too free in eating, drinking, and exerciſe; which are all in many caſes pernicious, more eſpecially where inflammation and ſuppuration have taken place. It is therefore the duty of the ſurgeon to reſtrict the patient for ſome time within certain bounds, till he finds by trials what the parts are capable of bearing without producing inflammation.

III. OF THE CURE OF STRICTURE BY ULCERATION.

The cure of a ſtricture by means of ulceration is likewiſe effected by a bougie; this method may be employed both in caſes where a bougie will paſs, and where it will not. In the firſt caſe there is not the ſame neceſſity for ulceration as in the ſecond, becauſe where a bougie will paſs there is no immediate danger ariſing from the ſtricture, which may therefore be dilated, as already deſcribed. But in caſe this method ſhould be preferred to a ſlow dilatation, which allows the parts time to adapt themſelves to their new poſition, the ſtricture may be deſtroyed by producing ulceration in the parts, eſpecially if they are not irritable, ſo as to admit of conſiderable violence.

When this is intended, the bougie ſhould be introduced as far into the ſtricture as poſſible, and the ſize of it increaſed as faſt as the ſenſations of the patient can well bear. This will produce ulceration in the part preſſed, which is a more laſting cure, becauſe more of the ſtricture is deſtroyed than when the parts are ſimply dilated, I believe however there are few patients that will ſubmit to this practice; and indeed few will be able to bear it; for I have ſeen it bring on violent ſpaſms on the part which produced ſuppreſſion of urine, and proved very troubleſome. Therefore as there is no abſolute neceſſity in ſuch caſes for purſuing this method, I do not recom-

mend

mend it as a general practice, although there are cases where it succeeds; and where this method is to be practised, it might probably not be amiss to accustom the passage to a bougie for some time before such violence is used.

If the smallest bougie which can possibly be made with some degree of strength cannot pass, dilatation becomes impracticable, and it is necessary that something else should be done for the relief of the patient; and the destruction of the stricture is to be effected some way or other. In many cases it may be proper to attempt this by ulceration of the part; for we find from experience, that a stricture may be removed by the simple pressure of a bougie. This effect must arise from the irritation of absorption being given to the diseased part, which from the stricture not being an original formed part, nor having any power of resistance equal to the original one, is more susceptible of ulceration, and thereby is absorbed. The bougies which are only to produce ulceration in consequence of their being applied to the stricture, need not be so small as in the former cases, as they are not intended to pass; and by being of a common size they will also be more certain in their application to the stricture. The force applied to a bougie in this case should not be great, for a stricture is the hardest part of the urethra; and if a bougie is applied with a considerable degree of pressure, and continued there, it sometimes happens that the end of the bougie slips off the stricture before there is time for ulceration, and makes it's way into the substance of the corpus spongiosum by the side of the stricture; and if the pressure be continued still longer, it will make a new passage beyond the stricture in the corpus spongiosum urethræ.* This more readily happens if the stricture be in the bend of the canal, as in such cases the bougie can hardly be applied exactly to it, not having the same curve; such mischief I have seen more than once; and sometimes the bougie has been pushed so far as to make it's way into the rectum.

It often requires a considerable time before the whole is so far ulcerated as to admit the bougie, and this tires the patient and almost makes him despair of a cure. In this process great attention should be paid to the seeming progress of the cure; for if it appears to the surgeon that he is gaining

* Vide plate II.

ground

ground by the bougie paſſing farther in, and yet the patient does not make water better in the leaſt, then he may be ſure that he is forcing a new paſſage.*

When the ſtricture is ſo far got the better of by theſe means as to admit a ſmall bougie, the dilatation is to be made as in the former caſe where a bougie paſſed at firſt. Whenever a bougie of a tolerable ſize paſſes with eaſe, and the parts and patient have become accuſtomed to them, it is no longer neceſſary that the ſurgeon ſhould continue to paſs them; the patient may be allowed to introduce them himſelf; and when he can do it readily, it may be truſted to him in common, as he can make uſe of them at the moſt convenient times, by which means they may be in general longer and oftener applied, the ſurgeon only ſeeing him occaſionally. This practice of the patient under a ſurgeon's eye, by which he is taught how to paſs them, becomes more neceſſary, as ſtrictures are diſeaſes that commonly recur, therefore no man who has ever had a ſtricture, and is cured of it, ſhould rely on the cure as laſting, but ſhould be always prepared for a return; and ſhould always have ſome bougies by him. He ſhould not go a journey even of a week without them; and the number ſhould be according to the time he is to be gone, or the place he is going to; for in many parts of the world he cannot be ſupplied with them. The bougies for ſuch purpoſe ſhould be of different ſizes, as it is uncertain in what degree the diſeaſe may return.

Bougies, in all caſes, from their ſhape, and from the action of the parts, readily ſlip out, which retards the cure; but it is much worſe when they paſs into the bladder; which can only take place in caſes where the ſtricture is in ſome meaſure overcome. The conſequence of a bougie paſſing into the bladder muſt at once appear in it's fulleſt force to every one; it ſubjects the patient in moſt caſes to be cut as for the ſtone; and indeed if it is either not ſoon thrown out, or cut out, it becomes the baſis of a ſtone. A young man was cut for a bougie only a fortnight after it had paſſed into

* This makes it neceſſary in all caſes of ſtrictures where bougies will not paſs, to be very particular in our inquiries, whether the patient has uſed bougies formerly, and whether there may not be reaſon to believe that they had taken a wrong direction.

the

the bladder; and it was almoſt wholly cruſted over with calculous matter. Bougies have been known to be forced out of the bladder along with the water by the action of that viſcus, and in ſeveral folds. It is probable that the bladder in a natural ſtate has not power ſufficient to perform ſuch an action; but we ſhall ſhow that in caſes of ſtrictures where the reſiſtance to the paſſing of the water is very much increaſed, the ſtrength of the bladder becomes proportionably greater; this happens principally in caſes of ſtrictures of long ſtanding.

Such accidents are often obſerved before the outer end of the bougie has got beyond the projecting part of the penis, but even then it is difficult of extraction. I have ſucceeded in ſome of theſe caſes by fixing the bougie in the urethra ſome way below it's end; for inſtance, in the perinæum, by preſſing againſt it with one hand, and puſhing back the penis upon the bougie with the other hand; then laying hold of the penis upon the bougie, removing the preſſure below, and drawing the whole up; and by performing theſe two motions alternately, I have been able to lay hold of the end of it. However this does not always ſucceed, for when the bougie is either ſmall, or becomes ſoft, it will not admit of the penis being puſhed down upon it without bending; or if the thick end of the bougie has got beyond the moveable, or projecting part of the penis, then this mode of treatment becomes impracticable. I have ſucceeded in theſe laſt caſes with the forceps for extracting the ſtone out of the urethra; but if it has got into the bend of the urethra, this practice will alſo fail; and in ſuch a ſtate it would be moſt adviſeable to paſs a catheter down to it, and cut upon that; and probably the above-mentioned forceps introduced through the wound might then lay hold of it's end; or by cutting a little further, ſo as to expoſe ſome part of the bougie, it might be eaſily extracted, without the neceſſity of cutting into the bladder; this part of the operation however would be very difficult in a fat or luſty man.

To prevent the inconveniency of the bougie coming out, or the miſchief of it's paſſing in, it is neceſſary to tie a ſoft cotton thread round that end of the bougie which is out of the urethra, and then round the root of the glans; this laſt part ſhould be very looſe, for an obvious reaſon; and the projecting part of the bougie ſhould alſo be bent down upon the penis, which makes it both leſs troubleſome, and more ſecure.

IV. OF THE APPLICATION OF CAUSTIC TO STRICTURES.

When a bougie can readily paſs there is no neceſſity for uſing any other method to remove the ſtricture: but there are too many caſes where a bougie cannot be made to paſs, or ſo ſeldom that it cannot be depended upon for a cure. This may ariſe from ſeveral cauſes. Firſt, the ſtricture may be ſo tight as not to allow the ſmalleſt bougie to paſs. Secondly, the orifice in the ſtricture may not be in a line with the urethra, which will make it uncertain, if not impoſſible, to paſs a bougie. Thirdly, there may be no paſſage at all, it having been obliterated by diſeaſe, and the urine paſſed by *fiſtulæ in perinæo*.

The firſt very rarely occurs, for if the paſſage in the ſtricture be in a line with the general canal, a ſmall bougie will commonly paſs, and although it may not readily do ſo upon every trial, it will be ſufficient to make way for another bougie, which is all that is wanted.

The ſecond caſe where the canal is not in a line with the common paſſage may ariſe from three cauſes. Firſt, when the ſtricture is in the bend of the urethra, although the paſſage through it may be in the centre of the canal, yet as the bougie cannot have the exact curve, it will be very uncertain in it's application. Secondly, from an irregularity in the formation of the ſtricture, which may throw the paſſage to one ſide, even in the ſtraight part of the urethra; and Thirdly, from ulceration having taken place, producing *fiſtulæ in perinæo*, which often make the canal irregular in it's courſe.

The third caſe where the application of the cauſtic may be neceſſary, is where there is no paſſage at all, which happens from ulceration and abſceſſes in the perinæum opening externally; and in the healing of them the paſſage is often cloſed up entirely. In all the above-mentioned caſes I have ſucceeded with the cauſtic beyond expectation.

If the obſtructions are any where between the membranous part of the urethra and the glans, where the canal is nearly ſtraight, or can eaſily be made

made ſo by the introduction of a ſtraight inſtrument, it becomes an eaſy matter to deſtroy them by cauſtic; but if beyond that, it becomes then more difficult; however at the beginning of the bend of the urethra the obſtruction may be ſo far got the better of as to admit of the paſſing of a bougie, or at leaſt to procure a tolerable free paſſage for the urine. I have ſeen ſeveral caſes where it was thought neceſſary to follow this practice, and it ſucceeded ſo well that after a few touches with the cauſtic the bougie could be paſſed, which is all that is wanted. The ſucceſs in theſe caſes was ſuch as would incline me to have recourſe to this practice very early, indeed whenever I could not paſs a ſmall bougie through the ſtricture; and I look upon the cauſtic as a much ſafer method than uſing preſſure with a bougie, for the reaſon before-mentioned, that is, the danger of making a new paſſage, without deſtroying in the leaſt any part of the obſtruction.

Moſt of the ſtrictures I ever examined after death, appeared to be in the power of ſuch treatment; however I have ſeen one or two caſes where the contraction was of ſome length and irregular, which would have puzzled me if I had attempted the cure with the cauſtic; becauſe I ſhould have been apt to ſuſpect that I was making a new paſſage by my gaining ground, and yet not relieving the patient, by the removal of the ſymptoms.

I have often tried this practice in ſtrictures where there were alſo fiſtulæ in the urethra, and where the water came through different paſſages. Such caſes I ſhould ſuſpect were not the moſt favourable, yet I ſucceeded in the greater part of them, that is, I got through the ſtricture and could paſs a bougie freely. I have ſeen ſeveral caſes of fiſtulæ of theſe parts, where the natural paſſage was obliterated by the ſtricture, in which I have ſucceeded with the cauſtic, and the fiſtulous orifices have readily healed up.

It does not happen always in caſes of obſtruction to the paſſage of the urine, that when the obſtruction is removed by the cauſtic, and the water of courſe paſſes freely, a bougie will alſo paſs. This I apprehend ariſes from the cauſtic not having deſtroyed the ſtricture in a direct line with the urethra; ſo that a bougie cannot catch the ſound urethra beyond. But this appears to me of little conſequence as it is as much in the power of the bougie to prevent a return at this part as if it paſſed on to the bladder; for if the water flows readily, it is certain that the cauſtic has gone beyond the ſtricture, although

though it may not be in a direct line, and that the only risk of a return of obstruction will be at the old stricture; but as a bougie can now pass beyond that part, it does as much good as if it passed into the bladder; for I have known several cases where the bougie appeared to have the same effect as if it had passed on to the bladder.

The application of the caustic need not be longer than a minute, and it may be repeated every day, or every other day, allowing time for the slough to come off. But there are other causes that may prevent the repetition of the caustic, besides waiting for the separation of the slough, for sometimes the use of it brings on irritation, inflammation, or spasm in the part, which frequently occasions a total suppression of urine for a time, against which all the means used commonly on such occasions to procure relief must be employed, and we must wait till these symptoms are gone off. If the patient can make water immediately after the application it will be proper, as it will wash away any caustic that may have been dissolved in the passage, which if left would irritate the parts; a little water injected into the urethra will answer the same purpose.

About the year 1752, attending a chimney-sweeper for a stricture, the first patient I ever had with this disease, and not finding that I gained any advantage after six months trial with the bougie, I conceived that I might be able to destroy the stricture by escharotics;* my first attempt was with red precipitate. I applied to the end of a bougie some salve, and then dipped it into red precipitate. This bougie I passed down to the stricture, but I found that it brought on considerable inflammation all along the inside of the passage, which I attributed to the precipitate being rubbed off in passing the bougie. I then had a silver canula made and introduced it down to the stricture, and through this canula passed the bougie with precipitate as before. Not finding however that he made water any better, and not yet being able to pass the smallest bougie through the stricture, I suspected that the precipitate had not sufficient powers to destroy it; I therefore took a small piece of lunar caustic and fastened it on the end of a wire with sealing wax, and introduced it through the canula to the stricture; after doing this three times

* Lately looking over some authors on this disease I find that this is not a new idea.

at

at two days interval, he came to me and told me that he made water much better; and in applying the caustic a fourth time my canula went through the stricture;[a] a bougie was afterwards passed for some little time till he was perfectly well.

Having succeeded so well in this case, I was encouraged to apply my mind to the invention of some instrument better suited to the purpose than the above-mentioned, which I have in some degree effected, although it is not yet perfectly adapted to all the situations of stricture in the urethra. The caustic should be prevented from hurting any other part of the canal; which is best done by introducing it through a canula to the stricture, making it protrude a little beyond the end of the canula, by which it acts only upon the stricture. The caustic should be fixed in a small port-crayon. It is necessary to have a piece of silver of the length of the canula, with a ring at one end, and a button at the other of the same diameter with the canula, forming a kind of plug, which should project beyond the end of the canula that enters the urethra, by which means it makes a rounded end; or the port-crayon may be formed with this button at the other end. The button being introduced into the canula, it should be passed into the urethra, and when got to the stricture the silver plug should be drawn, and the port-crayon with the caustic introduced in it's place; or if the plug and port-crayon are on the same instrument, then it is only withdrawing it, and introducing the port-crayon with the caustic, which will destroy the stricture. This plug, besides giving a smooth rounded end to the canula, answers another good purpose, by preventing the canula from being filled with the mucus of the urethra as it passes along, which mucus would be collected in the end of it, dissolve the caustic too soon, and hinder it's application to the stricture.[b]

If the stricture be in the bend of the urethra the canula may be bent at the end also; but it becomes more difficult to introduce a piece of caustic through such a canula, for the plug and port-crayon must also be bent at the end, which cannot be made to pass through the straight part of the canula;

[a] Wiseman had the same idea, but probably the clumsy way in which he attempted to put it in execution might be the reason why he seems not to have pursued it.

[b] Vide plate III, fig. 1.

canula; but this I have in ſome meaſure obviated by having the canula made flexible, except at the end where it is to take the curve.*

After the bougie can be made to paſs, the caſe is to be treated as a common ſtricture, either by dilating it ſlowly, or by quickly increaſing the ſize of the bougie, and thus continuing the ulceration.

There are ſometimes more ſtrictures than one; but it ſeldom happens that they are all equally bad; one only becomes the object of our attention. The ſmaller ones may however be ſufficient to hinder the paſſing the canula to the ſtricture which is to be deſtroyed by the cauſtic. When that is the caſe, thoſe ſmall ſtrictures are to be dilated with bougies, as in common, till they are ſufficiently large to allow the canula to paſs.

* Vide plate III, fig. 2 and 3.

CHAPTER

CHAPTER III.

OF STRICTURES IN WOMEN.

OBSTRUCTIONS to the water in women I believe generally arise from stricture, although not always; for I have known them produced by compression from some adjacent swelling; and they are common in utero-gestation, as also in dropsical or scirrhous ovaria; but such causes are commonly known long before this effect is produced, by which the suppression is easily accounted for: it may also arise from excrescences as in men.

How far a stricture in the urethra of this sex is really a consequence of a venereal inflammation I am not certain, but should suppose it was not; and for stronger reasons still than those given in speaking of the cause of strictures in men; for I can say, that in all the strictures I ever saw in women, none of them arose in consequence of this disease; at least I had no reason to believe that they did; and I have observed before, that in most women who have the venereal disease in the form of a gonorrhoea, it seldom attacks the urethra; therefore if we find a stricture in a woman who has had the disease we are not to impute it to that, at least till we know whether she had the disease in that canal; and even then it will remain doubtful.

Strictures are not near so common in women as in men, and this may be owing to the great difference there is in the length of the two canals; but more especially to the canal in women being more simple, and intended only for one purpose. The stricture in women does not produce such a variety of symptoms, or so much mischief, as in men, there not being so many parts to be affected.

I. OF

I. OF THE CURE OF STRICTURES IN WOMEN.

The cure of ſtrictures in the urethra of women is ſimilar to that in men; but it is rather more ſimple from the ſimplicity of the parts. There is however an inconvenience attending the paſſing the bougie in women, that does not take place in men, which is, that in moſt caſes it muſt be paſſed for them, it being hardly poſſible for a woman to introduce a bougie herſelf. The confinement of the bougie is alſo more difficult, for although they can eaſily be prevented from going into the bladder by bending the outer end down upon the mouth of the vagina; yet it is very difficult to prevent them from ſlipping out. It will be neceſſary to have a bandage of the T kind paſſing down between the labia over the bend of the bougie.

It appears to me that the cauſtic would anſwer extremely well in ſuch caſes, and therefore I ſhould prefer it to the bougie, both for convenience and efficacy.

II. OF THE GLEET IN CONSEQUENCE OF A STRICTURE.

I have already obſerved, that it happens generally, if not always, that there is a gleet when there is a ſtricture in the urethra. This I ſuppoſe ariſes from the irritation produced in the urethra beyond the ſtricture, by the urine in it's paſſage diſtending this part too much, which diſtention is increaſed by the increaſed ſtrength of the bladder. This ſymptom often leads us to the knowledge of a ſtricture, or at leaſt gives a ſuſpicion of ſuch a diſeaſe; and when a ſtricture is known to be the cauſe, no attempts ſhould be made to cure the gleet, for it is generally cured when the ſtricture is removed; but if it ſtill remains it may be cured as recommended in the common gleet, as probably ariſing from another cauſe than a ſtricture.

CHAPTER

CHAPTER IV.

OF STRICTURE ATTENDED WITH SPASMODIC AFFECTION.

THERE are very few ſtrictures that are not more or leſs attended with ſpaſms; but ſome much more than others; the ſpaſm being in ſome caſes more the diſeaſe than the ſtricture itſelf: but real ſtrictures are attended with occaſional contractions, which makes the paſſing of the urine much more difficult at one time than another. In all the caſes that I have ſeen of this kind, when not attended with ſpaſms, the diſeaſe is not formidable; but when the parts are in a ſpaſmodic ſtate the ſymptoms are as violent as in the ſimple ſtricture.

As this is a mixed caſe it has all the characters both of the permanent and ſpaſmodic ſtricture; for the urethra in ſuch caſes is in a ſtate ſimilar to what it is in the true ſpaſmodic kind, being very irritable, giving great pain in paſſing of the bougie, and often rejecting it altogether; as will be taken notice of when we ſhall treat of that diſeaſe.

Upon conſidering this ſubject we ſhould at firſt hardly be diſpoſed to believe that the ſpaſm in the urethra is in the ſtrictured part, which can ſcarcely be ſuppoſed capable of contraction; and it might therefore naturally be referred to the ſound part of the urethra, as being brought on by the waters not flowing freely; if this is a juſt mode of accounting for it, we muſt ſuppoſe that the contraction is behind the ſtricture, that being the only part dilated by the water; and ſuch urethras being very irritable, that part may contract ſo as to ſtop the flowing of the water altogether. But ſome circumſtances occurring in practice would incline us to believe that ſuch ſtrictures have the power of contraction; for we find the bougie graſped by the ſtricture when allowed to remain ſome time. And the circumſtance of the ſtrictured part refuſing the bougie at times is alſo a proof of the ſame.

There is ſometimes this ſingular circumſtance attending theſe caſes, that when there ariſes a gonorrhœa, or any other diſcharge of matter from the urethra, where none was before, or an increaſe of an old gleet, the paſſage becomes ſo free as to allow the urine to paſs as uſual: but theſe are uncertain, and only temporary reliefs; for whenever the diſcharge ceaſes the ſpaſmodic affection returns. I think it moſt probable that it is only the ſpaſm that is affected by the diſcharge, and not the real ſtricture. Two remarkable caſes of this kind fell under my obſervation, which I ſhall now relate.

A gentleman had for a long time a complaint in the urethra attended with a ſtricture, which was ſuppoſed to be originally from a venereal complaint: it was often attended with a diſcharge which always produced a ſlight fever on it's coming on; but while the diſcharge laſted the difficulty in making water was relieved, and that in proportion to the greatneſs of the diſcharge: and whenever he got a freſh gonorrhœa the ſame thing happened.

Another gentleman had a difficulty in making water, ſuppoſed to ariſe from a ſtricture; it was generally attended with ſuch a running as is common to ſtrictures: but when that diſcharge was much increaſed, then the ſtricture was leſs in proportion. During this complaint he contracted two different infections, both of which relieved him of the ſtricture for the time.

As this is a mixed diſeaſe it may be thought proper to paſs a bougie for the real ſtricture, and for the other to uſe the method hereafter recommended for the cure of ſpaſm.

It frequently happens in theſe mixed caſes, that a bougie does not immediately paſs, but is rejected by the ſpaſm; yet by letting it lie in the urethra almoſt cloſe to the ſtricture for ten, fifteen, or twenty minutes, it will often paſs. This is as it were ſtealing upon it; and the water ſhall flow although the bougie is not attempted to be paſſed on. Theſe however are only temporary modes of relief. In ſome inſtances the ſpaſm is almoſt as conſtant as the permanent ſtricture; in ſuch caſes paſſing a bougie into the urethra for three or four inches in length, covered by ſome irritating medicine, and keeping this in as long at each time as the patient can bear, will, if perſevered in for a few weeks, often prove a cure for the ſpaſmodic affection.

I. OF

CHAPTER V.

OF SOME CIRCUMSTANCES ATTENDING THE USE OF BOUGIES—THEIR FIGURE AND COMPOSITION.

IN cases of strictures where a bougie is used as a wedge, not as a stimulant, and where the stricture is so far overcome as to let a bougie pass on; the question is, whether it is better to pass the bougie the whole length of the urethra, so that the end shall be in the bladder, or only to pass it through the stricture a little way, so that the end shall remain in the urethra. Nothing but experience can determine this question, and in such cases I believe we seldom make a fair trial, generally pushing the bougie on to the bladder; though if we observe the consequences of the bougies not passing in those cases where they either cannot pass far beyond the stricture or not at all, we find no inconvenience arising from this circumstance, except where they are applied with too much force, so as to make a new passage. The common idea is, that it will be more hurtful to allow the end of the bougie to lie in the urethra than in the bladder; but I imagine this is more founded in theory than practice.

Some people have such a quantity of calculous matter in their urine; or so great a disposition in their urine to deposit it's calculous matter, that it only requires the presence of an extraneous body in the bladder to become an immediate cause of stone; for I have observed in some, that the end of a bougie cannot remain in the bladder a few hours without being covered with a crust of calculous matter. Such people I have generally advised to use as much exercise as all other circumstances will allow.

Bougies when first introduced often produce sickness, and sometimes even fainting. I have seen a patient become sick, the colour leave his face, a cold sweat

ſweat come on, and at laſt faint; but all theſe ſoon go off, and ſeldom return upon a ſecond or third trial.

They at firſt produce an irritation on the urethra, which gives pain in the time of making water, but goes off on repetition.

They produce a ſecretion of pus in thoſe caſes, where there was none, and generally increaſe the diſcharge where there is one previous to their application; but this effect gradually ceaſes.

It frequently happens that ſwellings in the lymphatic glands of the groin ariſe from the uſe of bougies, but I never ſaw them come the length of ſuppuration. As in moſt of theſe caſes there was a diſcharge of matter previous to the bougie being paſſed, they could hardly be owing to the abſorption of matter, but muſt have ariſen from ſympathy.

When treating of the ſtricture, I obſerved that it was often the cauſe of a ſwelling in one or both teſticles; and further, that the paſſing of a bougie often removed that complaint. I may now obſerve, that a very common conſequence of the paſſing of a bougie is a ſwelling of the teſticle, this alſo ariſes from ſympathy, and like the ſwelling of the glands, is a common effect of all irritations of the urethra.

It may not be improper here to add ſome obſervations on the figure and compoſition of bougies. They ought to be about two inches longer than the diſtance between the glans and the ſtricture, or more if they can paſs freely, ſo as always to allow an inch to bend upon the glans, and another to paſs beyond the ſtricture. The thickneſs is to be according to the ſize of the ſtricture; at firſt to be ſuch as will paſs with a ſmall degree of tightneſs, and this is to be followed up as the contracted part enlarges. But when the urethra has become of the natural ſize, then the bougie need not be increaſed, but it's uſe ſtill continued, as has been obſerved.

With regard to the ſhape, they ſhould not taper from end to end when very ſmall, but ſhould be nearly of an equal thickneſs till within an inch of their ſmalleſt end, after which they ſhould taper to a point, forming a round wedge fitted to paſs into the ſtricture; and this form gives them greater ſtrength than when made to taper from one end to the other.

The conſiſtence ought to vary according to the nature of the caſe, and ſize of the bougie. If the ſtricture be near the glans, a ſtiff bougie may be uſed,

uſed, and the whole may be made to taper gradually, becauſe a ſhort bougie will always have ſufficient ſtrength for any preſſure that is neceſſary; but if the ſtricture be deeper ſeated, as about the bulb, where the paſſage begins to take a curve, the bougie muſt be a little thicker in it's body to ſupport the neceſſary preſſure. If the ſtricture be any where in the bend of the urethra, or near the bladder, the bougie ſhould be very flexible, although this is contrary to our general poſition, becauſe in this caſe it muſt bend in order to take on the curve of the paſſage, which it ought to do with eaſe; for when it bends with difficulty it does not make it's preſſure upon the ſtricture, but upon the back part of the urethra, and therefore does not enter ſo eaſily; which circumſtance makes it more difficult to enter a ſtricture near the bladder, than near the glans.

In the compoſition of the bougie the conſiſtence is the moſt material thing to be conſidered, the medical properties, as far as known, being of little conſequence. The materials they are commonly made of are wax, oil, and litharge.

The litharge gives them ſmoothneſs, and takes off the ſtickineſs they would have if made of wax and oil only. A compoſition which anſwers well, is three pints of oil of olives, one pound of bees wax, and a pound and an half of red lead, boiled together upon a ſlow fire for ſix hours.

I. OF A NEW PASSAGE FORMED BY BOUGIES.

THE worſt conſequence ariſing from the improper uſe of the bougie, and the moſt dangerous is, where it makes a new paſſage.* I mentioned before that this generally aroſe from the attempt to produce ulceration by the application of the end of the bougie to the ſtricture in caſes where a bougie could not paſs; for in thoſe caſes where a bougie paſſes there can be no danger of ſuch an effect.

This new paſſage is ſeldom carried ſo far as to produce either an increaſe of the preſent diſeaſe, or a new one, although ſometimes it is; yet it prevents

* Vide plate II.

 the

the cure of the original disease, for it renders both the application of the bougie and caustic to the stricture so uncertain, that a continuance of either is dangerous, as they may increase the mischief, and at last produce very bad consequences.

This new passage is generally along the side of the old one, when in that part of the urethra which is on this side of the bend, and it is made in the spongy substance of the urethra; but when it is made at the beginning of the bend, then it passes on in a straight line through the body of the urethra, about the beginning of the membranous part, going through the cellular substance of the perinæum towards the rectum. When the new passage is made between the glans and the bend of the urethra, it may take place on either side of the canal equally, in the spongy substance of the urethra, between the canal and the skin of the penis, or scrotum; and it may be between the canal and the body of the penis. The situation of it will make some difference in the operation necessary for the cure of this complaint.

When a new passage is made I know of no other method of cure but to open the part externally; and the opening must be made in that part of the urethra which is most convenient for coming at the stricture; regard being had to the other external parts, such as the scrotum, &c. If the stricture be before the scrotum, the new passage will be there also, and therefore the operation must be made of course before that part; but if the stricture is opposite to the scrotum, the bottom of the new passage may also be opposite to this part; but if the new passage is of a considerable length, it's bottom or termination may be in the beginning of the perinæum; and in either situation the operation must be begun behind the scrotum, or indeed may be made a little way into it. But if the stricture and new passage are in the perinæum, then the operation is to be performed there.

The method of performing this operation is as follows: pass a staff, or any such instrument, into the urethra as far as it will go, which will probably be to the bottom of the new passage, and that we are certain is beyond the stricture; feel for the end of the instrument externally, and cut upon it, making the wound about an inch long, if the disease be before the scrotum; and an inch and an half, or more, if in the perinæum. If the new passage be between the urethra and the body of the penis, then you will most probably get into the found urethra before you come to the inftrument or new paffage; if fo it is not neceffary to go further to be able to get into the bladder, as we may be certain that this part of the urethra is behind the ftricture. Having proceeded fo far, take a probe, or fome fuch inftrument, and introduce it into the urethra by the wound, and pafs it towards the glans, which will be paffing it forwards towards the ftricture. If it meet with an obftruction there, we may be certain it is the ftricture, which is now to be got through, and which will afterwards be eafily enlarged. To complete the operation, I would advife the withdrawing the probe, and introducing in the fame manner a hollow canula forwards to the ftricture; then take another canula and introduce it from the glans downwards till the two canulas oppofe each other, having the ftricture between them; fome perfon laying hold of the urethra on the outfide, between the finger and thumb, juft where the two canulas meet, to keep them in their places; then through the upper canula introduce a piercer which will go through the ftricture, and pafs into the lower canula; this done, withdraw the piercer, and introduce a bougie into the fame canula, in the fame way, being fure it paffes into the lower canula, then withdraw the lower canula and the end of the bougie will appear in the wound; lay hold of the bougie there, and withdraw the upper canula over the bougie, leaving the bougie in the urethra; now the lower end of the bougie is to be directed into the urethra leading on to the bladder, and pufhed on to that vifcus. It may be further neceffary to lay the whole of the new paffage open, that it may all heal up; for it is poffible that this new paffage may often receive the bougie, which is to be applied in future, which would be troublefome, and might prove an obftruction to the cure.

If the new paffage be between the fkin and the canal of the urethra, after cutting down to the inftrument, you muft go further on in fearch of the natural canal, and when you have found it introduce a probe into it towards the glans to find the ftricture; and when this is done go on with the operation as above defcribed.

The bougie muft be left in the paffage, and as it may be found difficult afterwards to introduce another readily into the bladder, the longer the firft is allowed to remain fo much the more readily will the fecond pafs. I am

not

not yet certain but that it would be better to push on the hollow canula at first, and keep it there for some days, at least till the inflammation is over and the parts have adapted themselves to this body, which will make a bougie pass more easily afterwards. The bougies must be gradually increased in size, and continued till the wound is healed up.

The first time I ever saw a case of a new passage formed by the bougie was at the hospital for the third regiment of guards, about the year 1765, it was in a young soldier who had a stricture, for the cure of which he had bougies regularly passed for near half a year without any relief. They were encouraged to go on so long by appearing to gain ground on the stricture, for the bougie went further by two inches than at first; but it being suspected that there was something more than was then understood, I was consulted, and without foreseeing what was really the case, I proposed that an opening should be made into the urethra where the obstruction was, and carried further back if necessary, in search of the sound urethra, which was accordingly done in the following manner: the grooved staff was first passed as far down as it would go, which was to the bottom of the new passage, the scrotum was pulled up upon the penis, when the end of the staff was prominent towards the skin a little way above the perinæum, and there an incision was made on the end of the staff about half an inch long; this disengaged the end of the staff, which was pushed out at the wound, then search was made for the other orifice which led to the bladder, supposing that orifice to be the stricture, but none being to be found, we tried to trace it by blowing with a blow-pipe into the bottom and lower part of the wound, but no orifice could be observed; we then began to suspect that we were not in the urethra. To determine if we had been in the urethra, I began to dissect with care the parts at the bottom of the wound, and laid bare the musculi acceleratores. I then made an incision into the body of the urethra and came to the true canal, which was easily discovered. When this was done we passed a probe on to the bladder, then withdrew it and turned it, and passed it from this wound towards the glans penis, but found that it went not much more than two inches that way and then stopped. This struck us with a new idea of the case, for we were now sure that the end of the staff had not been in the urethra, but in a new passage made in the spongy part of the urethra, for two inches

inches beyond the ſtricture. We now paſſed a ſtaff by the glans down the urethra, and another up from the laſt wound, to ſee at what diſtance the ends of the two inſtruments were, which would give us the length of the ſtricture. We found by taking hold of the urethra between the finger and thumb on the outſide that the two ends were cloſe together. What was to be done next was our conſideration; it immediately ſtruck us that we might force our way through the ſtricture with ſafety. The gentleman who aſſiſted me in the operation paſſed a blow-pipe one-fifth of an inch in diameter, (being not ſufficiently furniſhed with inſtruments) from the wound forwards to the ſtricture, and then I took a ſilver canula open at both ends, which had an iron piercer longer than itſelf, and paſſed it down to the ſtricture from the glans; and now the end of the canula oppoſed the end of the blow-pipe, and they were almoſt cloſe upon one another. They were kept in this poſition with the finger and thumb applied on the outſide of the penis like ſplints on a broken bone. I then introduced the piercer and puſhed it on, which went through the ſtricture into the hollow of the blow-pipe. Great care was taken not to puſh too forcibly for fear the two ends of the hollow tubes ſhould ſlip by one another, which they would do if not held firmly, as actually happened twice in this caſe; but we ſucceeded the third time. I then puſhed on the canula through the ſtricture and with it puſhed out the blow-pipe. The next object was to paſs a hollow bougie along the urethra to the bladder, to do which the ſmall end of it was introduced into the canula, which being puſhed on forced out the canula at the wound; we then paſſed a director into the other orifice of the urethra, leading on to the bladder, and put the end of the bougie into the groove of the director, and puſhed it along the groove to the bladder, and before we withdrew the director we turned it round with it's back to the bougie, that the end of the bougie might not ſtop againſt the end of the groove, and ſo be pulled out again. After all this was done, one ſtitch was made in the urethra, but the external wound in the ſkin was left for the paſſage of the urine, that it might not inſinuate itſelf into the cellular membrane; we dreſſed the wound ſuperficially, and applied the T bandage, which was ſlit to go on each ſide of the ſcrotum, and juſt where it came to the ſcrotum we tied the two ends together, which ſupported the ſcrotum and kept it forwards on the penis, and the two ends that came from this knot on each ſide of the ſcrotum were tied to the circular part that came round the body. The patient had ſome ſlight fever for a day or two, and the urine came partly through the bougie and partly by the ſide of it through the wound. A ſwelling of one teſticle came on, likewiſe a ſwelling of the glands of the groins, pain in the belly, ſickneſs, and at times vomiting, all which ſymptoms were owing to ſympathy, and entirely went off in five or ſix days. The water in nearly the ſame time came entirely by the natural paſſage. The bougie was changed from time to time till the cure was compleated.

CHAPTER

CHAPTER VI.

OF DISEASES IN CONSEQUENCE OF A PERMANENT STRICTURE IN THE URETHRA.

STRICTURES in the urethra produce almost constantly diseases in the parts beyond them; that is, in the part of the urethra between the stricture and the bladder. They bring on in most cases a gleet, as has been described, and often considerable distention of this part of the canal; also inflammation and ulceration, and in consequence of them diseases in the surrounding parts, as in Cowper's glands, the prostate, and the surrounding cellular membrane, forming abscesses there, and at last ulceration, for the purpose of making a new passage for the urine. The bladder is also often affected, and sometimes the ureters, with the pelvis of the kidneys, and in some cases the kidneys themselves. All these are effects of every permanent obstruction to the urine; some of them are methods which nature takes to relieve the parts from the immediate complaints; such are the increase of the urethra beyond the stricture, and the enlargement of the ureters and pelvis of the kidneys, which are only to be considered as the parts accommodating themselves to the immediate consequence of the obstruction, which is the accumulation of urine. Of these complaints I shall take notice in their order.

I. OF THE ENLARGEMENT OF THE URETHRA.

THE urethra beyond the stricture I have observed is enlarged, because it is more passive than the bladder, and yields to the pressure of the urine. It is naturally passive while the bladder is acting, by which means it becomes distended in proportion to the force with which the bladder acts, and the

resistance

reſiſtance of the ſtricture. It's internal ſurface often becomes more irregular and faſciculated. It is alſo more irritable, the diſtention becoming often the immediate cauſe of ſpaſms in that part; and theſe ſpaſms are moſt probably excited with a view to counteract the effort produced by the action of the bladder.

II. OF THE FORMATION OF A NEW PASSAGE FOR THE URINE.

When the methods recommended above for the removal of ſtricture have either not been attempted, or have not ſucceeded, nature endeavours to relieve herſelf by making a new paſſage for the urine, which, although it often prevents immediate death, yet if not remedied is productive of much inconvenience and miſery to the patient through life. The mode by which nature endeavours to procure relief is by ulceration on the inſide of that part of the urethra, which is enlarged and within the ſtricture. The ulceration I believe commonly begins near or cloſe to the ſtricture, although the ſtricture may be a conſiderable way from the bladder; therefore we muſt ſuppoſe that there is ſome circumſtance beſides the diſtenſion of the urethra by the urine which determines the ulceration to a particular part; this circumſtance moſt probably ariſes immediately out of it's vicinity to the ſtricture, and may be called contiguous ſympathy. The ſtricture is often included in the ulceration, by which it is removed, the diſeaſe cured, and a ſtop ſometimes put to the further ulceration; but unluckily this is not always the caſe. We may obſerve that this ulceration is always on that ſide next to the external ſurface, as is common in abſceſſes.

As this ulceration does not ariſe from preceding inflammation; and as it cannot be ſaid that the urine acts exactly as an extraneous body, becauſe it is in it's natural paſſage, we find that there is but very little inflammation of the adheſive kind attending theſe ulcerations. We muſt allow however, that the urine produces the ulcerative diſpoſition here, like matter on the inſide of an abſceſs, although not ſo readily.

Whenever

Whenever therefore the internal membrane and ſubſtance of the urethra is removed by abſorption, the water readily gets into the looſe cellular membrane of the ſcrotum and penis, and diffuſes itſelf all over theſe parts, from their not having been previouſly united by the adheſive inflammation: and as the urine has conſiderable irritating powers when applied to the common cellular membrane, the parts inflame and ſwell conſiderably. The preſence of the urine prevents the adheſive inflammation from taking place; it becomes the cauſe of ſuppuration wherever it is diffuſed, and the irritation is often ſo great, more eſpecially in caſes where the urine has been allowed to become very ſtale, that it produces mortification in all the cellular membrane, and then in ſeveral places of the ſkin; all of which, if the patient lives, will ſlough away, making a free communication between the urethra and external ſurface, producing fiſtulæ in perinæo.

We may obſerve however, that this want of the adheſive inflammation in theſe ulcerations appears to be peculiar to that part of the urethra which lies between the membranous part and the glans penis; for we find from experience, that when this proceſs takes place farther back, viz. in the proſtate gland, that a circumſcribed abſceſs is generally formed. This may ariſe from the difference in texture of the cellular membrane of the parts, the firſt admitting of the diffuſions of the urine very readily from the looſeneſs of it's texture, the other producing adheſions before the urine is allowed to paſs; which adheſions afterwards exclude it.

It ſometimes happens that the urine gets into the ſpongy ſubſtance of the body of the urethra, and is immediately diffuſed through the whole, even to the glans penis, producing mortification of all theſe parts, which I have more than once ſeen.

When the urine has got into the cellular membrane, although the ulceration of the urethra is in the perinæum, yet it generally makes it's way eaſily forwards into the ſcrotum, that part being compoſed of the looſeſt cellular membrane in the body. When the ſeat of the ulceration is in the membranous or bulbous part of the urethra, and the pus and urine have found their way to the ſcrotum, there is always a hardneſs leading along the perinæum to the ſwelled ſcrotum, which is in the tract of the pus.

The ulceration cannot be prevented but by destroying the stricture; but when the water has got into the cellular membrane, which is the state we have been describing, the removal of the stricture will in general be too late to prevent all the mischief, although it will be necessary for the complete cure; therefore an attempt should be made to pass a bougie, for perhaps the stricture may be included in the ulceration, as was mentioned before, and thereby allow a bougie to pass. When this is the case, bougies must be almost constantly used to procure as free a passage forwards in the right way as possible. Where the bougie will not pass I am afraid that the use of the caustic, as described in the case of a stricture, will in many cases not be quick enough, and in others cannot be tried, as the situation of the stricture is often such as will not admit of it.

While the cure of the stricture is attempting, every method is to be used that removes inflammation, particularly bleeding; sitting over the steam of warm water gives great relief; but this is merely a palliative. The warm bath, opium, and the turpentines given by the mouth and also by the anus will assist in taking off any spasmodic affection; but all these are too often insufficient, and therefore immediate relief must be attempted, both to unload the bladder and prevent any further effusion of urine into the cellular membrane. This must be done by an operation which consists in making an opening into the urethra some where beyond the stricture, and the nearer to the stricture the better.

The method of performing the operation is first to pass a director or some such instrument into the urethra, as far as the stricture; then make the end of the instrument as prominent externally as possible so as to be felt, which in such a case is often difficult, sometimes impossible; if felt cut upon it till it is exposed, continue the incision a little further on towards the bladder, or anus, so as to open the urethra beyond the stricture; this will be sufficient to allow the urine to escape, and to destroy the stricture. If the instrument cannot be felt at first by the finger, cut down towards it, which will bring it within the feel of the finger, and then proceed as above-directed.

If the stricture in the urethra is opposite to the scrotum, it being impossible to make the opening there, it must be made in the perinæum, in which case there can be no direction given by an instrument, as one cannot be made to

pass

pass so far, therefore we must be guided by our knowledge of the parts. The opening being made, the stricture is to be searched for as described in the operation, in cases where a false passage has been made, by passing a probe from the wound forwards, towards the glans. The other steps of the operation will be nearly the same. In which ever way the operation is performed a bougie must be introduced, and the wound healed up over it. In my opinion a catheter answers this purpose better.

Great attention should be still paid to the inflammation which arises in consequence of the urine being diffused in the cellular membrane, as before described. Where this inflammation is attended with suppuration and mortification, it will be necessary as well in this case, as in that where no operation is required, to scarify the parts freely, to give an opening both to the urine and pus. Where mortification has taken place in the skin, the scarifications should be made in the mortified places, if it can be done with equal advantage, and this with a view to prevent irritation. Perhaps dressing the parts with opium might be of service.

In total suppressions of urine from whatever cause, the urine should never be allowed to accumulate, and should either be drawn off frequently, or a catheter should be kept continually in the urethra and bladder; because we should on no account allow the bladder to be distended beyond an easy state, for if it is, it always brings on debilitating and alarming symptoms, as paralysis of that viscus. Little regard is to be paid to the urethra in comparison of the bladder; but in many suppressions, as in cases of strictures, it becomes impossible to draw off the water. In some cases where the urethra is ulcerated, and the urine gets into the cellular membrane of the penis, and prepuce, so as to distend them much, producing a phymosis, it becomes impossible to find the orifice of the urethra. The following case illustrates most of the preceding facts.

A gentleman of a scrofulous habit had often had venereal gonorrhœas, which were generally severe, and commonly produced swellings, or knobs along the urethra, upon which account he was advised to avoid getting this disease as much as possible. When in the country in November 1782, he was attacked with a slight cold or fever, and a small discharge from the urethra, which he could not determine to be either venereal or not. In this state he

set

set out for London, but was taken ill on the road with a suppression of urine, which detained him two days at an inn. When he came to town, I found him with a good deal of fever, he spoke to me only of a discharge from the urethra; but as I did not conceive that the fever could arise from that cause, I desired him to be easy on that account. I ordered for that night six grains of James's powder: his physician saw him afterwards, and ordered for his fever what he thought proper. He was taken with a shivering fit which made us suspect it might terminate in an intermittent, and we waited for the result. He still complained of the discharge, and mentioned a soreness in the perinæum, both when he made water and when he pressed it externally. On examining the perinæum I found a fulness there, from which I suspected a stricture, and inquired particularly how he made water in common; he declared very well, which led me off from the true cause. We looked on this swelling as proceeding from an inflammation, either in consequence of the fever, the disposition of the part, or both, increased by sitting in a post-chaise for several days. The part was fomented, poulticed, and leeches applied several times. He had another shivering fit three days after the first, which if his disease had been an intermittent would have constituted a quartan; but he had another some hours after which made us give up our suspicions of an intermittent. We now began to suspect that matter was forming in this part, although I could never feel any thing like a fluctuation; nor was the pain of the throbbing kind, or so acute as we commonly find it in the suppurative inflammation. What in some degree surprised me was, that the swelling came forwards along the body of the penis towards the os pubis while it seemed to be diminishing in the perinæum. He now began to find a difficulty in making water, with a frequent desire, which increased till there was a total suppression. I pressed on the lower part of the belly to see if the urine was secreted and accumulated in the bladder, but I could not find any fulness, nor did he then feel pain on such pressure; however about twenty-four hours after he began to complain of a vast desire to make water, and a pain in the lower part of his belly, and on placing the hand there, a fulness of the bladder was readily felt. It was now clear that the water should be drawn off; but as I still suspected mischief in the urethra as a cause in his complaint, I took the necessary precautions. I provided myself

myſelf with catheters and bougies of different ſizes, and to be as much upon my guard as poſſible, I introduced a bougie of a ſmall ſize firſt, and found a full ſtop about the bulbous part of the urethra, I then took a ſmaller one, which paſſed but with difficulty. I afterwards paſſed a ſmall catheter on to the ſtricture, where it ſtopped, but as it was abſolutely neceſſary the water ſhould be drawn off, I uſed more force than I otherways would have done; it went on, but with difficulty, and I was not certain whether it was in the natural paſſage, or was making a new one. When I had got ſo far as to be in the bladder, (if I was in the right paſſage) I found that no water came, I therefore preſſed on the lower part of the belly, and the water immediately came out through the catheter, which ſhowed that the bladder had loſt it's power of contraction. The water was drawn off three times every day, that is, every eight hours, to give as much eaſe to the bladder as poſſible, but ſtill it was neceſſary to preſs upon the belly to aſſiſt the diſcharge of the urine; and it was upwards of a fortnight before the bladder began to recover it's power of contracting. The ſwelling in the perinæum ſtill continued, advancing along the body of the penis, and ſpreading a little on the pubis, it ſeemed to extend along the projecting part of the penis, and at laſt filled the whole cellular membrane of the prepuce, but did not in the leaſt affect the ſcrotum. This ſwelling appeared to be owing to the urine having found it's way into the cellular membrane of the perinæum, and from thence proceeding along the ſide of the penis. When the prepuce became much loaded with water, a very conſiderable phymoſis took place, which made the introduction of the catheter into the orifice of the urethra very uncertain, ſo much did the ſwelled prepuce project over the glans. I was obliged to ſqueeze the water back into the body of the penis, and introduce the finger, and feel for the glans, and on this finger introduce the catheter, and in a few minutes I generally hit the orifice.

The nature of the caſe was now plain, for ulceration had taken place beyond the ſtricture, and the ſwelling had ariſen from the urine having inſinuated itſelf into the cellular membrane of the perinæum; and as the urine paſſed out of the urethra it was puſhed forwards where the cellular membrane was looſeſt, till it got to the very end of the prepuce as beforementioned.

 By

By this time he was become extremely low and irritable, his pulſe quick and ſmall, his tongue brown, dry, and contracted, his appetite gone, with great drought, bad ſleep and the firſt ſtages of a delirium coming on. This diſcovery of the true ſtate of the caſe gave a change to the mode of treatment. Inſtead of evacuations to leſſen inflammation, bark, and cordials were given, with as much food as his ſtomach would bear; their effects on the conſtitution were almoſt immediate, and he began to recover, although but ſlowly. I made two punctures in the phymoſis at the extremity, with a view both to take off the tenſion and to evacuate the urine from the cellular membrane, between the penis and the ſkin.

Bliſters began to form on the ſkin of the penis, and at laſt mortification took place in ſeveral parts, eſpecially on the prepuce, which I divided at the mortified parts, and thereby the glans became expoſed ſo that the catheter could now be introduced eaſily.

Upon ſqueezing the ſwelling from the perinæum forwards along the penis, I could force out at the mortified parts, air, water, and ſome matter. The cellular membrane under the ſkin was almoſt wholly mortified. When bounds were ſet to the mortification, the ſloughing cellular membrane began to ſeparate, and a good deal was cut away to keep the parts clean, and to allow of a freer vent for the matter. Now that ſeparation was taking place I was clear that no more water from the bladder could inſinuate itſelf any further into the ſurrounding cellular membrane, therefore it was not neceſſary to paſs the catheter any more, and he was allowed to make water whenever he had a call; which when he did, the water came both ways, through the urethra, and through the cellular membrane, at the openings where the ſkin had ſloughed off. As the ſloughs ſeparated, they came forwards from behind, at the ſide of the ſcrotum, ſo that I could draw them out, and when moſt of the mortified cellular membrane was removed, I ſaw a part, about the ſize of a ſixpence, of the tendinous covering of the corpus cavernoſum dead, which was alſo allowed to ſlough off. Moſt of the water now came through the ſore. The parts became more painful, he was more reſtleſs, and one morning he had a ſhivering fit. I endeavoured to paſs a bougie down the ſore, between the ſkin and penis, but could not; in the evening of the ſame day a guſh of matter and blood came out of the ſore, which immediately

relieved

relieved him, and he began to mend again, and continued to do ſo, both in the parts and his general health, the water coming both ways, but often varying in quantity between the two paſſages; more and more however came the right way, till at laſt the new paſſage cloſed up entirely.

While the external parts were healing up, I paſſed a bougie occaſionally, to keep the paſſage clear and open. To find out the ſituation of the internal opening, I ordered him to preſs on different parts of the perinæum while he was making water, by which means he found that by preſſing upon a particular ſpot he could ſtop the water from flowing through the new paſſage. He was directed however not to preſs too hard, for fear of forcing together the ſides of the natural paſſage. Upon erections the penis was bent to the ſide that had ſuffered, but in time the parts gradually recovered their natural form.

III. OF INFLAMMATION IN THE PARTS SURROUNDING THE URETHRA.

Inflammation cauſed by the diſtention and irritation of the urethra often extends conſiderably further than the ſurface of this canal, for the ſurrounding parts become the ſeat of inflammation, the ſituation of which will commonly be according to the ſituation of the ſtricture. Thus we find the inflammation affecting the proſtate gland, the membranous part of the urethra, the bulb, and probably Cowper's glands, with other parts of the urethra between the bulb and the glans. But inflammation in the ſurrounding parts of the urethra is not always a conſequence of diſtenſion or ſtricture; it ariſes often from other irritations in this canal, ſuch as violent gonorrhœas, and very irritating injections. When inflammation attacks theſe parts it is of the true adheſive kind; and therefore when ſuppuration takes place an abſceſs muſt be formed unleſs the inflammation be reſolved. The matter, according to a general principle in abſceſſes, points externally; when the ſeat of the abſceſs is either in the proſtate gland, membranous part, or in the bulb, the matter will point in the perinæum; or the abſceſs may

may be formed forwards in the scrotum, or before it, according to the situation of the stricture.

The seat of these abscesses is generally so near the inner surface of the urethra, that the partition between them often gives way, and they open internally, as frequently happens in an abscess by the side of the rectum, so that the matter is at once discharged by the urethra or carried back into the bladder to be discharged with the urine. When the internal opening only takes place, I believe it is owing to the ulceration on the inner surface of the urethra having taken place, as has been already described, and in these cases also the stricture is sometimes involved in the abscess and ulceration, by which means the water will find a free passage forwards; but the urine has also a free passage into the abscess, which we may suppose retards it's healing, and often becomes the cause of it's opening externally; but here from the adhesive inflammation having taken place the urine cannot insinuate itself into the surrounding cellular membrane, so as to produce the consequences mentioned in treating of the way in which nature endeavours to relieve herself. In such cases we find upon pressing the abscess externally, the matter is squeezed into the urethra, and so out by the glans. It sometimes happens that a catheter can be introduced into the opening of such an abscess, by which means it can be washed by injecting something through the catheter, whereby probably it may be sooner healed. It more frequently happens that such abscesses open both internally and externally, discharging themselves both ways.

These ulcerations and suppurations of both kinds are to be considered as efforts of nature; or to speak more physiologically, as a natural consequence arising from such irritation, by which as the urine cannot pass by the old passage a new one is made to prevent further mischief.

Both these diseases when they open externally, if not properly treated, often lay the foundation for the complaint commonly called the fistula in perinæo; which is owing to the bottom of the abscess having a less disposition to heal than the external parts. It may be further supposed, that the urine passing into the abscess by the inner orifice, and making it's escape by the external, keeps up a constant irritation in the sore, which in some measure may prevent a union of the sides, and rather dispose them to form

themselves

themselves into a hard callous substance, whose inner surface looses the disposition for union, and assumes the nature of an outlet.

But it is more than probable that these abscesses not readily healing, depends upon the cause of their first action often continuing in full force, that is, a diseased state of the internal parts, as will be further illustrated when on the fistula in perinæo. They often heal up at the orifice in the skin, especially if the water has a free passage forwards; but if the internal opening is not perfectly consolidated, some water will insinuate itself into the old sore, become the cause of fresh inflammations and suppurations in the surrounding parts, which frequently open externally in different places, not following the old canal, although they sometimes communicate with it and form branches, as it were, from the principal trunk. I have seen the scrotum, perineum, and inside of the thigh, full of openings which were the mouths of so many sinuses leading to the first formed abscess When the abscess opens only externally, which is seldom the case, it is to be considered as a common abscess.

When these inflammations arise from stricture, the difficulty in making water is increased in the time of the inflammation, which is generally so great as to compress the sides of the urethra together for some way; besides the stricture itself will become tighter from being inflamed. Inflammation in these parts, even when it does not arise from a stricture, brings on a suppression of urine; but in such cases a bougie or catheter can be passed; the last of which, in cases of obstruction arising from contiguous swellings, as tumors, inflammations, and swelled prostate gland, is the proper instrument, as the sides of the urethra would be pressed together immediately upon withdrawing the bougie, by which the urine would be as much as ever prevented from following.

IV. OF THE TREATMENT OF THE INFLAMMATION IN THE SURROUNDING PARTS.

The inflammation of these parts is to be treated like other inflammations. Resolution is much to be wished for; but it is almost impossible it should take place where ſtricture is the cauſe. When the ſtricture is removed, either by ulceration or a bougie, we have only the inflammation to contend with; but this ſeldom happens, for the inflammation is but too often accompanied with ſuppuration.

When ſuppuration takes place the ſooner the abſceſs is opened externally the better, as that may in ſome caſes be the means, though ſeldom, of preventing it's opening internally; yet it may prevent the inner opening from becoming ſo large as it otherways might do. The opening externally ſhould be large; and if the ſtricture is not involved in the ſuppuration, then it muſt be deſtroyed; becauſe no cure can take place while the water paſſes through the new opening. I have ſucceeded with the cauſtic even in ſtrictures of long ſtanding.

When the ſtricture will admit of the paſſage of a bougie through it, it is to be kept almoſt conſtantly in the urethra, and to be withdrawn only at the time of making water; this will allow the urine to paſs more freely through the urethra, without eſcaping through the ſore. The ſore muſt be healed up from the bottom.

Hollow bougies are recommended in ſuch caſes, after the ſtricture is deſtroyed, to prevent the urine paſſing through the wound. This inſtrument admits of a conſtant dribbling of urine through it; but the bougie may be occaſionally ſtopped up, and the urine permitted to paſs when there is a deſire to make water. It becomes under certain circumſtances the worſt inſtrument poſſible, for if it's canal is not of a ſize ſufficient to let the water paſs as freely as the contraction of the bladder requires, the water will paſs eaſily by the ſide of the bougie to the abſceſs, and not getting forwards beyond the ſtricture flow out at the abſceſs: to avoid this effect as much as poſſible, the hollow bougies ſhould be as large as the ſtrictured part will allow, and it's ſides ſhould be as thin as poſſible, that it's paſſage may be the larger. The elaſtic gum has theſe two properties in a higher degree than the ſpiral wire covered with waxed cloth. But as I doubt very much the paſſage of the urine being an hinderance to the healing of the ſore, I am leſs ſolicitous about ſuch practice; for we find that after cutting for the ſtone the parts heal very readily; and even in this operation the external parts which are not diſeaſed heal up very readily. I ſuſpect

suspect that the want of disposition to heal arises from the strictures not being sufficiently subdued, or the deeper parts not being in a healthy state.

When these suppurations are left to themselves, and no method tried to remove the stricture, and of course nothing introduced into the urethra, the stricture sometimes closes entirely up, so that no water can pass forwards through the urethra; and therefore before any attempt can be made to heal the fistulous orifices, a passage must be made through the united parts. This cannot be done with a bougie; and if this union of the parts is before the bend of the urethra, which most commonly it is, nothing but the caustic can be applied with any prospect of success, as will be mentioned more fully in treating of the fistula in perinæo.

V. OF THE EFFECTS OF INFLAMMATION IN THE SURROUNDING PARTS UPON THE CONSTITUTION.

THE effects which these attempts to form a new passage for the urine have upon the constitution, are very considerable; much more so than what one would at first expect. Those cases appear to be most formidable which begin by ulceration on the inner surface of the urethra, and where the water diffuses itself into the cellular membrane of the scrotum and penis.

These where the inflammation is circumscribed are more the true abscess, and therefore do much less mischief to the parts than when the urine is diffused in the cellular membrane. In these last if not soon relieved, the patient sinks, and a mortification comes on. If before the patient sinks, a separation of the slough takes place, this separation performs the operation of opening, and the patient may recover. We should not I believe wait for such separation of the mortified part, but make an opening early, upon the first knowledge of a diffusion of water into the cellular membrane; and we should be guided as to situation by introducing a staff into the urethra on to the stricture. But in some cases this cannot be done, for when the urine gets into the corpus spongiosum, it produces mortification of all these parts, and renders the whole so indistinct that often no urethra can be found.

The

The effects that the circumscribed inflammation has upon the constitution, is generally not so serious as the above, for mortification as seldom takes place in this as in abscesses in general. When the abscess is from the bulb backwards, there is generally a smart sympathetic fever, because the abscess will be of considerable size before it gets to the skin of the perinæum, and is generally attended with great pain; but this pain goes off by the formation of the matter, especially if opened early.

As there is a great disposition for violent action, attended with great weakness in such cases, more especially in those of the first kind, it is adviseable to give the bark early, and in considerable quantity; but I apprehend it is necessary to give along with it sudorifics, as the saline draughts, or some of the preparations of antimony, as there is generally a good deal of fever. The bark gives strength, and also in some degree lessens irritability, and by that means lessens action; but it should be assisted by other medicines: opium will add to it's effects.

VI. OF FISTULÆ IN PERINÆO.

It often happens that the new passages for the urine do not heal on account of the stricture not being removed; and even when the stricture is removed, they frequently have no disposition to heal. In both cases they become fistulous, and produce fresh inflammations and suppurations, which do not always open into the old sore, but make new openings externally. These sometimes arise from the first external openings not being sufficiently large, so that they heal up long before the bottom, or long before the diseased urethra; and even when the external opening has been made as large as possible it will often heal sooner than the bottom, and become fistulous at last.

It is very common for these diseases to affect the constitution, so as to bring on agueish complaints. I have seen several affected with regular agues, where the bark has produced no effect; but whenever the obstruction has been got the better of, or the fistulous orifice opened and in a state of healing, these complaints have entirely gone off.

To

To cure this disease, it is necessary first to make the natural passage as free as possible, that no obstruction may arise from that quarter, and sometimes this alone is sufficient, for the urine finding a free passage forwards, is not forced into the orifice, and the parts lose the sensation of disease, or the necessity of keeping open; besides I apprehend that the bougie may bring on an inflammation on the urethra at this part, and produce adhesions there; but if this effect is not produced early, the bougie will rather do harm if applied too often, and too long at a time, as will be more fully explained. But this practice of dilating the stricture is not always sufficient; it is often necessary to perform some operation on those fistulæ, when they alone become the obstacle to the cure, which I shall now describe.

VII. OF THE OPERATION FOR FISTULÆ IN PERINÆO.

When the before-mentioned treatment is not sufficient for the cure of these new passages, a method should be followed similar to that used in the cure of a fistula in other parts, by laying it freely open to the bottom, and even making the orifice in the urethra a fresh sore if possible. This will be difficult in many situations of the internal opening; and the mode of opening and other circumstances attending the operation will vary according to the situation.

That as little of the sound part of the inner surface of the urethra may be opened as possible, and that the diseased part may be fully exposed, it is necessary to be well directed to the inner orifice for which we have commonly two guides, one is a staff introduced into the urethra as far as is thought necessary, or as far as it will go, which will only be to the stricture, where the stricture still exists, or it may pass on to the bladder in cases where the stricture has been destroyed; the other guide is a probe passed into the fistulous orifice. The probe should be first bent, that it may more readily follow the turns of the fistula, and introduced as far as possible; if it could be made to meet the staff so much the better, as then the operator could cut just what is necessary. If a straight probe could be made to pass, then perhaps a director might, if so, it is the best instrument for operating upon.

If neither the probe nor the director can be made to paſs on to the ſtaff, we muſt open as far as they go, and begin ſearching anew after the remainder of the paſſage with the ſame inſtrument, and purſue it till the whole fiſtulous canal is laid open. If there are any ſinuſes, they are to be laid open if poſſible; but it frequently happens that they cannot be followed by the knife, ſome running along the penis where the ſcrotum is attached, others paſſing on towards the pubis round the penis, while others are about the membraneous part of the urethra. In ſuch caſes I would not be delicate, I have ſeveral times introduced my finger into theſe ſinuſes, and have torn the parts ſo as to produce a conſiderable inflammation, by which means they often ſuppurate, granulate, and unite.

If the ſituation of the internal orifice is oppoſite to the ſcrotum, it will be difficult to get to it, but I imagine we may uſe great freedom with the external parts, whatever they are, for they are generally in a ſtate of calloſity, however this is to be done with judgment.

In caſes where the diſeaſe is before the membraneous part and the ſtricture is not removed, a ſtaff cannot be made to paſs on to the inner orifice. In ſuch the fiſtulous opening muſt be followed by introducing a probe or director into it, and dilating upon the inſtrument till the urethra beyond the ſtricture is found; and then a probe muſt be paſſed on towards the glans, to meet the end of the ſtaff at the ſtricture; ſimilar to what is done in the operation where a falſe paſſage has been made by the miſmanagement of the bougie; the ſtricture muſt then be deſtroyed, and a bougie paſſed, as was recommended in that operation.

If either the ulceration, or the abſceſs, is formed in or near the proſtate gland, then probably the ſtricture is near that part. In that caſe a ſtaff muſt be paſſed as far as poſſible, and a probe or director introduced into the external orifice, and the operation is to be directed accordingly. The difference of the operation in this caſe from the former will be, that we ſhall moſt probably be obliged to get into the urethra on both ſides of the ſtricture, therefore more of the canal muſt be expoſed.

As this operation is the opening of all the fiſtulous canals, and alſo the deſtruction of the ſtricture, if there has been one, an inſtrument now can in every caſe be paſſed into the bladder. It will moſt probably always be proper to introduce an instrument into the bladder, and keep it there almost constantly, so as to preserve the passage of the urethra in a regular form, while the openings made are healing; and probably the catheter will be by much the best instrument, because it it is not necessary to be withdrawn whenever the necessity to make water comes on, which a bougie must, and it's introduction again is often not practicable, for it's end will be apt to get into the wounds, &c.

In such cases as require a hollow canula to be left in the bladder for the purpose of taking off the water, whether a catheter or hollow bougie, it is absolutely necessary it should be fixed there, or else it will in common come out by the actions of the part. To effect this it is necessary to fix that end of the instrument out of the penis to some part of the body that is the least moveable: what will answer extremely well is the common belt-part of the bag truss, with only two thigh-straps fixed behind and made to tie or buckle before; and two or three very small rings or short tapes fixed to those straps; where they pass between the thigh and scrotum they should not be at a great distance from one another where they are fixed behind to the belt, for otherwise they are much altered in tightness by the motion of the thigh. If they have a flat spring in them so much the better.*

. The common bag truss for the scrotum answers extremely well, first by fixing two or three rings on each side of it along the side of the scrotum, and with a piece of small tape the ring of the canula can be fastened to any one of those rings that is most convenient for it's situation.

Whatever instrument is used for the purpose of keeping the passage clear and open while the sores are healing, whether the sores are in consequence of this operation, or in consequence of the causes of the fistulæ, which I have described, there is a limited time in many cases for it's continuance; for if continued beyond a certain period, it frequently acts contrary to what was intended; at first it often assists the cure, but towards the last it may obstruct the healing of the sores by acting at the bottom of the wound as an extraneous body. Therefore whenever the sores become stationary I would advise the withdrawing of the instrument, and the intro-

* Mr. Vanbutchell's springs would answer very well.

ducing

during it only occasionally. The catheter will probably be still the best instrument for this purpose, as it will pass more readily, and draw off the water at the same time; however I have often used a bougie, and by great care have passed it with success; and probably it will be proper to use it every now and then, even when all is healed, to know if the passage keeps well.

The sore and the wound are to be at first dressed down to the bottom as much as possible, which will prevent the reunion of the parts just divided, and make the granulations shoot from the bottom so as to consolidate the whole by one bond of union.

When the urethra has suffered so much that abscesses have formed beyond the scrotum, the patient should ever after take great care to avoid a fresh gonorrhœa, for he seldom in that case escapes a return of the same complaints; and indeed if he is not careful in many other respects he is liable to returns of the same disease. If notwithstanding this precaution he should contract a gonorrhœa, every thing heating is to be carefully avoided, particularly irritating injections.

The following case shows that keeping extraneous bodies in the urethra prevents wounds made into the canal from healing.

A man, aged twenty-six, came into St. George's Hospital, March 2, 1783. He had laboured under a fistula in perinæo for near two years, arising from a stricture attended with great pain and difficulty in making water. Four fistulous orifices were to be observed in the perinæum and scrotum. The smallest bougie could not be made to pass into the bladder after repeated trials. The caustic was then applied but without success.

[illegible] operation for the fistula in perinæo was performed, September 19. [illegible] catheter was first introduced as far as it would go, as a director, and all [illegible] were laid open to that catheter, which exposed near an inch in [illegible] of that instrument; then the catheter was in part withdrawn to expose that part of the urethra which was laid bare. The blood being sponged off, the orifice in the stricture was next searched for, and when found it was dilated. The catheter was now pushed on to the bladder, although with some difficulty, and the end of it was then fastened to a roller which went round the thighs; and the wound was distended with lint. He took an anodyne

anodyne draught after the operation, and another at night. September 20, he had ſome pain in the head from the opiates, his pulſe was natural, and he had ſlept tolerable well.

21ſt. This day the catheter ſlipped out, and the ſecond introduction of it gave conſiderable pain. The anodyne was repeated.

October 1. The catheter was ſtill to be ſelt by introducing a probe into the wound.

From this time to the 25th, nothing material happened, excepting a piece of lint of the firſt dreſſing coming away through the urethra.

November 20. The wound having for ſome time been ſtationary, and ſhowing no diſpoſition to heal, I conceived that the catheter was now acting as an extraneous body at the bottom of the wound, and therefore deſired that it might be withdrawn, and paſſed occaſionally; and no ſooner was the wound free from it but it put on a healthy look; and by the 10th of December no urine came through the wound, but paſſed tolerable well through the urethra; and on the 12th the wound was quite healed, and his water came from him in a pretty full ſtream, and without pain, although we could never paſs either catheter or bougie afterwards, probably from the new and old paſſages being irregular.

CHAPTER VII.

OF SOME OTHER AFFECTIONS OF THE URETHRA.

THE ſubſtance of the urethra is muſcular, and it is therefore capable of contracting it's canal, ſimilar to an inteſtine, ſo much ſo as to ſhut it up entirely. This makes it ſubject to diſeaſes peculiar to muſcle in general; which is indeed the only proof we have of it's being muſcular.

I. OF THE SPASMODIC AFFECTIONS OF THE URETHRA.

IN a ſound ſtate of parts theſe muſcles are never excited to violent actions, acting ſimply as ſphincter muſcles; but when irritated they are capable of acting violently, as is beſt ſeen in ſome caſes upon the firſt uſe of injections, the urethra often refuſing the injection entirely: this ſeems rather to be a ſalutary motion to hinder things from getting into the bladder; but there are often ſpaſmodic contractions of theſe muſcular fibres in different parts of the canal ſhutting up the paſſage and obſtructing the courſe of the urine, often not allowing a drop to paſs. That this alſo is owing to ſpaſm upon the muſcular fibres is evident, becauſe a large bougie will ſometimes paſs when it is at the worſt. When the contraction is near the bladder it is called a ſtrangury, and is often produced in a ſound ſtate of parts by irritating medicines, the power of which fall upon theſe parts, as cantharides; and when this part is in an irritable ſtate the ſpaſm may be brought on by a vaſt number of things, ſuch as moſt of the peppers, fermented liquors of all kinds, violent exerciſe, &c.

The urethra in caſes of ſpaſmodic ſtricture is more irritable than in the true ſtricture, which irritation indeed is in a great meaſure the cauſe of the ſpaſm. Spaſmodic ſtrictures often bear ſo ſtrong a reſemblance to the

cramp,

cramp, that one would be apt to attribute them to the same cause as that which produces cramp. In such cases the spasm also goes off by tickling the part, similar to the removal of cramp.

In all cases of very irritable urethras, where spasm very readily take place, the person should never long retain his urine when he has an inclination to make it; for I have seen cases where this alone has brought on the spasm; and indeed these parts when in perfect health will be thrown into a spasmodic affection if the urine is too long confined in the bladder; while at the same time a certain fulness of the bladder, or a small degree of retention of the urine will make the bladder contract with more force; and the urethra will for the same reason relax more freely; therefore in cases where there is a tendency to strangury there is seldom any harm in waiting a little after the inclination comes on.

I may be allowed here to caution surgeons who have not had opportunities of seeing many of these cases, when they meet with permanent strictures which are becoming troublesome, attended with frequency in making water, and a difficulty in passing it often threatening strangury, not to advise, or rather not to allow, their patients to take long journeys either on horseback or in carriages, more especially in the winter when the weather is cold; for I have known many patients labouring under such complaints taken ill in the middle of a journey and obliged to stop for days upon the road, and who have continued in misery the remainder of the journey; and after having arrived at the place of their destination, have been laid up for months, and have suffered from most of the before-mentioned complaints.

II. OF THE CURE OF THE SPASMODIC AFFECTION OF THE URETHRA.

It may not be improper to premise, that in diseases of the actions only of the urethra and bladder, whether spasmodic, and proceeding from too great irritability, or paralytic, although two opposite diseases; irritations on other parts have often wonderful effects on both, equally diminishing the action in the one, and increasing it in the other. The proof of this will appear

appear in treating of the irritable and paralytic urethra and bladder; for in either part, and in either caſe, we find bliſters applied to the lower part of the ſmall of the back or the perinæum, as alſo many other applications to this part, often producing great effects.[*]

As ſpaſm ſimply is not an alteration of ſtructure, but is only a diſeaſed or preternatural action ariſing from ſome irritation, it may be made to ceaſe inſtantaneouſly. In whatever part of the urethra the ſpaſm is, if time will allow, it is proper to try internal medicines, and alſo external applications, to remove it. The internal medicines that may be ſaid to act immediately are opiates and turpentines,[†] given either by the mouth or the anus; but they are more immediate in their effects in the form of clyſter, eſpecially the opium. It is very poſſible that camphire might be of uſe in ſtranguries ariſing from ſpaſm, as well as in thoſe produced by cantharides. Bark is often had recourſe to in ſpaſmodic affections, in which it is thought to be of ſervice; but in ſuch affections of the urethra I think I have ſeen it frequently do harm.

The external applications are the ſteam of warm water with ſpirits, the pediluvium, the warm bath, bladders of warm water applied to the perinæum, and ſimilar applications. The crumb part of a new baked loaf, warm from the oven, applied to the perinæum, has been found to give eaſe.

I have known a bliſter applied to the loins in a great meaſure remove the ſpaſm from the urethra; and the ſame put upon the perinæum is fully as effectual. But in moſt caſes theſe methods are too tedious; therefore when the caſe has been of ſome ſtanding before aſſiſtance has been called

[*] That the parts concerned in the expulſion of the urine (as the bladder and urethra) ſympathiſe ſtrongly with the ſkin of the perinæum, I believe is commonly ſuppoſed, from applications being often made to that part in caſes of ſtoppages of urine. This ſympathy not only takes place in the diſeaſed actions of thoſe parts, ſo as to bring about a natural action, but often becomes a ſtimulus to natural actions where there is no diſeaſe.

A gentleman who had no complaint in theſe parts, had a ſmall fiſtula at the ſide of the rectum, for which he often had occaſion to ſit over the ſteam of warm water and vinegar; and this application to the perinæum never failed of making him make water.

[†] Dr. Home, in his experiments on this medicine, found that large doſes brought on the ſtrangury in women.

for

for, and requires immediate relief, recourse should be had to the catheter or bougie immediately.

If the contraction is near the bladder, the catheter will answer best; but in most cases the bougie will be sufficient, and is a much safer instrument; for in many hands the catheter is a very dangerous one, requiring a dexterity only to be got by a thorough knowledge of the course of the canal, and a habit of passing it. The bougie has likewise this advantage, that in many cases where the part spasmodically affected will not allow it to pass, it may be allowed to lie close to the stricture; for it is not always necessary for the bougie to pass through the constricted part; as I have seen where a bougie has only passed a little way into the urethra, and by letting it stay there till the desire of making water has come on, the water, on withdrawing the bougie, has followed very freely. In such cases, even when the bougie passes into the bladder, it is necessary to let it stay in the passage till the inclination to make water comes on, and then to withdraw it; if the water does not follow on the first attempt, it will be proper to make another, or if only part follows the bougie, it will be necessary to introduce it again. This circumstance of the water following the bougie with more certainty if it is allowed to stay till the inclination comes on, is a proof that the disposition in the bladder for contracting, removes in some degree the disposition for contraction in the urethra.

Some attention is necessary with respect to the passing of the bougie in these cases, for the urethra being more irritable than common, it often resists the bougie before it reaches the true spasmodic part; when this is the case force is not to be used, but we should rather wait a little with patience, and then make another attempt to push it on. Dipping the end of the penis in very cold water often removes the spasm, and the water flows immediately and freely.

In most cases there is an uneasy sensation at the end of the penis, which leads the patient to rub those parts, and sometimes, though rarely, during the friction, the water will pass. Gently irritating injections only thrown in a little way, often give ease. They act I suppose somewhat like the bougie that does not pass, by irritating one part of the urethra the other relaxes. They act in some cases as a preventive.

 III. OF

III. OF THE PARALYSIS OF THE URETHRA.

In oppoſition to the foregoing diſeaſe, there is the want of power of contraction of the urethra; but this is not ſo frequent a caſe as the former. This diſeaſe is attended with ſymptoms contrary to thoſe of the foregoing; the bladder is hardly allowed to be filled ſo as to give the ſtimulus of repletion; but the water dribbles away inſenſibly as faſt as ſecreted by the kidneys; or if the bladder is filled ſo as to receive the ſtimulus for expulſion, then it immediately takes place, and the water flows, if the perſon does not act with the muſculi acceleratores; but ſometimes in ſuch caſes the power of contraction of theſe muſcles is loſt, and then the water will flow, whether the perſon will or not, there being little or no power of retention. There is great difference in the degrees of violence of this diſeaſe.

IV. CURE OF THE PARALYSIS OF THE URETHRA.

It is to be cured by ſtimulants, as a bliſter to the loins, or a bliſter to the perinæum. Putting the feet into cold water may be uſeful. Cantharides taken internally, fifteen or twenty drops once or twice a day, according to their effects, are of ſingular ſervice in ſome caſes.

A man came to St. George's Hoſpital with this complaint. I ordered him the before-mentioned medicine, and it had ſuch an effect as to bring on the contrary diſeaſe, or a ſpaſmodic affection of the urethra, ſo that he could not make water when he had the inclination; but an injection of opium removed this complaint, and he was then well. In this caſe a few drops leſs, probably would have effected a cure without any inconvenience.

Spices, and ſteel medicines are of ſervice; and from what was ſaid before of the bark I ſhould ſuppoſe it a good medicine. Electricity may alſo be tried. Waſhing the parts with cold water may probably be of ſervice.

V. OF

V. OF CARUNCLES OR EXCRESCENCES IN THE URETHRA.

Strictures are not ſuppoſed to be the only cauſes of obſtruction to the paſſage of urine in this canal; excreſcences or caruncles are likewiſe mentioned by authors as happening frequently. From the familiarity with which they talk of them, and the few inſtances in which they really occur, one would ſuſpect that this cauſe of obſtruction was originally founded in opinion, and not obſervation, and afterwards handed down as matter of fact. If caruncles had been at firſt deſcribed from actual examination of caſes, the language would have accorded with the appearances, and they would have been conſidered as ſeldom the cauſes of obſtruction compared with ſtrictures. However they do ſometimes happen, although but rarely. I have in all my examinations of dead bodies ſeen only two, and theſe were in very old ſtrictures, where the urethra had ſuffered conſiderably. They were bodies riſing from the ſurface of the urethra like granulations, or what would be called polypi in other parts of the body. It is poſſible they may be a ſpecies of internal wart, for I have ſeen warts extend ſome way into the beginning of the urethra, having very much the appearance of granulations. Moſt probably it will not be poſſible in the living body to diſtinguiſh caruncles, excreſcences, or riſings in the urethra, from a ſtricture; for I cannot conceive that they can produce any new ſymptoms, or peculiar feel to the examiner.

VI. OF THE CURE OF THE EXCRESCENCE OR CARUNCLE.

I ſhould very much ſuſpect that this diſeaſe is not to be cured by the bougie; at leaſt dilatation in ſuch caſes is not to be attempted, as there is no contraction. If therefore the bougie is of any uſe, it muſt be in making the carnoſity ulcerate from it's preſſure, which probably may be done by a large bougie preſſing upon it with conſiderable force. But if this ſhould not have the

the desired effect, I should certainly recommend or use the caustic, if the parts were so situated as to admit of the application; and from such practice I should not doubt of a cure. But the difficulty lies in distinguishing the disease from a true stricture; for although authors talk of caruncles as common, and give us the method of treatment, yet they have not told us how we are to distinguish them from strictures.

I have never met with a caruncle in women.

CHAPTER

CHAPTER VIII.

OF THE SWELLED PROSTATE GLAND.

ANOTHER difeafe of the parts furrounding the urethra which is often very formidable, is a fwelling of the proftate gland; it is of more ferious confequence than any of the former caufes of obftruction, becaufe we have fewer methods of cure, for we cannot deftroy it as we can the ftricture, nor can nature relieve herfelf by forming new paffages; we have however often the means of temporary relief in our power, which is not the cafe in the ftricture, for moft commonly we can draw off the water by the catheter.

The fwelling of the proftate gland is moft common in the decline of life, feldom happening to young men. The ufe of this gland is not fufficiently known to enable us to judge of the bad confequences that attend it's difeafed ftate abftracted from fwelling. It's fituation is fuch, that the bad confequences of it's being fwelled muft be evident, as it may be faid to make a part of the canal of the urethra, and therefore when fo difeafed as to alter it's fhape and fize, it muft affect that canal. When it fwells it does not leffen the furface of the urethra at the part fimilar to a ftricture; on the contrary it rather increafes it; but the fides of the canal are compreffed together, producing an obftruction to the paffage of the urine, from which an irritation takes place in the bladder that brings on all the fymptoms in that vifcus that ufually arife from a ftricture or ftone. From the fituation of the gland which is principally on the two fides of the canal, and but little if at all on the fore part, as alfo very little on the pofterior fide, when it fwells it can only be laterally, whereby it preffes the two fides of the canal together, and at the fame time ftretches it from the anterior edge or fide to the pofterior, fo that the canal inftead of being round, is flattened into a narrow groove. Sometimes the gland fwells more on one fide than the other, which makes an obliquity in the canal paffing through it.

Befides this effect of the lateral parts fwelling, a fmall portion of it which lies behind the very beginning of the urethra fwells forwards like a point as it were into the bladder, acting like a valve to the mouth of the urethra, which can be feen even when the fwelling is not confiderable, by looking upon the mouth of the urethra from the cavity of the bladder in a dead body. It fometimes increafes fo much as to form a tumor,* projecting into the bladder fome inches. This projection turns or bends the urethra forwards, becoming an obftruction to the paffage of a catheter, bougie, or any fuch inftrument; and it often raifes the found over a fmall ftone in the bladder, fo as to prevent it's being felt. The catheter fhould for this part be more curved than is neceffary for the other parts of the urethra. In fuch cafes I have frequently paffed firft a hollow elaftic catheter till it came to this point, and if it chanced to go over it is very well; but if it does not, a ftillet or brafs wire properly curved to go over the proftate gland is to be paffed down. The advantages of this method are, that if the hollow catheter paffes, no more is neceffary, and if it does not, the curved wire will pafs along the hollow bougie much eafier both to the furgeon and patient than it would have done if it had been introduced at firft with the hollow bougie over it; for it would be forcing by it's end to adapt the urethra to the curve, whereas when introduced afterwards the ftillet is only acting on the infide of the hollow bougie, which the patient hardly feels.

A gentleman had been often founded for a ftone and yet no ftone could be found; but it afterwards appeared that there was a ftone together with the fwelling of the proftate gland, which had been the caufe of his death.

John Doby, a poor penfioner in the charter-houfe, had been feveral years afflicted with the ftone in the bladder, and was relieved from all the fymptoms by an enlargement of this part of the proftate gland, preventing the ftones from falling down upon the neck of the bladder and irritating thefe parts. A twelvemonth after the fymptoms of the ftone had gone off he was attacked with a ftrangury, to relieve which, many ineffectual attempts were made both with the bougie and catheter, but it foon proved fatal.

* Vide plates V and VII.

Upon

Upon examination of the parts in the dead body, the proſtate gland was found enlarged to a ſize ſix times greater than what it is in common, and the urethra paſſing through it was a ſlit about an inch and half in length, the two ſides of which were cloſe together, the upper end towards the pubes and the lower towards the rectum. This ſlit was formed by the ſides of the proſtate gland only ſwelling, and the right ſide was the moſt enlarged, having it's ſurface next the urethra rounded or convex, and the left ſide was exactly fitted to it, having it's ſurface hollowed in the ſame proportion. The ſmall projecting point of the gland was ſo much enlarged, as to come forwards into the cavity of the bladder and fill up entirely the paſſage at the neck of it. The bladder itſelf was very much enlarged and thickened in it's coats, and contained above twenty ſtones, moſt of them lying behind the projecting proceſs of the proſtate gland, and the reſt lodged in ſmall ſacs, made by the internal membrane being puſhed ſome little way between the faſciculi of muſcular fibres.

The proſtate gland when ſwelled, generally becomes conſiderably firmer in it's conſiſtence. The effects of theſe ſwellings are very conſiderable, for they ſqueeze the ſides of the urethra cloſe together, and the projecting point hinders in ſome degree the urine from entering the paſſage, and in many caſes ſtops it entirely. Further, the increaſed firmneſs of the ſubſtance of the gland hinders it from yielding to the force of the urine, ſo that little or none can paſs. It will be unneceſſary to relate the particular ſymptoms which this diſeaſe occaſions; they are ſuch as ariſe from any ſtoppage of urine, producing an irritable bladder.

When a difficulty in making water takes place, a bougie is the inſtrument the ſurgeon will naturally have recourſe to, and if he finds the paſſage clear, which he often will, in ſuch caſes he may very probably ſuſpect a ſtone. If ſearch is made and no ſtone felt, he ſhould naturally ſuſpect the proſtate gland, eſpecially if the ſound or inſtrument he ſearched with, meets with a full ſtop, or paſſes with ſome difficulty juſt at the neck of the bladder. He ſhould examine the gland. This can only be done by introducing the finger into the anus, firſt oiling it well, placing the fore part of the finger towards the pubis; and if the parts as far as the end of the finger can reach are hard, making an eminence backwards into the rectum, ſo that the finger is obliged

obliged to be moved from ſide to ſide, to feel the whole extent of ſuch a ſwelling, and it alſo appears to go beyond the reach of the finger, we may be certain the gland is conſiderably ſwelled, and is the principal cauſe of thoſe ſymptoms.

In thoſe caſes where only the ſides of the gland are principally ſwelled, either a catheter or bougie can be eaſily paſſed, but the projecting point often prevents this relief. It is with great difficulty that a catheter or bougie can be got to paſs over it when of a conſiderable ſize, as it gives too quick a turn to the paſſage. It is neceſſary in theſe caſes to be very careful, eſpecially with the catheter; the flexible is the beſt; but even that inſtrument will often ſtick againſt this proceſs, and by puſhing it on, the point will be rather bent backwards than forwards, ſo that it cannot paſs.

I have known caſes where the common catheter has been puſhed through this projecting part into the bladder, and the water then drawn off; but in one patient the bleeding from the wound paſſed into the bladder and increaſed the quantity of matter in it, the uſe of the catheter was attempted a ſecond time, but not ſucceeding I was ſent for. I paſſed the catheter till it came to the ſtop, and then ſuſpecting what was the caſe, that this part of the proſtate projected forwards, I introduced my finger into the anus, and found that gland very much enlarged. By depreſſing the handle of the catheter which of courſe raiſed the point, it paſſed over the projection, but unfortunately the blood had coagulated in the bladder, which filled up the holes in the catheter ſo that I was obliged to withdraw it, and clear it repeatedly. This I practiſed ſeveral days, but ſuſpecting that the coagulum muſt in the end kill, I propoſed cutting him as if for the ſtone; but he died before it could be conveniently done, and the diſſection after death explained the caſe to be what I have now deſcribed.

In ſome of thoſe caſes where this part of the gland ſwells into the bladder in form of a tumor, the catheter has been known not to bring off the water at times when it appeared to have paſſed; and upon the death of the patient when the parts were examined, it was imagined that the catheter had made it's way into the tumor ſo has to have been buried in it at thoſe times.

From the knowledge of the above facts, and from the mode of accounting for the ſymptoms, whenever I find the urine does not flow immediately upon introducing

introducing the catheter into the bladder, I have pushed it on and depressed the handle so as to reach the fundus of the bladder with the end of the catheter, and have always succeeded.

For the more ready introduction of the instrument, a catheter made flexible at the point only for about an inch, is perhaps best, as it is more under the command of the hand than when wholly flexible.

If the bougie be used, it should be first warmed and then very much bent at the point, and allowed to cool in this position, and passed quickly with the concave side upwards, before it loses the bend in it's passage. But the bougie does not answer so well as the catheter, because upon withdrawing the bougie the sides of the gland soon close again. I have known where the water has passed by the side of the bougie with more freedom than when it was pulled out, because the bougie gave a straightness to this part of the canal which it had not when the bougie was withdrawn. The following case is a strong instance of the inconveniences arising from such a disease of the prostate gland.

A gentleman was attacked with a suppression of urine; a catheter could not be passed, but a bougie passed very readily and relieved him. He continued well for five years; but the same complaint returned, the bougie could not be passed, and the disease was supposed to be a stricture. A catheter however passed, although with a good deal of difficulty; and the bougie, though often tried, could not be passed, excepting once, just after using the catheter. I was sent for, and tried the bougie with as little success, and was obliged to have recourse to the catheter. I passed it with great ease, and the water was drawn off. The late Mr. Tomkyns, who had Daran's bougie, was sent for; but he was not more successful, and was obliged to have recourse to the catheter; but such violence was used as to cause a good deal of blood to come from the urethra, and after all it was not passed. I was sent for again, and passed the catheter, but with much more difficulty than before, which made me believe that the passage had been a good deal torn. Upon taking out the catheter I passed a large bougie into the bladder with great ease; this I allowed to remain for three days, and he made water tolerably freely by the side of it. The moment I drew out the bougie I attempted to pass another, but did not succeed although

I gave it the natural bend of the paſſage. Upon withdrawing thoſe bougies that did not paſs, I obſerved that all of them had a bend at the point, contrary to the direction of the paſſage; this made me ſuſpect that the place which ſtopped the bougie was on the poſterior ſurface, and that by puſhing it on, it bent forwards into the paſſage, and of courſe the point turned back. I therefore took a thick bougie; and before I introduced it I bent the point almoſt double, as mentioned before, ſo that it could not catch at the poſterior ſurface of the urethra, where I ſuppoſed the ſtop to be; this point of the bougie rubbed all along the anterior and upper ſurface of the urethra, by which means it avoided catching on the poſterior ſurface, and it paſſed with great eaſe into the bladder. He made water by the ſide of the bougie, as before. He had been for ſome time troubled with fits of an intermittent, which at firſt were very irregular, but became afterwards more regular. In one of the cold fits, the bougie being in the urethra, gave him at that time great pain, and obliged him at laſt to pull it out, on which he had immediate eaſe. The ſenſation was as if it ſtretched the paſſage too much, and in pulling it out it ſeemed to come with difficulty. This looks as if there was a contraction of the urethra, as well as of the veſſels of the ſkin, in the cold fit, ſo that this diſpoſition runs deep. By giving the bougie this bend he was able for the future to paſs them with great eaſe. I may juſt obſerve, that by introducing the finger into the anus the proſtate gland was found much enlarged.

Many patients while labouring under any of the before-mentioned diſeaſes of the urethra, and ſometimes even after they have been cured of them, find great pain in throwing forwards the ſemen; they expreſs themſelves as if it ſcalded. This ariſes from the very irritable ſtate the muſcles of this part are in, giving great pain by their own action.

I. OF THE TREATMENT OF THE SWELLED PROSTATE GLAND.

THE methods practiſed in the above caſes afforded only temporary relief; yet ſuch muſt be had recourſe to in order to prevent the conſequences of retaining

retaining the urine too long. As a temporary relief from pain, as alſo to remove ſpaſm, opiate clyſters ſhould be thrown up once or twice a day. A certain cure I am afraid is not yet known.

I have ſeen hemlock of ſervice in ſeveral caſes, which was given upon a ſuppoſition that thoſe caſes had ſomething ſcrofulous in them.

I have recommended ſea bathing, and have ſeen conſiderable advantages from it, and in two caſes, a cure of ſome ſtanding. It is upon the ſame principle of the ſcrofulous nature of the complaint that I ſuſpect hemlock has done good.

In one caſe in which I was was conſulted, the ſurgeon had found the burnt ſponge reduce the ſwelling of the gland very conſiderably: this medicine is alſo uſed upon the ſame principle. I ſhould be inclined to try the mezereon in ſuch caſes.[a]

This diſeaſe, like the ſtricture, produces complaints in the bladder; but in this the bladder is generally more irritable, perhaps from the cauſe being nearer to that viſcus.

Diſeaſes of the veſiculæ ſeminales are very familiarly talked of, but I never ſaw one. In caſes of very conſiderable induration of the proſtate gland and bladder, where the ſurrounding parts have become very much affected, I have ſeen theſe bags alſo involved in the general diſeaſe; but I never ſaw a caſe where it appeared that they were primarily affected.

[a] In a caſe of a ſwelled proſtate gland, with ſymptoms of an irritable bladder, in a young gentleman about twenty years of age, Mr. Earle tried a bliſter to the perinæum; but not finding the deſired effect, and conceiving a greater irritation and diſcharge to be neceſſary, he paſſed a ſeton in the direction of the perinæum. The orifices were about two inches diſtant from each other. The ſymptoms of irritability in the bladder began to abate, and in time went entirely off. Upon examination of the proſtate gland, from time to time, it was found to decreaſe gradually till it was nearly of the natural ſize. The ſeton was continued ſome months, and upon withdrawing it the ſymptoms began to revive again. It was adviſed to introduce it again, which was accordingly done, but without the former good effects.

CHAPTER

CHAPTER IX.

OF THE DISEASES OF THE BLADDER, PARTICULARLY FROM THE BEFORE-MENTIONED OBSTRUCTIONS TO THE URINE.

ALL the diseases of the urethra, as also the diseases of those parts belonging to this canal, which are capable of affecting it, such as the prostate gland, I have now treated of; and shall next consider the effects of them upon the bladder; as also the diseases of that viscus, independent of affections of the urethra.

The disease of the bladder arising from obstruction alone, is increased irritability, and it's consequences, by which the bladder admits of little distention, becomes quick in it's action, and thick and strong in it's coats. But prior to the description of the effects of the diseases of the urethra on the bladder, it will be necessary for the better understanding of the whole to make some remarks upon those diseases of the two parts, in which we find that each affects the other; and these I shall consider without having any regard to the cause, but only the general effects when diseased. It may be observed, that every organ in an animal body is made up of different parts, whose functions or actions are totally different from each other, although all tend to produce one ultimate effect. In most, if not in all, when perfect there is a succession of motions, one naturally arising out of the other, which in the end produces the ultimate effect; and an irregularity alone in these actions will constitute disease, at least produce very disagreeable effects, and often totally frustrate the final intention of the organs.

I may be allowed also to premise, that the natural width of the urethra gives such a resistance to the force or power of the bladder in expelling the urine, as is easily overcome by the natural action of the bladder; but when the canal is lessened, either by stricture, spasm, swelled prostate gland, or any

any other means, this proportion is loſt, by which means the bladder finds greater difficulty than natural, and is of courſe thrown into an increaſed action to overcome the reſiſtance, which becomes a cauſe of the irritability and increaſed ſtrength of this viſcus in ſuch diſeaſes.

It is to be underſtood, that in a ſound ſtate of theſe two parts, the bladder and urethra, the contraction of the one produces a relaxation of the other, and vice verſa; ſo that their natural actions are alternate, and they may be conſidered as antagoniſt muſcles to one another. Thus when the ſtimulus of expulſion of the urine takes place in the bladder, which immediately produces contractions in it, the urethra relaxes, by which means the urine is expelled from the bladder and allowed to paſs through the urethra; and when the action ceaſes in the bladder, the urethra contracts again like a ſphincter muſcle,* for the purpoſe of retaining the urine which flows into the bladder from the kidneys till it gives the ſtimulus for expulſion again.

But in many diſeaſes of theſe two parts this neceſſary alternate action is not regularly kept up, the one not obeying the ſummons of the other. This irregularity ariſes perhaps oftner from diſeaſe in the urethra, than in the bladder; for the action of the urethra depends upon the actions of the bladder; and if it is not diſpoſed to obey the notices of the bladder, then there muſt be an irregularity as to time, which produces very troubleſome ſymptoms.

We find in many diſeaſes of the urethra, ſuch as ſtrictures and ſpaſms, as alſo in diſeaſes of certain parts belonging to this canal, ſuch as the proſtate, and Cowper's glands, that there is a greater diſpoſition in this canal for contraction, than common, ſo that when the bladder has begun to act, the water is not allowed to flow, the urethra not immediately relaxing; and the moment ſuch a ſymptom takes place, every other power takes the alarm, and is brought in to aſſiſt the bladder, ſuch as ſtraining violently with the

* It may be remarked, that many ſphincter muſcles have two cauſes of action; one which may be called involuntary, depending on the natural uſes and actions of the parts; the other is voluntary, where a greater degree of action can be produced by the command of the will: and when a diſeaſed action takes place, it is probably of this voluntary action, for it is an increaſed action over the natural, which the voluntary is.

abdominal muſcles, and muſcles of reſpiration, from all which there is violent pain in the parts immediately concerned, eſpecially in the glans penis.

This diſeaſe has different degrees of violence. When ſlight, the diſtance in time between the contraction of the bladder, and the relaxation of the urethra is but ſhort, only giving a momentary pain and ſtraining, and the urethra relaxes, and the water flows according to the dilatation of the urethra, which in many of theſe caſes is but very ſmall. In others the diſtance of time is very long, many ſtraining for a conſiderable time before a drop will come; and what does come is often only in drops; and ſometimes before the whole urine can be expelled in this way, the ſpaſm of the urethra comes on again, and there is a full ſtop which gives excruciating pain for a while; but at laſt the bladder is as it were tired, and ceaſes to act. But as the urine in ſuch caſes is ſeldom all diſcharged, and often but a very little of it, the ſymptoms ſoon recur; and in this way, with a call to make water perhaps every hour out of the four and twenty, the patient drags on a miſerable life.

The bladder, in all caſes of obſtruction, whether conſtant, as in the permanent ſtricture, or ſwelled proſtate gland, or only temporary, as in the ſpaſmodic ſtricture, is generally kept diſtended, but much more ſo in the permanent ſtricture; and when the irritation of fulneſs comes on, which is very frequent, the contraction of that viſcus becomes violent, in proportion to the reſiſtance: the ſympathetic contraction of the muſcles of the abdomen takes place, and is alſo violent, yet the water at ſuch times ſhall only dribble, and be diſcharged in ſmall quantity; and in the ſpaſmodic ſtricture often not a drop ſhall paſs, ſo that the bladder is never entirely empty; and what does paſs is no more than what is ſufficient to take off the irritation of fulneſs; by which means theſe actions become more frequent, and conſequently there is almoſt always a conſtant oozing of urine from the penis between the times of making water. This however is not always the caſe, for the bladder ſometimes is ſo irritable as not to ceaſe acting till it has evacuated the whole water; and even then it is not at eaſe, but ſtill ſtrains though there is nothing to throw out, the action of the bladder becoming a cauſe of it's own continuance.

In

In all ſuch affections of the bladder there is a ſenſation of pain and itching combined in the glans penis.

If the ſymptoms are more urgent than a ſtricture or diſeaſe of the proſtate gland will well account for, a ſtone is to be ſuſpected.

I. OF THE TREATMENT WHERE THE ACTIONS OF THE URETHRA AND BLADDER DO NOT EXACTLY ALTERNATE.

THE cure where the diſeaſe ariſes from ſpaſm alone, conſiſts in removing the diſpoſition to over-action in the urethra, and the irritable diſpoſition of the bladder when the urethra does not obey it. Perhaps opiate clyſters as a temporary relief, are the very beſt; I have known a bliſter to the loins, or to the perinæum remove the ſpaſm in a great meaſure from the urethra.

When the circumſtance of the ultimate actions of theſe parts not being regular ariſes from ſtricture, ſwelled proſtate gland, or any mechanical obſtruction to the urine, then that cauſe muſt be removed, as has been fully deſcribed in the treatment of theſe diſeaſes.

II. OF THE PARALYSIS OF THE BLADDER FROM OBSTRUCTION TO THE PASSAGE OF THE URINE.

WE may obſerve that the bladder is a part eaſily deprived of it's power of contraction, for we find in many debilitating diſeaſes and long illneſſes from any cauſe, as fever, gout, and conſiderable local diſeaſes which debilitate, that the bladder often becomes paralytic, and the water muſt be drawn off. We may alſo obſerve when the bladder has been diſtended conſiderably from whatever cauſe, ſo as to have it's contractile power deſtroyed, that there is a conſiderable extravaſation of blood from the inner ſurface of the bladder, ſo that the water which is evacuated is often extremely bloody. I have ſeen in caſes where the patient has died with this obſtruction upon him, that the inner membrane of the bladder has been almoſt black, being loaded with extravaſated extravafated blood, but this fymptom of bloody urine goes off; as the bladder acquires again it's powers of action.

In the difeafes of the urethra, before-defcribed, when not properly attended to, or in time, and in cafes of ftricture where nature has not been able to relieve herfelf, the water muft of courfe be retained in the bladder, which is perhaps always productive of another difeafe, that is, the lofs of the power of contraction of that vifcus. Although this one effect, the retention of urine, arifes from very different caufes, as before-related, yet immediate relief muft be given in all of them, which can only be effected by the evacuation of the water. According to the nature of the obftruction, the mode of evacuation will be different, and will be of two kinds, one by the natural paffage by means of an hollow tube, the other by an artificial opening made into the bladder.

If the caufes of fuppreffion are either fpafmodic affections of the urethra, a fwelled proftate gland, inflammation in the furrounding parts of the urethra, or tumors preffing upon it, as happens in pregnant women, immediate relief may be procured by means of a catheter, becaufe under fuch circumftances a catheter will moft probably pafs, the fides of the canal being merely forced together by fpafm, or external preffure.

A bougie, although it will alfo pafs under fuch circumftances will not anfwer fo well, becaufe a bougie muft be withdrawn before the water can flow, which will allow the caufe of the obftruction to have again it's full force; and if the fpafm fhould not now exift, yet the bougie will not anfwer, unlefs there be a power of action in the bladder; for it is with difficulty the urine can be made to pafs through the urethra, by preffing the abdomen only.

When the catheter is paffed, it will be neceffary to make the patient ftrain with his abdominal mufcles, as alfo with his mufcles of refpiration, to fqueeze out the water, the bladder having no power of contraction, and even this will not be fufficient, for it will be neceffary to prefs on the region of the pubis with the hand to make the water flow.

In cafes where there is a confiderable degree of debility in the bladder, or in thofe cafes where there is a confiderable ftrangury and of long ftanding, and where a fmall quantity of urine in the bladder gives the ftimulus of

fulnefs

fulness to that viscus, which is always attended with considerable urgency to make water; and where only very small quantities are evacuated the bladder not being emptied at each time of making it, and when a catheter either rigid or flexible can with readiness be passed, the question is, what is the best way upon the whole to evacuate the water? There are three ways in which it can be done, one, by allowing the parts to do their own business as much as they can, and this at first sight might be supposed to be the very best, but it is in some cases the very worst, for the frequency of the inclination to make water, arising from the water not being wholly evacuated each time, the evacuation not readily taking place, increases the effort and for a few minutes produces excruciating pain, keeping up a considerable and almost constant irritation in all those parts, which few can bear. Another method is, to draw off the water each time with a catheter, but this in many cases is next to impracticable; for supposing the operation to be performed only twice or three times in the day, we shall find that this is oftener than what should be done. The third method is, to leave the catheter almost constantly in the bladder.

Which of these three methods gives on the whole the least irritation must depend upon circumstances attending different cases. Where the frequency and the urgency is great, and the flowing of the water difficult, either the second or the third is to be pursued; and when the symptoms are such that a catheter must be passed very often, I believe it had better be left in, only taking it out occasionally: I think this is supported by observation and experience.

It sometimes happens in cases of swelled prostate gland, that the catheter cannot be passed without the utmost difficulty, and when this has been the case I have left it in the bladder, for fear of not being able to pass it again, and continued it there till the bladder has sufficiently recovered it's tone, which is known by it's being able to throw the urine through the catheter; after which that instrument may be withdrawn.

If the spasm, in such cases as arise from that cause, should still continue after the bladder has recovered it's tone, we must continue the use of the catheter. But it often happens that the spasm leaves the urethra before the bladder recovers it's power of contraction, the diseafe becoming then fimply a paralyfis of that vifcus.

One of the firft fymptoms of the bladder beginning to regain it's power of contraction is, the fenfation of fulnefs, or an inclination to make water, and when that fenfation comes on the patient fhould be allowed to make water but not to force it, for that circumftance alone will bring on the fpafm if the urethra is not very ready to dilate. I have feen however in fome cafes, that a flight fenfation is not altogether to be depended upon, for it required a little retention more effectually to ftimulate the bladder to action, and then the water has paffed more freely.

The fpafmodic contraction of the urethra does not appear to give up it's action fimply upon the ftimulus or inclination to make water, and not till the bladder begins to have the power of contraction; for in cafes where the bladder is paralytic, and yet fenfible of the ftimulus arifing from being full, as it does not contract, the urethra does not relax, and the water cannot be made to pafs.

It would appear that as the bladder recovers of the paralyfis it is not able to contain fo much water as ufual, therefore the patients are obliged to make water often, and of courfe in fmall quantities.

III. OF THE CURE OF THE PARALYSIS OF THE BLADDER, FROM OBSTRUCTION ARISING FROM PRESSURE OR SPASM.

THE removal of the caufes of the paralyfis of the bladder was fully defcribed when we were treating of the difeafes which produce that complaint, and the immediate relief, when the bladder is rendered inactive, has juft now been confidered; the paralyfis itfelf is therefore the only remaining thing to be attended to. In this difeafe there are often contrary indications of cure, for a fpafm is very different from a paralyfis; and if the fuppreffion is from fpafm, and that ftill continues, then what may be good for the paralyfis, may be bad for the fpafm. As in fuch cafes the water can be drawn off, the bladder fhould be firft attended to. Stimulants and ftrength-

eners

eners are uſeful; bliſters to the loins to rouze the bladder to action, and bliſters to the perinæum, to take off the ſpaſm from the urethra, often ſucceed. Electricity is ſometimes of ſingular ſervice, when applied in ſuch caſes to the perinæum. Through the whole of the cure the urine muſt be drawn off frequently, becauſe the bladder ſhould not be allowed to be diſtended, which otherways would be the conſequence; and the ſenſation ariſing from the diſtention of that viſcus is a very oppreſſive one.

A gentleman was at times attacked with a difficulty in making water, which he paid no attention to, as it had always gone off; but at laſt he was taken ſo bad as to be obliged to have recourſe to the catheter, which afforded only a temporary relief. The ſpaſm continued, and I was ſent for; when I paſſed the catheter, I was obliged to preſs the lower part of the abdomen to ſqueeze out the water, for the bladder appeared to give but little aſſiſtance. I ordered a bliſter to the loins which gave ſome power of contraction to the bladder, and took off ſome of the ſpaſm in the urethra, but ſtill he was very little relieved; I then directed a bliſter to be applied to the perinæum, which immediately removed his complaint.

CHAPTER

CHAPTER X.

OF A SUPPRESSION OF URINE—AND OPERATIONS FOR THE CURE OF IT.

IN cafes of total fuppreffion of urine arifing from ftrictures or other caufes where a catheter cannot be paffed, and where every other method recommended is impracticable, an artificial opening muft be made into the bladder for the evacuation of the water. There are three places where this opening may be made, and each has had it's advocates. This operation has not been confidered in all it's circumftances in different patients, fo as to direct the young furgeon in the variety of cafes that may occur; for under fome circumftances the operation is more advifable in one place than another; and indeed it may fometimes be next to impoffible to perform it in a particular part.

The opening may be made firft, in the perinæum, where we now cut for a ftone; fecondly, above the pubis, where cutting for the ftone was formerly practifed; and thirdly, from within the rectum, where the bladder lies in contact with the gut.

The firft queftion which naturally occurs is, which of thofe fituations is the moft proper for the fafety of the patient, the evacuation of the water, and the conveniency of operating, when no particular circumftance forbids either of the fituations?

On the firft view of the fubject, one would be apt to prefer that above the pubis, or from the rectum, as the bladder is nearer to either, and the parts more adapted to an operation, than from the perinæum, where we muft cut at random. Thefe two fituations, although the moft proper in this refpect, under certain circumftances, yet may become the moft improper, for they are fubject to greater changes than the perinæum.

The

The reafons that may render it very improper above the pubis are, the perfons being very fat, or the bladders not diftending fufficiently fo as to rife above the pubis, which is common enough in difeafes of thofe parts.

In very fat people it will be found that the fubftance to be cut through may be three, or four inches, which will not only make the operation very unpleafant, but often improper; for fuch thicknefs of parts will make the fwell of the bladder very obfcure and uncertain; in many of thofe cafes of obftruction the bladder being fo difeafed as to allow of but little diftention, and in fuch the fymptoms of diftention come on very early, perhaps where there is only a few ounces of water collected. But if the retention has been for fome confiderable time, as twenty-four hours, then we may fuppofe that the bladder has allowed of diftention to a much greater degree, which may in fome cafes be afcertained by introducing the finger into the rectum.

But where the bladder diftends, and the parts are fo thin that it can be plainly felt above the pubis, I fee no material objection to this fituation; and it has this advantage over the operation by the rectum, that a catheter can more eafily be introduced, and kept in, which will be neceffary to be done till the caufe is removed.

It may be neceffary here to mention fome precautions refpecting the keeping the inftrument in the bladder; as alfo the beft kind to be ufed. It muft be a hollow tube, and fhould reach as far as the pofterior furface of the bladder, for upon the contraction of that vifcus it's anterior part recedes backwards and downwards from the abdomen towards it's fixed point, which may draw the bladder off from the tube. But as the diftance between the fkin of the abdomen and pofterior furface of the bladder cannot be exactly afcertained, the canula may be either too long, or too fhort; if too long, it's end may prefs upon the pofterior furface of the bladder and produce ulceration there, and in time work it's way into the rectum. To avoid this mifchief, as alfo the inconveniences arifing from it's being too fhort, and the bladder flipping off from it's end, I would recommend the tube to be made with a curve, and to lie with it's convex fide on the pofterior part of the bladder, which being a large furface, and following nearly the fame curve as the canula, lefs mifchief is to be expected. The openings into the canula may be made on the concave fide.

 Probably

Probably it might be attended with more ſafety, as alſo eaſe to the patient, to have the curved end of the catheter introduced into the urethra from the bladder. The paſſing of it into the urethra is very impracticable, and we know that ſuch a body lying in the urethra is not productive of any miſchief. A common catheter paſſed in this way enters ſo far as to bring the handle almoſt flat to the belly, at moſt only a little bolſter between the catheter and belly is neceſſary, and then with a piece of tape fixed to the handle of the catheter it might be faſtened to the body, or a ſhort catheter might be made with ears to fix the tape to.* In caſes where the canula has remained in ſome time, the artificial paſſage will become in ſome degree permanent, ſo that it may be taken out occaſionally, and cleaned from any ſtony matter that may be attached to it. To avoid this part of the operation it has been recommended to have two canulas, one within the other, that by drawing out the inner it might be cleaned, and again introduced; but in moſt caſes it will alſo be neceſſary to withdraw the outer one, as it's external ſurface will contract a cruſt.

The ſecond method, or puncture by the anus, will more commonly admit of being performed than that above the pubis; for it does not require that diſtention of bladder which the other does, therefore not ſo often impracticable from that cauſe; and perhaps the only obſtacle here is a ſwelled proſtate gland. In many of theſe caſes of diſeaſes of the urethra, the proſtate gland is very much ſwelled, which I can conceive may make the proper place for the puncture very uncertain; for the proſtate gland in ſuch caſes will be preſſed down towards the anus, before the bladder, and will be the firſt thing felt by the finger. Care muſt therefore be taken to diſtinguiſh the one from the other, which can only be done by getting the finger beyond the proſtate gland, which may not be practicable; and if practicable, it may not be an eaſy matter to diſtinguiſh the one from the other, as a thickened and diſtended bladder may ſeem to be a continuation of the ſame tumor. However if the

* Where this operation is performed in conſequence of a ſtricture, I have conceived that by paſſing it into the urethra from the bladder till it came to the ſtricture, and then paſſing another ſtraight canula from the glans down the urethra, that the two might nearly meet, only having the ſtricture between them; and a piercer might be paſſed down and forced into the end of the one from the bladder, and afterwards either a bougie or hollow catheter introduced.

objections

objections given to the performing of it above the pubis exist, I should prefer operating by the rectum, for although the probability of succeeding here may not be apparently greater than above the pubis, yet the chances are in it's favour.

I must however observe here, that the objections which I have started, are only raised in my own mind from my knowledge of the diseases of those parts, and not from cases of suppression of urine under all the before-mentioned circumstances having occurred to me in practice.

A case of a total suppression of urine arising from stricture, where no instrument could be passed by the natural passage, and where a puncture was made into the bladder, from the rectum, with success, is related in the Philosophical Transactions, by Dr. Hamilton of Kings Lynn in Norfolk.*

What led Dr. Hamilton to do it here, was a difficulty which was found in passing the clyster-pipe into the rectum, which induced him to introduce his finger into the anus, and he found the bladder so prominent in the rectum as to give the hint of performing the operation there.

The man was put into the same position as in the operation for the stone, and a trochar was introduced upon the finger into the anus, and thrust into the lower and most prominent part of the tumor, in the direction of the axis of the bladder, and upon withdrawing the piercer the water flowed out through the canula.

A straight catheter was then introduced through the canula, least the orifice in the bladder should be drawn off from the canula.

Then the canula was pulled out over the catheter, which was left in till the whole water was evacuated, and was then withdrawn.

The bladder, notwithstanding of this perforation, retained the water as usual, till the inclination to make it came on; and when he performed the action of making water, the orifice in the bladder seemed to open, and it rushed out by the anus. This continued about two days, when the water began to find it's natural passage, and a bougie was introduced into the bladder, through the urethra, which gave a free passage for the water, and of course less came by the anus; so that on the sixth day after the operation

* Philosophical Transactions for the Year 1776, vol. 66, page 578.

the whole came by the natural paſſage. The man continued the uſe of the bougie till the ſtricture was dilated.

Dr. Hamilton further remarks, that in thoſe caſes of ſuppreſſion of urine, in general, he has found that calomel and opium, in large doſes, anſwer better than any thing he has tried.

He is convinced from repeated trials, that the ſpecific efficacy is in the calomel, as large doſes of opium alone have proved ineffectual; but he does not ſay that calomel alone will anſwer. He orders ten grains of calomel with two of opium, to be repeated in ſix hours if it has not anſwered in that time; and he ſays he has ſeldom been obliged to give a third doſe.

This method of tapping the bladder was firſt ſuggeſted by Monſ. Fleurant, ſurgeon to the Charité, at Lyons, in the year 1750. The operation was performed at that time, and an account of it was afterwards publiſhed by Monſ. Pouteau, in 1760, with the hiſtory of three caſes, in all which the operation was performed by Monſ. Fleurant. The propriety of performing the operation in this part occurred to him in a manner ſimilar to that before-related of Dr. Hamilton; for in introducing the finger into the rectum to examine the ſtate of the bladder in a caſe where he was going to puncture in the perinæum, he found the bladder ſo prominent there, and ſo much within the reach of his inſtrument that he immediately altered his intention, and performed it in this part. He very readily drew off the water, and kept the canula in, with a T bandage, till the urine came the right way, and then withdrew it, and all terminated well. But there was a good deal of trouble on account of the canula being left in on going to ſtool, as alſo from the conſtant dribbling of the water through it, all of which was prevented in Dr. Hamilton's caſe, by removing the canula immediately upon the evacuation of the water. This was productive of another good effect, which was the retention of the urine till the ſtimulus of fulneſs was given, and then it paſſed through the artificial as it would through a natural paſſage. Should this be a conſtant effect in conſequence of performing the operation here, I think it muſt be owned to be an unexpected circumſtance which at firſt could not have been imagined.*

* A hiſtory, with a deſcription of this operation, is publiſhed by Mr. Reid, ſurgeon of Chelſea, in 1778.

In

In another patient of Monf. Fleurant's, the canula was kept in the anus and bladder thirty-nine days, without any inconveniency; fo that the objection to this part of the operation cannot be material.

Pouteau mentions one cafe where he performed this operation, in the year 1752, and the man died.*

He fays, I was called to vifit a poor man fuffering under a retention of urine, fo obftinate and violent that it had already the fymptoms of what is called a reflux of urine into the blood; and the complaint had continued more than three days. An empiric, to whofe care he had been entrufted, after having very improperly given him the moft powerful diuretics, had likewife the rafhnefs to fearch him. It appears probable that thefe attempts which were made without fuccefs muft have increafed the mifchief. A catheter could not be paffed into fuch parts by unfkilful hands, without increafing the inflammation. I only made three flight efforts to effect a paffage into the bladder by the urethra, which appeared to be much difeafed, as well by the effufion of blood, as the extreme pain thefe attempts produced. I determined at once to do as before, and plunged my trochar by the rectum into the bladder. The fuccefs was exactly the fame; the bladder was entirely emptied, and I allowed the canula to remain there a whole night and a day, during which time the urine flowed without intermiffion. Every thing went on without any accident which could be fuppofed connected with the operation; and death, which happened next day, was entirely independent of it.

One muft fuppofe with Pouteau, that the death of the patient could not have arifen from this operation, but from the preceding difeafes.

The bags called veficulæ feminales, and the hæmorrhoidal veffels, have been mentioned as parts in danger of being wounded in the operation, and thereby proving troublefome; but if either of them were wounded, no inconveniency could arife. To avoid the veficulæ feminales, it is recommended to perforate high up, and directly in the middle of the bladder, between the two fides, and this fituation is at the fame time the one where

* Pouteau Melanges de Chirurgie, printed at Lyons, 1760, page 506, 507, and 508.

the hæmorrhoidal veſſels are the ſmalleſt, and therefore it is of leſs conſequence if they are wounded.

It muſt appear from the following caſe, ſent me by a gentleman, that a communication being kept up between the bladder and rectum, is only inconvenient, and not ſo much ſo as might be expected.

With reſpect to the ſailor who paſſed his urine by the rectum, I have examined the few papers by me, but cannot find the particular remarks I made; however, as the caſe was ſingular, I recollect the man told me, that a few years before, (this was at Madras hoſpital, in December 1779) he had the venereal diſeaſe, very bad, and long; that the urine came by the anus, but this paſſage healed up, and it came by the penis, and continued to do ſo till he caught the diſeaſe again, when the urine found it's way a ſecond time by the anus, and came that way for years. When he firſt came under my care, in the hoſpital at Bombay, February 1779, he felt no uneaſineſs or inconvenience from this manner of paſſing his urine; whenever he had an inclination to make water he ſat down. I often made him lie upon his breaſt, with his legs drawn up, and the ſtream came through the anus with great force.

In other caſes, in conſequence of abſceſſes forming between the bladder and rectum, where they have not healed up, there has been a reciprocal paſſing of the contents of theſe cavities from the one to the other.

It only remains to ſpeak of the puncture in the perinæum. An obſtruction to the urine taking place in the natural paſſage prevents us from introducing an inſtrument in moſt of thoſe caſes, and deprives us of all the advantages we could receive from it as a guide in the operation; yet there may be caſes of ſtricture, where by cutting into the urethra, beyond the ſtricture, the water will flow; but this muſt be done without any guide or direction, and requires a nice and accurate knowledge of the parts; or if the obſtruction ariſes from the valvular projection of the proſtate gland, a ſtaff may be paſſed as far as this projection, and cut upon as for the ſtone, only making a ſmaller inciſion, uſing a ſmall gorget, or in the room of that, a trochar of a particular form might be run along it into the bladder; for although the ſtaff does not enter the bladder, yet the diſtance to paſs through without this guide is but ſmall. If this cannot be done, a ſmall and deep inciſion incifion may be made in the perinæum, with an impofthume lancet towards the bladder; the point of the trochar is to be introduced by this, paffing at the fame time the fore-finger of the other hand into the anus, which will be a guide both for the direction of the inftrument, as alfo to avoid it's point paffing into the rectum; with thefe precautions the error cannot be great.

I muft own however, that I have not feen cafes enough to enable me to give all the varieties that commonly happen, and of courfe to give all the advantages and difadvantages of each method.

I. OF ALLOWING A CATHETER TO REMAIN IN THE URETHRA AND BLADDER.

In cafes of debility of the bladder, and where a catheter paffes with difficulty, or with great uncertainty, and in cafes where it muft be ufed frequently, and for a length of time, it will be neceffary to keep an inftrument in the urethra and bladder, fo as to allow the water to pafs through it freely. A common catheter, or one made of the elaftic gum are perhaps the beft inftruments of any; but they muft be fixed in the canal; this will be beft done by it's outer end being tied to fome external body, as I fhall now defcribe. When the catheter is fairly in the bladder, the outer end is rather inclined downwards, nearly in a line with the body, take the common ftrap or belt-part of a bag-trufs, and have two thigh-ftraps either fixed to it or hooked to it; let a ftrap come round each thigh and forwards by each fide of the fcrotum, to be faftened to the belt where the ears of the bag are ufually fixed. Have a fmall ring or two fixed to each ftrap juft where it paffes the fcrotum or root of the penis; then take a piece of fmall tape, and fix the ends of the catheter to thofe rings, which will keep it in the bladder. A bit of rag about four or five inches long, with a hole at the end of it, paffed over the exterior end of the catheter, and the loofe end allowed to hang in a bafon, placed between the thighs, will catch the water which cannot difengage itfelf from the catheter, and keep the patient dry; or if another curved pipe is introduced into the catheter it will anfwer equally well.

Under

Under ſuch treatment the bladder will never be allowed to be diſtended; and when the patient wants to have the bladder in ſome degree emptied, he has only to ſtrain with his abdominal muſcles, by which means he will be able to throw out a great deal at each time.

As the bladder begins to recover it's actions, the patient will find that an inclination to make water will come on, and at thoſe times he will alſo find that the water will come from him without ſtraining with the abdominal muſcles; when this takes place readily the catheter may be taken out, and it will be found that he will be able in future to make water of himſelf. If it is neceſſary to keep in the catheter a conſiderable time, it will be the cauſe of a great deal of ſlime and mucus being formed in the urethra and bladder; but I believe this is of no conſequence. I have known a catheter kept in this way for five months without any inconveniency whatever.

In all caſes where it is neceſſary to keep an extraneous body for a conſiderable time in the bladder, whether in an artificial paſſage or the natural one, it will be proper a few days after it's firſt introduction to withdraw it and examine whether it is incruſting, or filling up in it's cavity with the calculous matter of the urine; if after remaining in the bladder for ſome days it has contracted none, we need be under no apprehenſions of it's doing it; but if, as frequently happens, it ſhould have a conſiderable quantity collected, then it will be neceſſary to have it occaſionally withdrawn and cleaned; the beſt method probably of doing this is to put it in vinegar, which will ſoon diſſolve the ſtony matter.

II. OF THE INCREASED STRENGTH OF THE BLADDER.

The bladder in ſuch caſes as before-deſcribed, having more to do than common, is almoſt in a conſtant ſtate of irritation and action; by which, according to a property in all muſcles, it becomes ſtronger and ſtronger in it's muſcular coats; and I ſuſpect, that this diſpoſition to become ſtronger from repeated action, is greater in the involuntary muſcles than the voluntary; and the reaſon why it ſhould be ſo is I think very evident; for in the involuntary muſcles the power ſhould be in all caſes capable of overcoming the

the refiftance; as the power is always performing fome natural and neceffary action, for whenever a difeafe produces an uncommon refiftance in the involuntary parts, if the power is not proportionably increafed the difeafe becomes very formidable; whereas in the voluntary mufcles there is not that neceffity, becaufe the will can ftop whenever the mufcles cannot follow; and if the will is fo difeafed as not to ftop, the power in voluntary mufcles fhould not increafe in proportion.

I have feen the mufcular coats of the bladder near half an inch thick, and the fafciculi fo ftrong as to form ridges on the infide of that cavity;[a] and I have alfo feen the fafciculi very thin, and even wanting in fome parts of the bladder, fo that a hernia of the internal coat had taken place between the fafciculi, and formed pouches.[b] Thefe pouches arife from the thin parts not being able to fupport the actions of the ftrong; as happens in ruptures at the navel, or rings of the abdomen.

III. OF THE DISTENTION OF THE URETERS.

It fometimes happens that the irritation from the diftention of the bladder, and the difficulty in throwing out it's contents, is fo great, that the urine is prevented from flowing freely into that vifcus from the ureters, which become thereby preternaturally diftended. The pelvis of the kidneys, and infundibula are alfo enlarged; but how far this dilatation of the ureters and pelvis is really owing to a mechanical caufe I am not fo clear; or whether it is not a difpofition for dilatation arifing out of the ftimulus given by the bladder. In fome cafes of long ftanding, where the bladder was become very thick, and had been for a long time acting with great

[a] This appearance was long fuppofed to have arifen from a difeafe of this vifcus; but upon examination I found that the mufcular parts were found and diftinct; that they were only increafed in bulk in proportion to the power they had to exert; and that it was not a confequence of inflammation, for in that cafe parts are blended into one indiftinct mafs.

[b] This is perhaps the caufe of the ftone being often found in a pouch formed in the bladder; for the bladder in cafes of ftone is often very ftrong, which arifes from the violent contraction of that vifcus caufed by the irritation of the ftone on the fides of it; and alfo from the ftone being often oppofed to the mouth of the urethra in the time of making water.

violence, it had affected the mamillæ, ſo that the ſurface of theſe proceſſes produced a matter, and perhaps even the ſecreting organs of the kidneys, ſo that the urine ſecreted was accompanied with a pus, ariſing from the irritation being kept up in all theſe parts.

The urine in the above caſes is generally ſtale, even before it is thrown out of the bladder, which when joined with the circumſtance of the linen being conſtantly kept wet, by the almoſt continual diſcharge of urine, (which of itſelf would produce a ſtaleneſs of urine, in theſe parts) becomes very offenſive, and it is hardly poſſible to keep the patient ſweet.

IV. OF IRRITABILITY IN THE BLADDER INDEPENDENT OF OBSTRUCTIONS TO THE PASSAGE OF THE URINE.

ANOTHER diſeaſe of the bladder, connected with our preſent ſubject is, where that viſcus becomes extremely irritable, and will not allow of it's uſual diſtention. The ſymptoms of this diſeaſe are very ſimilar to thoſe ariſing from obſtructions to the paſſage of the urine in the urethra, but with this difference, that in the preſent diſeaſe the urine flows readily, becauſe the urethra obeys the ſummons and relaxes; however there is often conſiderable ſtraining, after the water is all made, ariſing from the muſcular coat of the bladder ſtill continuing it's contractions.

This irritabilty of the bladder often ariſes from local cauſes, as a ſtone, cancer, or tumors forming on the inſide, all of which produce irritability of this viſcus. In ſuch caſes, the ſtraining is violent, for the cauſe ſtill remains which continues to give the ſtimulus of ſomething to be expelled, and the bladder continues to contract till tired, as in the caſes of ſimple irritability; and then there is a reſpite for a time; but this reſpite is of ſhort duration, for the urine is ſoon accumulated.

This diſeaſe will kill in the end, by producing waſting and hectic-fever.

V. OF

V. OF THE CURE OF SIMPLE IRRITABILITY OF THE BLADDER.

When the ſymptoms ariſe from irritability alone, and not from a ſtone, or any local affection, the nature of the complaint may not at firſt be ſo obvious; temporary relief may however be procured by opium, which is moſt effectual in ſlight and recent caſes; and if it be applied as near to the part as poſſible, it's effects will be more evident; and therefore it may be given by clyſter as well as by the mouth.

I ſhould however be inclined to rely more on a bliſter applied to the perinæum, than any other method of cure; or to the lower part of the ſmall of the back, or upper part of the ſacrum, if more convenient.

In all caſes where there is an irritation of the bladder the patient ſhould never endeavour to retain his water beyond the inclination to make it. It hurts the bladder and increaſes it's irritability; and indeed I am apt to think that this circumſtance even in ſound parts, is often a prediſpoſing cauſe of diſeaſe in this viſcus and it's appendage, the urethra; for I have known ſeveral caſes where it has brought on the ſpaſmodic ſtricture in the urethra, in ſound parts; and it is frequently an immediate cauſe of ſtrangury in thoſe who have either a ſtricture, or a diſpoſition to ſpaſms in thoſe parts.

A gentleman in perfect health, from retaining his urine beyond the inclination in the play-houſe, had all the ſymptoms of an irritable bladder brought on, and continued for ſeveral years, rendering him miſerable.

VI. OF A PARALYSIS OF THE ACCELERATORES MUSCLES.

In many irritations of the bladder, the urethra not only relaxes directly on the ſtimulus to make water being felt in that viſcus, as has been deſcribed, but a paralyſis ſometimes takes place in the voluntary muſcles of thoſe parts, ſo that the will cannot command them to contract to hinder the inconveniences that may attend an immediate evacuation of that fluid. If we

attempt

attempt to ſtop the water, which is an act of the will, we cannot, the acceleratores muſcles will not obey, and the water flows.

A bliſter applied to the perinæum will have conſiderable effects in removing this complaint.

CHAPTER

CHAPTER XI.

OF THE DISCHARGE OF THE NATURAL MUCUS OF THE GLANDS OF THE URETHRA.

THE ſmall glands of the urethra, and Cowper's glands, ſecrete a ſlimy mucus ſimilar to the white of an egg not coagulated. This ſeldom appears externally, or flows from the urethra, but during the indulgence of laſcivious thoughts, and is ſeldom or never attended to, excepting by thoſe who are under apprehenſions either of a gonorrhœa coming on, or imagine the laſt infection is not gone off entirely, and ſuch patients are kept in conſtant terror by this natural diſcharge. They often find it in ſuch quantity as to leave ſpots on the ſhirt, but without colour; and often after toying, the lips of the urethra are as it were glewed together by it, from it's drying there, which appearances alarm the mind of the patient without cauſe. Although this is only a natural diſcharge, and is now ſecreted under the ſame influence which naturally produces it, it muſt at the ſame time be owned, that it is commonly much increaſed in thoſe caſes of debility ariſing from the mind, which is probably not eaſily to be accounted for; it would ſeem that the conteſt between the mind and the body increaſes this ſecretion, for it cannot be conſidered as a diſeaſe of the parts.

I. OF THE DISCHARGE OF THE SECRETIONS OF THE PROSTATE GLAND AND VESICULÆ SEMINALES.

THIS complaint is imagined to be the conſequence of the venereal diſeaſe in the urethra; but how far this is really the caſe is not certain; though moſt probably it is not. It is a diſcharge of mucus by the urethra which generally comes away with the laſt drops of urine, eſpecially if the bladder is irritable; and ſtill more at the time of being at ſtool, particularly if the patient be coſtive; for under ſuch circumſtances the ſtraining or actions of the muſcles of thoſe parts are more violent. It has generally been ſuppoſed that this diſcharge is ſemen, and it is the diſeaſe called a ſeminal weakneſs; but it appears from many experiments and obſervations, that the diſcharge is undoubtedly not ſemen. It is only the mucus ſecreted either by the proſtate gland, by thoſe bags improperly called veſiculæ ſeminales, or both; and it may not be improper to give here the diſtinguiſhing marks between theſe two fluids. Firſt; I may obſerve the diſcharge in queſtion is not of the ſame colour with the ſemen, and is exactly of the colour of the mucus of the proſtate gland, and of thoſe bags. It has not the ſame ſmell, and indeed it hardly has any ſmell at all. The quantity evacuated at one time is often much more conſiderable than the evacuation of ſemen ever is; and it happens more frequently than it could poſſibly do were the diſcharge ſemen. It is a diſeaſe that often attacks old men, where one can hardly ſuppoſe much ſemen to be ſecreted; and we find that thoſe who are affected with this diſeaſe are no more deficient in the ſecretion and evacuation of the ſemen in the natural way than before they had the diſeaſe. If the mind be at eaſe this ſhall take place immediately after a diſcharge of this fluid, as well as before, which could not be the caſe were it ſemen. Further, if thoſe that labour under this complaint are not connected with women they are ſubject to nocturnal diſcharges from the imagination, as perſons are who are perfectly ſound; and indeed moſt patients when made acquainted with theſe circumſtances become very ſenſible that it is not the ſemen.

It is not clear what the diſeaſed ſtate of the parts is upon which this diſcharge depends, whether there is a larger ſecretion of this mucus than natural, or whether it is entirely owing to a preternatural, uncommon action of thoſe parts; and if this laſt, why theſe parts ſhould be put into action when the bladder, rectum, and abdominal muſcles are thrown into action to expel their contents, is not eaſily explained. It is plain that the moſt violent actions of theſe parts are neceſſary to produce this evacuation; for it does not come with the firſt of the urine, nor in general when they go with eaſe to ſtool.

As

As it was thought to be a seminal discharge, it was imagined to arise from a weakness in the organs of generation; and as frequent discharges of the semen in the natural way generally weaken, it was therefore imagined that this discharge must also weaken very considerably; and the imagination will operate so strongly as to make the patients believe they really are weakened. Whether the cause of such a discharge is capable of weakening, I will not pretend to say; but I believe that the discharge simply does not. Fear, and anxiety of mind may really weaken the patient. In the cases I have seen of this kind, the mind has been more affected than the body.

From my own practice, I can hardly recommend any one medicine, or way of life, for removing this complaint. In one case I found considerable benefit from giving hemlock internally.

The idea that has been formed of the disease leads to the practice generally used and recommended, such as giving strengthening medicines of all kinds, as bark, &c. but I never saw any good effects from any of them; and I should rather be inclined to take up the soothing plan to prevent all violent actions. Keeping the body gently open will in some degree moderate the discharge, and probably may effect a cure in the end.

CHAPTER

CHAPTER XII.

OF IMPOTENCE.

THIS complaint is by many laid to the charge of Onanifm at an early age; but how far this is juft, it will in many cafes be difficult to determine; for upon a ftrict review of this fubject, it appears to me to be by far too rare to originate from a practice fo general.

How far the attributing to this practice fuch a confequence, is of public utility, I am doubtful, particularly as it is followed moft commonly at an age when confequences are not fufficiently attended to, even in things lefs gratifying to the fenfes; but this I can fay with certainty, that many of thofe who are affected with the complaints in queftion are miferable from this idea; and it is fome confolation for them to know that it is poffible it may arife from other caufes. I am clear in my own mind that the books on this fubject have done more harm than good. I think I may affirm that this act in itfelf does lefs harm to the conftitution in general than the natural. That the natural with common women, or fuch as we are indifferent about, does lefs harm to the conftitution than where it is not fo felfifh, and where the affections for the woman are alfo concerned. Where it is only a conftitutional act it is fimple, and only one action takes place; but where the mind becomes interefted, it is worked up to a degree of enthufiafm, increafing the fenfibility of the body and difpofition for action; and when the complete action takes place it is with proportional violence; and in proportion to the violence is the degree of debility produced, or injury done to the conftitution.

In the cafes of this kind that have come under my care, although the perfons themfelves have been very ready to fuppofe that the difeafe arofe from the caufe here alluded to; yet they did not appear to have given more into the practice than common; and in particular, the worft cafe I have ever feen was where but very little of this practice had ever been ufed, much lefs leſs than in common among boys or lads. The only true objection to this ſelfiſh enjoyment is the probability of it's being repeated too frequently.

Nothing hurts the mind of a man ſo much as the idea of inability to perform well the duty of the ſex. If his ſcrotum hangs low it makes him miſerable; he conceives immediately that he is to be rendered incapable of performing thoſe acts in which he prides himſelf moſt. It is certain that the relaxation, or contraction of the ſcrotum, is in ſome degree a kind of ſign of the conſtitution; but it is of the conſtitution at large, not of thoſe parts in particular. Nurſes are ſo ſenſible of the contraction of that part being a ſign of health in the children under their care, that they take notice of it. The relaxation of it in them cannot be ſuppoſed to ariſe from inability to perform thoſe acts at one time more than another. The face is one of the ſigns of the conſtitution, and has as much to do with thoſe peculiar acts as the ſcrotum. However we muſt allow that this part is much more lax than what we ſhould conceive was intended by nature, even in young men who are well in health; but as this is very general, I rather ſuſpect that it ariſes from the circumſtances of the part being kept too warm, and always ſuſpended, the muſcles hardly ever being allowed to act, ſo that they have leſs force. How far it is the ſame in thoſe countries whoſe dreſs does not immediately ſuſpend thoſe parts, I have not been able to aſcertain. Warmth appears to be one cauſe, for we find that cold has always an immediate effect; but this is perhaps owing to it's not being accuſtomed to cold, which if it were, it might poſſibly become as regardleſs of it as it was of warmth. What the difference is in this part, in a cold and warm climate, all other circumſtances the ſame, I do not know. But whatever may be the cauſe, if it is really in common more lax than intended by nature, it is of no conſequence as to the powers of generation. The teſticles will ſecrete whether kept high or low.

I. OF IMPOTENCE DEPENDING ON THE MIND.

As the parts of generation are not neceſſary for the exiſtence or ſupport of the individual, as what relates to food and ſleep, but have a reference to ſomething elſe in which the mind has a principal concern, a complete action in thoſe parts cannot take place without a perfect harmony of body and of mind; that is, there muſt be both a power of body, and diſpoſition of mind; for the mind is ſubject to a thouſand caprices which affect the actions of theſe parts.

Copulation is an act of the body, the ſpring of which is in the mind; but it is not volition; and according to the ſtate of the mind ſo is the act performed. To perform this act well, the body ſhould be in health, and the mind ſhould be perfectly confident of the powers of the body; the mind ſhould be in a ſtate entirely diſengaged from every thing elſe; it ſhould have no difficulties, no fears, no apprehenſions; not even an anxiety to perform the act well; for even this anxiety is a ſtate of mind different from what ſhould prevail; there ſhould not be even a fear that the mind itſelf may find a difficulty at the time the act ſhould be performed. Perhaps no function of the machine depends ſo much upon the ſtate of the mind as this.

The will, and reaſoning faculty, have nothing to do with this power; they are only employed in the act, ſo far as voluntary parts are made uſe of; and if they ever interfere, which they ſometimes do, it often produces another ſtate of the mind which deſtroys that which is proper for the performance of the act; it produces a deſire, a wiſh, a hope, which are all only diffidence and uncertainty, and create in the mind the idea of a poſſibility of the want of ſucceſs, which deſtroys the proper ſtate of mind, or neceſſary confidence.

There is perhaps no act in which a man feels himſelf more intereſted, or is more anxious to perform well, his pride being engaged in ſome degree, which if within certain bounds would produce a degree of perfection in an act depending upon the will, or an act in voluntary parts; but when it produces a ſtate of mind contrary to that ſtate on which the perfection of the act depends, a failure muſt be the conſequence.

The body is not only rendered incapable of performing this act, by the mind being under the above influence, but alſo by the mind being perfectly confident of it's power, but conſcious of an impropriety in performing it; this in many caſes producing a ſtate of mind which ſhall take away all power. The ſtate of a man's mind reſpecting his ſiſter takes away all power.

power. A confcientious man has been known to lofe his powers on finding the woman he was going to be connected with unexpectedly a virgin.

Shedding tears arifes entirely from the ftate of the mind, although not fo much a compound action as the act in queftion; for none are fo weak in body that they cannot fhed tears; it is not fo much a compound action of the mind and ftrength of body, joined, as the other act is; yet if we are afraid of fhedding tears, or are defirous of doing it, and that anxiety is kept up through the whole of an affecting fcene, we certainly fhall not fhed tears, or at leaft not fo freely as would have happened from our natural feelings.

From the above account of the neceffity of having the mind independent, refpecting the act, we muft fee that it may very often happen that the ftate of mind will be fuch as not to allow the animal to exert it's natural powers: and every failure increafes the evil. We muft alfo fee from this ftate of the cafe, that this act muft be often interrupted; and the true caufe of this interruption not being known, it will be laid to the charge of the body or want of powers. As thefe cafes do not arife from real inability, they are to be carefully diftinguifhed from fuch as do; and perhaps the only way to diftinguifh them is, to examine into the ftate of mind refpecting this act. So trifling often is the circumftance which fhall produce this inability, depending on the mind, that the very defire to pleafe fhall have that effect, as in making the woman the fole object to be gratified.

Cafes of this kind, we fee every day; one of which I fhall relate as an illuftration of this fubject, and alfo of the method of cure.

A gentleman told me, that he had loft his powers in this way. After above an hour's inveftigation of the cafe, I made out the following facts; that he had at unneceffary times ftrong erections, which fhowed that he had naturally this power; that the erections where accompanied with defire, which are all the natural powers wanted; but that there was ftill a defect fomewhere, which I fuppofed to be from the mind. I inquired if all women were alike to him, his anfwer was no; fome women he could have connection with, as well as ever. This brought the defect, whatever it was, into a fmaller compafs; and it appeared that there was but one woman that produced this inability, and that it arofe from a defire to perform the act with

with this woman well; which desire produced in the mind a doubt, or fear of the want of success, which was the cause of the inability of performing the act. As this arose entirely from the state of the mind, produced by a particular circumstance, the mind was to be applied to for the cure; and I told him that he might be cured, if he could perfectly rely on his own power of self-denial. When I explained what I meant, he told me that he could depend upon every act of his will, or resolution; I then told him, if he had a perfect confidence in himself in that respect, that he was to go to bed to this woman, but first promise to himself, that he would not have any connection with her, for six nights, let his inclinations and powers be what they would; which he engaged to do; and also to let me know the result. About a fortnight after he told me that this resolution had produced such a total alteration in the state of his mind, that the power soon took place, for instead of going to bed with the fear of inability, he went with fears that he should be possessed with too much desire, too much power, so as to become uneasy to him, which really happened; for he would have been happy to have shortened the time; and when he had once broke the spell, the mind and powers went on together; his mind never returning to it's former state.

II. OF IMPOTENCE FROM A WANT OF PROPER CORRESPONDENCE BETWEEN THE ACTIONS OF THE DIFFERENT ORGANS.

I formerly observed when treating of the diseases of the urethra, and bladder, two parts concerned in the actions of each other, that every organ in an animal body, without exception, was made up of different parts, whose functions, or actions, where totally different from each other, although all tending to produce one ultimate effect. In all such organs when perfect, there is a succession of motions, one naturally arising out of the other, which in the end produces the ultimate effect; and an irregularity alone in these actions, will constitute disease, at least will produce very disagreeable effects, and often totally frustrate the final intention of the organ. I come now to apply

apply the above principle to the actions of the testicle and the penis; for we find that an irregularity in the actions of these parts sometimes happens in men, producing impotence, and something similar probably may be one cause of barrenness in women.

In men the parts subservient to generation may be divided into two, the essential, and the accessory. The testicles are the essential; the penis, &c. the accessory. As this division arises from their uses or actions in health, which exactly correspond with one another; a want of exactness in the correspondence, or susceptibility of those actions may also be divided into two. First; where the actions are reversed, the accessory taking place without the first or essential, as in erections of the penis, where neither the mind, nor the testicles, are stimulated to action; and the second, is where the testicle performs the action of secretion too readily for the penis, which has not a corresponding erection. The first is called priapism; and the second is what ought to be called seminal weakness.

The mind has considerable effect on the correspondence of the actions of these two parts; but it would appear in many instances, that erections of the penis depend more on the state of the mind, than what the secretion of the semen does; for many have the secretion, but not the erection; but in such, the want of erection appears to be owing to the mind only.

Priapism often arises spontaneously, and often from visible irritation of the penis, such as the venereal gonorrhœa, especially when violent. The sensation of such erections is rather uneasy than pleasant, nor is the sensation of the glans at the time similar to that arising from the erections of desire but more like to the sensation of the parts immediately after coition.

Such as arise spontaneously are of more serious consequence than those from inflammation, as they proceed probably from causes not curable in themselves, or by any known methods.

The priapism arising from inflammation of the parts, as in a gonorrhœa, is attended with nearly the same symptoms, but generally the sensation is that of pain, proceeding from the inflammation of the parts. It may be observed that what is said of priapism, is only applicable to it, when a disease in itself, and not as a symptom of other diseases, which it frequently is.

The common practice in the cure of this complaint is to order all the nervous and strengthening medicines, such as bark, valerian, musk, camphire, and also the cold bath. I have had experience of the good effects of the cold bath; but sometimes it does not agree with the constitution, in which cases I have found the warm bath of service. Opium appears to be a specific in many cases, from which circumstance I should be apt, upon the whole to try a soothing plan.

Seminal weakness, or a secretion and emission of the semen without erections, is the reverse of a priapism, and is by much the worst disease of the two. There is great variety in the degrees of this disease, there being all the gradations from the exact correspondence of the actions of all the parts to the testicles acting alone; in every case of the disease there is too quick a secretion and evacuation of the semen. Like to the priapism it does not arise from desires and abilities, although when mild it is attended with both, but not in a due proportion; a very slight desire often producing the full effect. The secretion of the semen shall be so quick that simple thought, or even toying shall make it flow.

Dreams shall produce this evacuation repeatedly in the same night; and even when the dreams have been so slight, if there have been any, that there has been no consciousness of them when the sleep has been broken by the act of emission. I have known cases where the testicles have been so ready to secrete, that the least friction on the glans has produced an emission: I have known the simple action of walking, or riding, produce this effect, and that repeatedly, in a very short space of time.

A young man, about four or five and twenty years of age, not so much given to venery as most young men, had these last-mentioned complaints upon him. Three or four times in the night he would emit; and if he walked fast, or rode on horseback, the same thing would happen. He could scarcely have connection with a woman, before he emitted, and in the emission, there was hardly any spasm. He tried every supposed strengthening medicine, as also the cold bath, and sea-bathing, but with no effect. By taking twenty drops of laudanum, on going to bed, he prevented the night emissions; and by taking the same quantity in the morning, he could walk or ride, without the before-mentioned inconvenience. I directed this practice

to

to be continued for ſome time, although the diſeaſe did not return, that the parts might be accuſtomed to this healthy ſtate of action; and I have reaſon to believe the gentleman is now well. It was found neceſſary as the conſtitution became more habituated to the opiate to increaſe the doſe of it.

The ſpaſms upon the evacuation of the ſemen in ſuch caſes are extremely ſlight, and a repetition of them ſoon takes place; the firſt emiſſion not preventing a ſecond, the conſtitution being all the time but little affected.* When the teſticles act alone, without the acceſſory parts taking up the neceſſary and natural conſequent action, it is ſtill a more melancholy diſeaſe; for the ſecretion ariſes from no viſible, or ſenſible cauſe, and does not give any viſible or ſenſible effect, but runs off ſimilar to involuntary ſtools, or urine. It has been obſerved that the ſemen is more fluid than natural in ſome of theſe caſes.

There is great variety in the diſeaſed actions of theſe parts, of which the following caſe may be conſidered as an example.

A gentleman has had a ſtricture in the urethra for many years, for which he has frequently uſed the bougie, but of late has neglected it. He has had no connection with women for a conſiderable time, being afraid of the conſequences. He has often in his ſleep involuntary emiſſions, which generally awake him at the paroxyſm; but what ſurpriſes him moſt is, that often he has ſuch, without any ſemen paſſing forwards through the penis, which makes him think that at thoſe times it goes backwards into the bladder. This is not always the caſe, for at other times the ſemen paſſes forwards. At the time he has thoſe uncommon paroxyſms, he has the erection, the dream, and is awaked with the ſame mode of action, the ſame ſenſation, and the ſame pleaſure, as when the ſemen paſſes through the urethra, whether dreaming or waking. My opinion is, that the ſame irritation takes place in the bulb of the urethra without the ſemen, that takes place there when the ſemen enters, in conſequence of all the natural preparatory ſteps, whereby the very ſame actions are excited as if it came into the paſſage; from which

* It is to be conſidered that the conſtitution is commonly affected by the ſpaſms only, and in proportion to their violence, independent of the ſecretion and evacuation of the ſemen.

In ſome caſes even the erection going off without the ſpaſms on the emiſſion, ſhall produce the ſame debility as if they had taken place.

one

one would ſuppoſe that either ſemen is not ſecreted, or if it be, that a retrograde motion takes place in the actions of the acceleratores muſcles; but if the firſt be the caſe, then we may ſuppoſe that in the natural ſtate the actions of thoſe muſcles do not ariſe ſimply from the ſtimulus of the ſemen in the part; but from their action being a termination of a preceding one making part of a ſeries of actions. Thus they may depend upon the friction, or the imagination of a friction on the penis, the teſticles not doing their part, and the ſpaſm in ſuch caſes ariſing from the friction and not from the ſecretion.

In many of thoſe caſes of irregularity, when the erection is not ſtrong, it ſhall go off without the emiſſion; and at other times an emiſſion ſhall happen almoſt without an erection; but theſe ariſe not from debility, but affections of the mind.

In many of the preceding caſes, waſhing the penis, ſcrotum, and perinæum, with cold water, is often of ſervice; and to render it colder than we find it in ſome ſeaſons of the year, common ſalt may be added to it, and the parts waſhed when the ſalt is almoſt diſſolved.

CHAPTER

CHAPTER XIII.

OF THE DECAY OF THE TESTICLE.

IT would appear from some circumstances, that the parts of generation are not to be considered as necessary parts of the animal machine, but only as parts superadded for particular purposes; and therefore only necessary when those particular purposes are to be answered; for we may observe, that they are later of coming to maturity than any other parts, and are more liable to decay. Thus far in their natural properties they are different from most other parts of our body, the teeth only excepted, which are similar in some of those circumstances.

The testicles appear to be more subject to spontaneous disease than any other part of the body; but what is the most singular thing of all, is the wasting of those bodies. One or both testicles shall wholly disappear, like to the thymus gland, or membrana pupillaris, &c. in the infant. This we do not find in any parts of the body which are essential to it's œconomy; excepting the parts are of no further use, and might become hurtful in the body, as the membrana pupillaris; but the testicles do not undergo this change as if in consequence of an original property stamped upon them, as is the case of the thymus gland, whenever the age of the person is such as to render them useless; but are liable to it at any age, and therefore the disposition is in the testicles themselves, independent of any connection with the animal œconomy. An arm, or leg, may lose it's action, and may waste in part, but never wholly.

Testicles have been known to waste in cases of rupture, probably from the constant pressure of the intestine. Mr. Pott has given us cases of this kind. I have seen in hydrocele the testicle almost wasted to nothing, probably from the compression of the water; but in all these the causes of wasting are obvious, and would probably produce similar effects in other parts of the body under the same circumstances; but a testicle without any previous diſeaſe waſtes wholly; or at other times it inflames, either ſpontaneouſly, or from ſympathy with the urethra, becomes large, and then begins to ſubſide, as in the reſolution of common inflammation of the body, but does not ſtop at the former ſize, but continues to decay till it wholly diſappears. The following caſes are inſtances of this.

Caſe I. A gentleman about nine years ago had a gonorrhœa, with a buboe, which ſuppurated. A ſwelling of one of the teſticles came on, for which he uſed the common methods of producing reſolution, and ſeemingly with ſucceſs. All the other ſymptoms being removed he thought himſelf quite well; but ſome time after, he found that the teſticle which had been ſwelled was become rather ſmaller than the other, which made him now pay attention to it; this decreaſe continued till it waſted entirely. For ſome years paſt there has been no appearance of a teſticle. He is not in the leaſt different in inclination, or powers, from what he was before.

Caſe II, communicated by Mr. Nanſan. "A gentleman, aged about eighteen, who never had any venereal complaint, has had two different attacks of the ſame nature, one in each teſticle. February 3, 1776, after ſkating a few hours, without having to his knowledge received any injury from it, he was ſeized with a violent pain and inflammation of the left teſticle, which in a few days increaſed much in ſize. A ſurgeon being ſent for, followed the uſual treatment in ſuch caſes of inflammation. In about ſix weeks the inflammation and ſwelling gradually ſubſided, ſome hardneſs only remaining. A mercurial plaiſter was now applied, which after being worn for ſome time was left off. The teſticle ever ſince has continued gradually to decreaſe, and is no larger than a horſe bean; indeed the body of the teſticle is quite decayed, nothing remaining but what ſeems part of the epididymis. It appears to have no ſenſe of pain, except when preſſed, and is very hard and uneven on it's ſurface. The ſpermatic chord is not in the leaſt affected.

October 20, 1777, he was ſeized in the ſame manner in the right teſticle, without any apparent cauſe, whereupon I was applied to. He was immediately bled, took an opening mixture, after that a ſaline mixture with tartar emetic; and a fomentation and embrocation of ſpiritus mindereri, and ſpiritus vini, was uſed. On the 27th a cataplaſm was applied of lin-ſeed

meal

meal and aqua vegeto-mineralis. This treatment was perfifted in till about the middle of November. The inflammation went off, and the tefticle feemed much in the natural ftate. On December 19, I was applied to again; it feemed to be growing hard, and decreafing in fize, much in the fame manner as the other had done, which made him very unhappy. I ordered him fome pills with calomel and tartar emetic, in hopes of increafing the fecretion of the glands in general, and making fome change in the tefticle. At firft this method feemed to be of fervice, but foon loft it's effects, and the tefticle began to decreafe juft as the other did." Mr. Adair and Mr. Pott were confulted with me, but nothing could be thought of that could give any hopes of fuccefs. I advifed him to try electricity, and to employ the parts in their natural ufes, as much as inclination led him, with a view of putting a ftop to the unnatural actions; but all was to no purpofe, the tefticle continued to decreafe till not a veftige was left.

Cafe III, communicated by Dr. Cothorn of Worcefter.

"A young man, aged fixteen, was fuddenly feized with great coldnefs and fhivering, attended with frequent rigors. During this paroxyfm which continued three hours, his pulfe was fmall and contracted, and fo exceedingly quick that the ftrokes of the artery were with difficulty counted. This period was fucceeded by an intenfe heat, and a ftrong, hard, full pulfe, on which account he was copioufly bled; a dofe of cooling phyfic was immediately adminiftered, and a clyfter thrown up to promote it's more fpeedy effects. In the evening the bleeding was repeated. All this day he complained of excruciating pain in his loins, and the fide of his belly defcending down into the fcrotum. On examining the part affected, I faw an appearance of inflammation in the groin of the left fide, and a great tenfion about the ring of the abdominal mufcles, with an enlargement of the tefticles. Thefe parts were now ordered to be fomented with a difcutient fotus ftrongly impregnated with crude fal ammoniac, and to be bathed with fpiritus mindereri, and fpiritus volat. aromat. before the application of each ftupe; and he was directed to take fix grains of the pulv. antimonialis, with fifteen grains of nitre every three hours; his food to be thin gruel, with fruit and lemon juice, and his drink barley-water with fugar and nitre. Notwithftanding this antiphlogiftic plan of frequent cooling phyfic, anodynes, three emetics,

emetics, and thirteen blood lettings, the fever continued, and the pain, inflammation and tumor increaſed till the eighth day, including the firſt day of ſeizure; when ſeeing no hope of diſcuſſing the tumor, the teſticle being nearly as large as a child's head, I attempted by emollient fotuſes, and maturating cataplaſms, to bring it to ſuppuration. On the 10th, a fluctuation was perceptible; and on the 12th, much more ſo, the ſcrotum having then put on a livid appearance. I uſed every poſſible argument for permiſſion to open it, but he being now quite eaſy would not admit it. On the 15th, the patient was again attacked with rigors, coldneſs and ſhivering, ſucceeded by a great feveriſh heat, which ſoon terminated in a profuſe ſweat, yet no pain attended this paroxyſm. In the evening however the tumor was ſo prominent that I was of opinion it would open ſpontaneouſly before morning, when I hoped to obtain his conſent to enlarge the aperture; but this not happening, and all remonſtrance and intreaties relating to the neceſſity of an inciſion proving ineffectual, I contented myſelf with giving the bark with elixir of vitriol. From this time, after every fever paroxyſm, the teſticle was obſerved to decreaſe; not being permitted to make an inciſion, and his ſtrength and appetite continuing good, I began to entertain hopes of ſucceſs without it, and adviſed him to perſiſt in the uſe of the tonic and antiſeptic plan, with the addition of ſtupes wet with the decoction of bark, to be conſtantly applied; by which means at the end of thirty days from the firſt ſeizure the pus was totally abſorbed. The teſticle then appeared to be of the ſize of a hen's egg, and was as hard as a ſchirrus. I directed it to be rubbed night and morning, with equal parts of the unguent. mercur. fort. and liniment. volat. camphorat. and ordered internally ſome mercurial alteratives, with a decoction of bark. By theſe aids his night ſweats, and every other diſagreeable ſymptom, gradually abated; he gathered ſtrength, fleſh and ſpirits, very faſt, and the diſeaſed teſticle went on conſtantly decreaſing, though very ſlowly, for near twelve months; at the expiration of which time there was no other appearance of it than a confuſion of looſe fibres, obvious to the feeling, in the upper part of the ſcrotum. About a month ago the patient conſented to my examining it. Of the teſticle there was not the leaſt veſtige, neither could I perceive the tunica vaginalis on that ſide in the groin; but upon the

the os pubis, and a little under it, I could embrace with my fingers and thumb the chord, and diſtinguiſh the veſſels, which were without the leaſt degree of hardneſs or ſchirroſity; and if I preſſed one in particular, I gave him exquiſite pain for a moment. He is in perfect health, a ſtrong, robuſt conſtitution, and has fine healthy children; the only change he perceived in the conſtitution was a propenſity to grow fat, which neither temperance, nor violent exerciſe on horſeback, daily, with little reſt, will prevent.

PART IV.

CHAPTER I.

OF CHANCRE.

I Have been hitherto speaking of the effects of this poison, when applied to a secreting surface and without a cuticle, of the intention of nature in producing these effects, and of all the consequences, both real and supposed: I now mean to explain it's effects when applied to a surface that is covered with a common cuticle, as the common skin of the body, which on such a surface will be found to be very different from those I have been describing. But I may be allowed here to remark, that the penis, the common seat of a chancre, is like every part of the body liable to diseases of the ulcerative kind; and from some circumstances, rather more so than other parts; for if attention is not paid to cleanliness, we have often excoriations, or superficial ulcers, from that cause; also, like almost every other part that has been injured; these parts when once they have suffered from the venereal disease are very liable to ulcerate anew. Since then this part is not exempted from the common diseases of the body, and as every disease in this part is suspected to be venereal, great attention is to be paid in forming our judgment of ulcers there.

Venereal ulcers commonly have one character, which however is not entirely peculiar to them, for many sores that have no disposition to heal, which is the case with a chancre, have so far the same character. A chancre has commonly a thickened base, and although in some the common inflammation spreads much further, yet the specific is confined to this base. The future, or consequent ulcers, are commonly easily distinguished from the original, or venereal, which will be described hereafter.

It

It is an invariable effect, that when any part of an animal is irritated to a certain degree, that it inflames and forms matter, the intention of which is to remove the irritating cause. This process is easily effected when it is on a surface whose nature is to secrete; but when on a surface whose nature is not to secrete, it then becomes more difficult, for another process must be set up, which is ulceration. This is not only the case in common irritations, but also in specific irritations from morbid poisons, as the venereal disease and smallpox. The variolous matter, as well as the venereal, produces ulcers on the skin; but when it affects secreting surfaces a diseased secretion is the consequence; and this is different in different parts; on the tongue, inside of the mouth, uvula and tonsils, the coagulable lymph is thrown out in form of sloughs, somewhat similar to the putrid sore throat; but in the fauces and all down the œsophagus, a thickish fluid in appearance like matter is secreted. When the irritation is applied to a surface whose cuticle is thin, and where there is a secretion naturally, as the glans penis, or inside of the prepuce, there it sometimes only irritates, so as to produce a diseased secretion, as was described; but this is not always the effect of such irritation on such surfaces, they are often irritated to ulceration, producing a chancre.

The poison has in general either no disposition or not sufficient powers to blister or excoriate the common skin, for if it did the symptoms most probably would be at first nearly the same if not exactly so with a gonorrhœa; that is a discharge of matter from a surface without a cuticle newly inflamed; for it is reasonable to suppose, that the poison would produce on that excoriated surface a secretion of matter, which would be at first a gonorrhœa, and which very probably would afterwards fall into the second mode of action or ulceration, and then become a chancre.

There are three ways in which chancres are produced. First, by the poison being inserted into a wound. Secondly, by being applied to a non-secreting surface; and thirdly, by being applied to a common sore. To whichever of these three different surfaces it is applied, the pus produces it's specific inflammation and ulceration, attended with a secretion of pus. The matter produced in consequence of those different modes of application is of the same nature with the matter applied, because the irritations are the same in both.

The

The poiſon much more readily contaminates if it is applied to a freſh wound, than to an ulcer, in this reſembling the inoculation of the ſmallpox. Whether there are any parts of the ſkin, or any other part of the body, more ſuſceptible of this irritation than others in conſequence of local application is not yet aſcertained.

This form of the diſeaſe, like the firſt, or gonorrhœa, is generally caught on the parts of generation, in conſequence of a connection between the ſexes; but any part of the body may be affected by the application of venereal matter, eſpecially if the cuticle is thin.

I have ſeen a chancre on the prolabium, as broad as a ſixpence, caught the perſon did not know how.* The penis, and particularly the prepuce, being the parts moſt commonly affected by this form of the diſeaſe, are ſo conſtructed as to ſuffer much from it, eſpecially when they are very ſuſceptible of ſuch irritation; for the conſtruction alone produces many inconveniences, beſides conſiderable pain, while under the diſeaſe, and in general retards the cure.

The chancre is not ſo frequent an effect of the poiſon as the gonorrhœa; and I think very good reaſons may be aſſigned for it, although there are more modes than one of catching it, as I juſt now mentioned; but the parts in two of them, to wit, the wound, and the ſore, are ſeldom in the way of being infected; therefore when it is caught it is commonly by the ſame mode of application with that of the gonorrhœa; but as the cuticle cannot be affected by this poiſon, this covering acting as a guard to the cutis, it is often prevented from coming in contact with it; and indeed it is almoſt ſurpriſing that the cutis ſhould ever be affected by it, where it has ſuch a covering, excepting about the glans, the inſide of the prepuce, or other parts of the body, where this covering is thin. The proportion the caſes of gonorrhœa bear to thoſe of chancre is as four or five to one.

When it is caught in men, it is generally upon the frænum, glans penis, prepuce, or upon the common ſkin of the body of the penis; and ſometimes on the fore part of the ſcrotum; but I think moſt frequently on the frænum,

* That this ſore was a chancre I made no doubt, for beſides it's diſeaſed appearance, he had a bubo forming in one of the glands under the lower jaw, on the ſame ſide.

It is moſt probable that he caught it by his own fingers being the conveyers.

and in the angle between the penis, and glans. It's affecting these parts arises from the manner in which it is caught, and not from any specific tendency these parts have to catch it more than others; and it's affecting the frænum, &c. more frequently than the other parts of the penis arises from the external form of this part, which is irregular, and allows the venereal matter to lie undisturbed in the chinks; by which means it has time to irritate, and inflame the parts, and to produce the suppurative, and ulcerative inflammation in them. But as this matter is easily rubbed off from prominent parts, by every thing that touches them, it is a reason why such parts in general so often escape this disease.

The distance of time between it's application, and it's effects, upon the part is uncertain; but upon the whole it is rather longer of appearing than the gonorrhœa; however this depends in some measure on the nature of the parts affected. If it be the frænum, or the termination of the prepuce into the glans that is affected, the disease will in general appear earlier; these parts being more easily affected than either the glans, common skin of the penis, or scrotum; for in some cases where both the glans and prepuce were contaminated from the same contamination, it has appeared earlier on the prepuce.

I have known cases where the chancres have appeared twenty-four hours after the application of the matter, and I have known them seven weeks. A remarkable case of this kind was in a gentleman who had not touched a woman for seven weeks, when a chancre appeared, which was very probably the reason of the poison contaminating at all, for it is probable, the having connection with another woman might have proved a prevention, by freeing the parts from the venereal matter. That this was a venereal chancre was proved, by his having had the lues venerea from it, and being under a necessity of taking mercury. An officer in the army had a chancre broke out upon him two months after he had had any connection with a woman. After the last connection he marched above an hundred miles, the chancre broke out, and only gave way to mercury.

This, like most other inflammations which terminate in ulcers, begins first with an itching in the part; if it is the glans that is inflamed, generally a small pimple appears full of matter, without much hardness, or seeming

inflammation,

inflammation, and with very little tumefaction, the glans not being so readily tumefied from inflammation as many parts are, especially the prepuce; nor are the chancres attended with so much pain or inconvenience, as those on the prepuce; but if upon the frænum, and more especially the prepuce, an inflammation more considerable than the former soon follows, or at least the effects of the inflammation are more extensive and visible. Those parts being composed of very loose cellular membrane, afford a ready passage for the extravasated juices; continued sympathy also more readily takes place in them. The itching is gradually changed to pain; the surface of the prepuce is in some cases excoriated, and afterwards ulcerates: in others a small pimple, or abscess appears, as on the glans, which forms an ulcer. A thickening of the part comes on, which at first, and while of the true venereal kind, is very circumscribed, not diffusing itself gradually and imperceptibly into the surrounding parts, but terminating rather abruptly. It's base is hard, and the edges a little prominent. When it begins on the frænum, or near it, that part is very commonly wholly destroyed, or a hole is often ulcerated through it, which proves rather inconvenient in the cure, and in general it had better in such cases, be divided at first.

If the venereal poison should be applied to the skin, where the cuticle is more dense than that of the glans penis, or frænum, such as that upon the body of the penis, or forepart of the scrotum; parts which are very much exposed to the application of this matter, then it generally appears first in a pimple, which is commonly allowed to scab, owing to it's being exposed to evaporation. This scab is generally rubbed off, or pushed off, and one larger than the first forms. I think there is less inflammation attending these last than those on the frænum and prepuce, but more than those upon the glans.

When the disease is allowed to go on, so as to partake of the inflammation peculiar to the habit, it becomes in many instances more diffused, and is often carried so far, as to produce disagreeable symptoms, as phymosis, and sometimes paraphymosis; greatly retarding the cure; but still there is a hardness peculiar to this poison, surrounding the sores, especially those upon the prepuce.

When these ulcers are forming, and after they are formed, or in the state of inflammation, it is no uncommon thing for the urethra to sympathise with

with them, and give a tickling pain, eſpecially in making water; but whether there is ever a diſcharge in the urethra from ſuch a cauſe I will not determine; but if a diſcharge never takes place but when the diſeaſe really attacks the urethra, it would make us ſuppoſe that this ſympathy is not really inflammatory; or if it is carried ſo far as to produce inflammation, yet that it is not of the ſpecific kind. However it is poſſible in thoſe caſes where there is a gonorrhœa preceded by a chancre, that this gonorrhœa may ariſe from ſympathy, and is not a diſeaſe proceeding from the original contamination, nor from the matter of the chancre. That the ſenſation in the urethra, in thoſe inſtances where there is no diſcharge, is from ſympathy, and not from the urethra being attacked with the diſeaſe at the time that the matter laid the ground-work for the chancre, is evident from the following obſervation. I have ſeen it happen more than once, when the ſeat of the chancre had broke out a ſecond time, and where no new or freſh infection had been caught, that the patient complained of the ſame tickling and ſlight pain in the urethra before any diſcharge had taken place in the beginning ulcerations. From the ſame connection of parts I have ſeen a chancre coming upon the glans abſolutely cure both a gleet and an irritation all along the paſſage of the urethra. So great was the previous irritation in this caſe, that I ſuſpected a ſtricture; but on paſſing a bougie found none.

In conſequence of the urethra ſympathiſing with the chancre, the teſticles and ſcrotum will further ſympathiſe with the urethra, and become affected. I have ſeen this ſympathy extend over the whole pubes, and ſo ſtrong that touching the hairs gently on the pubes has given diſagreeable ſenſations, and even pain.

In ſpeaking of the local, or immediate effects of the venereal diſeaſe, I mentioned that they were ſeldom wholly ſpecific, and that they partook both of the ſpecific and the conſtitutional inflammation; and therefore it is always very neceſſary to pay ſome attention to the manner in which chancres firſt appear, and alſo to their progreſs; for they often explain the nature of the conſtitution at the time. If the inflammation ſpreads faſt, and conſiderably, it ſhows a conſtitution more diſpoſed to inflammation than natural. If the pain is great it ſhows a ſtrong diſpoſition for irritation. It alſo ſometimes happens

happens that they begin very early to form floughs; when this is the cafe they have a ftrong tendency to mortification.

Thefe additional fymptoms mark the conftitution and direct the future mode of treatment.

Where there is a confiderable lofs of fubftance, either from floughing or ulceration, a profufe bleeding is no uncommon circumftance, more efpecially if the ulcer is on the glans; for it would appear that the adhefive inflammation does not fufficiently take place there to unite the veins of the glans fo as to prevent their cavity from being expofed, and the blood is allowed to efcape from what is called the corpus fpongiofum urethræ. The ulcers, or floughs, often go as deep as the corpus cavernofum penis, where the fame thing happens.

I. OF THE PHYMOSIS AND PARAPHYMOSIS.

These difeafes arife from a thickening of the cellular membrane of the prepuce, in confequence of an irritation capable of producing confiderable and diffufed inflammation, which when it does happen is generally in confequence of a chancre in this part. This irritation however, and inflammation fometimes attacks the prepuce, even when the difeafe is in the form of what I fufpect to be a gonorrhœa of the glands and prepuce,* fometimes even in the common gonorrhœa, but moft frequently of all from a chancre in the prepuce. When this difeafe or tumefaction takes place in confequence of a chancre, I fufpect that there is an irritable difpofition in the habit; for it is plain there is more than the fpecific action, the inflammation extending beyond the fpecific diftance.

It may be obferved here, that the prepuce is no more than a doubling of the fkin of the penis when not erected, for then it becomes too large for the penis, by which provifion the glans is covered and preferved when not neceffary to be ufed, whereby it's feelings are probably more acute. When the penis becomes erect it in general fills the whole fkin, by which the

* See page 41, where this gonorrhœa is mentioned.

doubling forming the prepuce in the non-erect ſtate is unfolded, and is employed in covering the body of the penis.

The diſeaſes called phymoſis and paraphymoſis, being a thickening of the cellular membrane of this part, they will commonly be in proportion to the inflammation and diſtenſibility of the cellular membrane of the part. The inflammation often runs high, and is frequently of the eriſypelatous kind; beſides, in ſuch parts where the cellular membrane is ſo very looſe, the tumefaction is conſiderable, the end of the prepuce being a depending part the ſerum is accumulated in it, which in many inflammations is allowed to paſs from the inflamed to ſome more depending part, as in an inflammation of the leg or thigh, where the foot commonly ſwells or becomes œdematous in conſequence of the deſcent of the ſerum extravaſated above.

A natural contraction of the aperture of the prepuce is very common, and ſo ſtrong in ſome, that thoſe under ſuch conſtruction of parts have a natural and conſtant phymoſis. Such a ſtate of parts is often attended with chancres, producing very great inconveniences in the time of the cure, and in thoſe caſes of conſiderable diffuſed inflammation, a diſeaſed phymoſis ſimilar to the other is unavoidably the caſe; and whether diſeaſed or natural it may produce the paraphymoſis ſimply by the prepuce being brought back upon the penis; for this tight part acting as a ligature round the body of the penis, behind the glans, retards the circulation beyond the ligature, producing an œdematous inflammation on the inverted part of the prepuce. When the paraphymoſis takes place in conſequence of a natural tightneſs only, although attended with chancres, yet it has nothing to do with the conſtitution, this being only accidental; however, in either caſe, a paraphymoſis is to be conſidered as in ſome degree a local violence.

This natural phymoſis is ſo conſiderable in ſome children as not to allow the urine to paſs with eaſe, but in general becomes larger and larger, as boys grow up, by frequent endeavouring to bring it over the glans, which effect often prevents the bad conſequences that would otherways enſue in it when affected with diſeaſe.

This part of the prepuce, although in moſt men it is looſe enough to produce no inconvenience in a natural ſtate, yet it ſometimes contracts without any viſible cauſe whatever, and becomes ſo narrow as to hinder the water

water from getting out, even after it has got free of the urethra, so that the whole cavity of the prepuce shall be filled with the urine, giving great pain. The cases that I have seen of this kind have been principally in old men.

When the prepuce is in it's natural position it then covers entirely the glans, and is commonly a little loose before it; but when it begins to swell and thicken, more and more of the skin of the penis is drawn forwards over the glans, and the glans at the same time is pushed backwards by the swelling against it's end. I have seen the prepuce projecting from such a cause more than three inches beyond the glans, and it's aperture much diminished.

It often becomes in some degree inverted by the inner skin yielding more than the outer, having a kind of neck where the outer skin naturally terminates. From the tightness and distension of the parts in a state of tumefaction it becomes impossible to bring it back over the penis, so as to invert it, and expose the sores on the inside.

Such a state of the prepuce is very often productive of bad consequences, especially when the chancres are behind the glans, for the glans being between the orifice of the prepuce and the sores, it there fills up the whole cavity of the prepuce, between the chancres and opening, and often so tightly that the matter from the sores behind cannot get a passage forwards between the glans and prepuce, by which means there is an accumulation of matter behind the corona glandis, forming an abscess which produces ulceration upon the inside of the prepuce; this abscess opens externally, and the glans often protruding through the opening throws the whole prepuce to the opposite side, the penis appearing to have two terminations.

On the other hand, if the prepuce is loose, wide, and is either accustomed to be kept back in it's sound state, or is pulled back to dress the chancres, and is allowed to remain in this situation till the above tumefaction takes place, then it is called a paraphymosis; or if the prepuce is pulled forcibly back after it is swelled, it is then brought from the state of a phymosis, as beforedescribed, to that of a paraphymosis.

This lastdescribed situation of the prepuce is often much more troublesome, and often attended with worse symptoms than the former, especially if it should have been changed from a phymosis to a paraphymosis. The reason

reaſon of which is, that the aperture of the prepuce is naturally leſs elaſtic than either the internal inverted part, or the external ſkin; therefore when the prepuce is pulled back upon the body of the penis that part graſps it tighter than any other part of the ſkin of the penis, and more ſo in proportion to the inflammation; the conſequence of which is, the ſwelling of the prepuce is divided into two, one ſwelling cloſe to the glans, the other behind the ſtricture or neck. This ſtricture is often ſo great as to interrupt the free circulation of the blood beyond it, which alſo aſſiſts in increaſing the ſwelling, adds to the ſtricture, and often produces a mortification of the prepuce itſelf, by which means the whole diſeaſed part, together with the ſtricture, is ſometimes removed, forming what may be called a natural cure.*

In many caſes the inflammation not only affects the ſkin of the penis, in which is included the prepuce, but it attacks the body of the penis itſelf, often producing adheſions, and even mortification in the cells of the corpus cavernoſum, either of which will deſtroy the diſtenſibility of that part ever after, giving the penis a curve to that ſide in it's erections. This ſometimes takes place through the whole cellular ſubſtance of the penis, producing a ſhort and almoſt inflexible ſtump.

The adheſions of thoſe cells are not confined to the venereal inflammation as a cauſe; we ſometimes ſee them taking place without any viſible cauſe whatever, and often in conſequence of other diſeaſes.

A gentleman, ſixty years of age, who has been lame with the gout theſe twenty years paſt, but has for theſe eighteen months had the penis contracted on the left and upper ſide, ſo as to bend that way, very conſiderably in erections, which erections are more frequent than common.

Quere: Is the gout the cauſe of this, by producing adheſions of the cells of one corpus cavernoſum, ſo as not to yield to, or allow of the influx of blood on that ſide? And is the irritation of the gout the cauſe, of the frequency of the erections?

* A young man came into St. George's Hoſpital, with a paraphymoſis in conſequence of chancres on the inſide of the prepuce. All the parts before the ſtricture formed by the prepuce mortified and dropped off. I ordered nothing to be done but to dreſs it with common dreſſings, and it healed very readily, and he left the Hoſpital cured of the local complaint. Whether or not abſorption had taken place, previous to the mortification, I do not know, as I never heard more of him.

CHAPTER

CHAPTER II.

OF CHANCRE IN WOMEN.

WOMEN are ſubject to chancres, but from the ſimplicity of the parts the complaint is often leſs complicated than in men. For in this ſex we have only the diſeaſe and conſtitutional affection, no inconvenience ariſing from the formation of the parts.

When the matter is introduced into the vagina or urethra, it there irritates a ſecreting ſurface, as has been deſcribed when treating of the diſeaſe in general, and of women in particular; but when it is lodged in the inſide of the ſkin of the labia, nymphæ, &c. ſimilar to the glans penis, they are often only affected with gonorrhœa; but like the parts in men they are alſo capable of ulceration; theſe ulcerations are generally more numerous in women, becauſe the ſurface upon which they can form is much larger. We find them on the edge of the labia, ſometimes on the outſide, and even on the perinæum.

Theſe ulcers that are formed on the inſide of the labia, nymphæ, &c. are never allowed to dry or ſcab; but thoſe on the outſide of the labiæ, &c. are ſubject to have the matter dry upon them, which forms a ſcab, ſimilar to thoſe on the body of the penis or ſcrotum.

The venereal matter from ſuch ſores is very apt to run down the perinæum to the anus, as in a gonorrhœa, and excoriate the parts, eſpecially about the anus where the ſkin is thin, often producing chancres in thoſe parts.

Chancres have been obſerved in the vagina, which I ſuſpect not to have been original ones, but to have ariſen from the ſpreading of the ulcers on the inſide of the labia.

This form of the diſeaſe like the gonorrhœa, both in women and in men is entirely local, the conſtitution having no connection with it but ſympathetically, and I believe much more ſeldom in this than in the former.

CHAPTER III.

GENERAL OBSERVATIONS ON THE TREATMENT OF CHANCRES.

THE inflammation from the venereal poiſon when it produces ulceration generally if not always continues till cured by art, which I obſerved was not the caſe with the gonorrhœa. It will perhaps not be an eaſy taſk to account for this material difference in the two kinds of diſeaſe; but I am inclined to think that as the inflammation in the chancre ſpreads, it is always attacking new ground, which is a ſucceſſion of irritations, and is the cauſe that it does not cure itſelf.

Chancres, as well as the gonorrhœa, are perhaps ſeldom or never wholly venereal; but are varied by certain peculiarities of the conſtitution at the time. The treatment therefore of them, both local and conſtitutional, will admit of great variety; and it is upon the knowledge of this variety, that the ſkill of the ſurgeon principally depends. On this account the concomitant ſymptoms are what require particular attention. Mercury is the cure of the venereal ſymptoms abſtractedly conſidered; but there is no one ſpecific for the others, the treatment of which muſt vary according to the conſtitution. From hence we muſt ſee that no one kind of medicine joined with mercury will be likely to ſucceed in all caſes, although the different pretended ſecrets are of this kind. Some caſes not requiring any thing except mercury, others requiring a ſomething beſides, according to their nature, which in many caſes it will not be an eaſy matter to find out, from the appearances of the chancre itſelf, but which muſt be diſcovered by repeated trials.

Probably from the beforementioned circumſtances it is, that a chancre is in common longer in healing than moſt of the local effects from the conſtitutional diſeaſe, or lues venerea; at leaſt longer than thoſe in the firſt order of of parts; and this is found to be the case notwithstanding that the cure of a chancre may be attempted both constitutionally, and locally, while the lues venerea can in common only be cured constitutionally. It is commonly some time before a chancre appears to be affected by the medicine. The circulation shall be loaded with mercury for three, four, or more weeks before a chancre shall begin to separate it's discharge from it's surface, so as to look red, and show the living surface; but when once it does change, it's progress towards healing is more rapid. A lues venerea shall in many cases be perfectly cured before chancres have made the least change.

Upon the same principle some attention should be paid to internal medicines; and it should be considered, whether weakening, strengthening, or quieting medicines should be given; for sometimes one kind, sometimes another, will be proper.

Chancres admit of two modes of treatment; the object of one, is to destroy, or remove them by means of escharotics, or by extirpation; that of the other, is to overcome the venereal irritation by means of the specific remedy for that poison.

I have endeavoured to show that chancres are local complaints; this opinion is further confirmed by their being destroyed or cured by merely a local treatment. But in chancres, as well as in a gonorrhœa, it has been disputed whether mercury should ever be applied locally to them or not; some having objected to it, while others have practised it, and probably the dispute is not yet generally settled.

Upon the general idea I have endeavoured to give of the venereal disease, it can be no difficult task to determine this question.

It is to be observed that in the cure of chancres we have two points in view, the cure of the chancre itself, and the prevention of a contamination of the constitution.

The first, or the cure of the chancre, is to be effected by mercury applied either in external dressings, or internally through the circulation, or in both ways. The second object, or preservation of the constitution from contamination is to be obtained, first by shortening the duration of the chancre, which shortens the time of absorption, and also by internal medicine, which must be in proportion to the time that the absorption may have been going on.

If the power of a chancre to contaminate the conſtitution, or which is the ſame thing, if the quantity abſorbed is as the ſize of the chancre, and the time of abſorption, which moſt probably it is, then whatever ſhortens the time muſt diminiſh that power, or quantity abſorbed; and if the quantity of mercury neceſſary to preſerve the conſtitution is as the quantity of poiſon abſorbed, then whatever leſſens the quantity abſorbed muſt proportionally preſerve the conſtitution. For inſtance, if the power of a chancre to contaminate the conſtitution in four weeks is equal to four, and the quantity of mercury neceſſary to be given internally, both for the cure of the chancre and the preſervation of the conſtitution, is alſo equal to four, then whatever ſhortens the duration of the chancre muſt leſſen in the ſame proportion the quantity of the mercury; therefore if local applications along with the internal uſe of mercury will cure the chancre in three weeks, then only three-fourths of the mercury is neceſſarily wanted internally. Local applications therefore, ſo far as they tend to ſhorten the duration of a chancre, ſhorten the duration of abſorption, which alſo ſhortens the neceſſity of the continuance of an internal courſe of mercury, all in the ſame proportion. For example, if four ounces of mercurial ointment will cure a chancre and preſerve the conſtitution in four weeks, three ounces will be ſufficient to preſerve the conſtitution if the cure of the chancre can be by any other means forwarded ſo as to be effected in three weeks. This is not ſpeculation, but the reſult of experience, and the deſtruction of chancres confirms it.

I. OF THE DESTRUCTION OF A CHANCRE.

The ſimpleſt method of treating a chancre is by deſtroying or extirpating it, whereby it is reduced to the ſtate of a common ſore or wound, and heals up as ſuch. This only can be done on the firſt appearance of the chancre, when the ſurrounding parts are not as yet contaminated; becauſe it is abſolutely neceſſary that the whole diſeaſed part ſhould be removed, which is done with difficulty when it has ſpread conſiderably. It may be done either by inciſion or by cauſtic. If the chancre appears upon the glans, touching it with the lunar cauſtic is preferable to inciſion, becauſe the

hæmorrhage

hæmorrhage by ſuch a mode would be conſiderable, from the cells of the glans.

The common ſenſation of the glans is not very acute, therefore the cauſtic will give but little pain. The cauſtic to be uſed ſhould be pointed at the end like a pencil, that it may only touch thoſe parts that are really diſeaſed; this treatment ſhould be continued till the ſurface of the ſore looks red and healthy after having thrown off the laſt ſloughs; after it has arrived at this ſtate it will be found to heal like any other ſore produced from a cauſtic.

If the ſore is upon the prepuce, or upon the common ſkin of the penis, and in it's incipient ſtate, the ſame practice may be followed with ſucceſs; but if it has ſpread conſiderably it is then out of the power of the cauſtic, when only applied in this ſlow manner, to go ſo deep as to keep pace with the increaſing ſore; but it is very probable that the lapis ſepticus may anſwer very well in ſuch caſes. When this cannot be conveniently uſed, inciſion will anſwer the purpoſe effectually.

I have diſſected a chancre out, and the ſore has healed up without any other treatment but common dreſſings.

However, as our knowledge of the extent of the diſeaſe is not always certain; and as this uncertainty increaſes as the ſize of the chancre, it becomes neceſſary in ſome degree to aſſiſt the cure by proper dreſſings, and therefore it may be prudent to dreſs the ſore with mercurial ointment.

From ſuch treatment there is but little danger of the conſtitution being infected, eſpecially if the chancre has been deſtroyed almoſt immediately upon it's appearance, as we may then reaſonably ſuppoſe there has not been time for abſorption.

But as it muſt be in moſt caſes uncertain whether there has been abſorption or not, this practice is not always to be truſted to; and from that circumſtance perhaps never ſhould; and therefore even in thoſe caſes where the chancre has been removed almoſt immediately, it would be prudent to give ſome mercury internally; the quantity ſhould be proportioned to the time and progreſs of the ſore; but if it has ſpread to a conſiderable ſize before extirpation, then mercury is abſolutely neceſſary, and perhaps not a great deal is gained by the extirpation.

II. OF THE CURE OF CHANCRES—LOCAL APPLICATIONS.

The cure of a chancre is a different thing from it's destruction, and consists in destroying it's venereal disposition and action, and then the parts heal of course as far as they are venereal.

Chancres may be cured in two different ways, either by external applications or internal applications through the circulation. The same medicine is necessary for both these purposes, that is mercury.

I have shown that a gonorrhœa and a chancre have so far the same disposition as to form the same kind of matter; yet I have also observed that mercury has no more power in curing the gonorrhœa than any other medicine; and therefore it might be supposed that mercury would have no effect in the present complaint; but we find that in a chancre it is a specific, and will cure every one that is truly venereal; but as other dispositions take place so other assistance is often necessary, as will be taken notice of in the history of the cure.

The action of this medicine must be the same in whatever way it is given, for it's action must be upon the vessels of the part, in one way acting only externally, in the other internally.*

For external local applications, mercurial ointments are the common dressings; but if the mercury were joined with watry substances instead of oily, by mixing with the matter the application would be continued longer to the sore, and would prove more effectual. This is an advantage that poultices have over common dressings. I have often used mercury rubbed down with some conserve in the room of an ointment, and it has answered

* This is well illustrated by the application of some medicines locally to parts whose actions are immediate and visible; and by throwing the same medicine into the constitution the same immediate and visible effect is produced; for instance, if ten grains of Ipecacuanha is thrown into the stomach of a dog, it will in a short time make it vomit, from it's local applications to that viscus; and if a solution of five grains is thrown into a vein, it will produce vomiting before we can conceive it to have got to the vessels of the stomach. The same effects are produced from an infusion of jalap thrown into the veins that are commonly produced when taken into the stomach and bowels.

extremely

extremely well. Calomel ufed in the fame way, and alfo the other preparations of mercury mixed with mucilage or with honey anfwers the fame purpofe. Such dreffings will effect a cure in cafes that are truly venereal; but perhaps we feldom have a conftitution fo free from any tendency to fome difeafe as to be capable of taking on the venereal action fimply by itfelf.

Some will take on an indolent difpofition, to counteract which the actions fhould be increafed by joining with the mercury fome warm balfam in a fmall proportion, or as much red precipitate as will only ftimulate without acting as an efcharotic; and fometimes both may be neceffary.

Calomel mixed with fome falve, or any other fubftance which will fufpend it, is more active than common mercurial ointment, and in fuch cafes as require ftimulating applications it will anfwer better.

Many other applications are recommended, fuch as folutions of blue vitriol, verdigreafe, calomel, with the fpiritus nitri dulcis, and many others.

But as all of thefe are only of fervice in remedying any peculiar difpofition of the parts, having no fpecific power on the true venereal action; and as fuch difpofitions are innumerable, it becomes almoft impoffible to fay what will cure every difpofition; fome will anfwer in one ftate of the fores, fome in another. It may be found oftentimes that the parts affected are extremely irritable; in fuch cafes it will be neceffary to mix the mercury with opium, or perhaps preparations of lead, as white or red lead, to diminifh the action of the parts.

The oftner the dreffings are fhifted the better, as the matter from the fore feparates the application from the difeafed parts, by which means the effects are loft or diminifhed. Three times every day in many cafes is not oftner than neceffary, efpecially if the dreffings are of the unctuous kind, for they do not mix like watry dreffings with the matter, fo as to impart fome of their virtues to it, which would in a proportional degree affect the fore.

Chancres after having their venereal taint corrected often become ftationary, and having acquired new difpofitions increafe the quantity of difeafe in the part, as will be taken notice of hereafter. When they become ftationary only they may often be cured by touching them flightly with the lunar cauftic. They feem to require that the furface which had been

been contaminated, or the new fleſh which grew upon that ſurface ſhould be either deſtroyed or altered before it can cicatriſe; and it is ſurpriſing often how faſt they will heal after being touched, and probably once or twice may be ſufficient.

III. OF THE TREATMENT OF PHYMOSIS IN CONSEQUENCE OF, OR ATTENDED WITH CHANCRE.

FROM the hiſtory which I have given of the diſeaſe we muſt ſee that a phymoſis may be of two kinds, one natural with the diſeaſe ſuperadded, the other brought on by diſeaſe. The firſt may be increaſed by the diſeaſe; but if otherways it is not ſo troubleſome as the other. Such as ariſe from the diſeaſe I have obſerved depend upon the peculiarity of the conſtitution. In either caſe it is often not practicable to apply dreſſings to the chancres on the inſide of the prepuce.

A phymoſis ſhould be prevented if poſſible, therefore upon the leaſt ſigns of a thickening of the prepuce, which is known by it's being retracted with difficulty and pain, the patient ſhould be kept quiet; if in bed ſo much the better, as in an horizontal poſition the end of the penis will not be ſo depending, but may be kept up. If lying in bed cannot be complied with, then the end of the penis ſhould be kept up to the belly if poſſible, but this can hardly be done when the perſon is obliged to walk about; for the extravaſated fluids deſcending and remaining in the prepuce, contribute often more to render the prepuce incapable of being drawn back than the inflammation itſelf.

When the diſeaſed phymoſis completely takes place the ſame precautions may be followed; but as the ſores cannot be dreſſed in the common way, we muſt have recourſe either to dreſſings in form of injections, or the operation for the phymoſis. If injections only they ſhould be often repeated, as they are only temporary applications.

The dreſſings in form of injections ſhould be mercurial, either crude mercury rubbed down with a thick ſolution of gum arabic, which will aſſiſt in retaining ſome of the injection between the glans and prepuce; or calomel with

with the ſame, with a proportion of opium. In the proportions of theſe no nicety is required; but if a ſolution of corroſive ſublimate is made uſe of as an injection, ſome attention is to be paid to it's ſtrength. About one grain of this to an ounce of water will be as much as the ſenſation of the part will allow the patient to bear; and if this gives too much pain it may be lowered by adding more water.

After the parts are as well cleaned as poſſible with this injection, it will be neceſſary to introduce other mercurial applications of ſome kind to remain there till the parts want cleaning again, which will be very ſoon; ſuch as are mentioned before will anſwer this purpoſe very well: but I have my doubts about the propriety of uſing any irritating medicines or injections in ſuch caſes.

Every time of making water the patient may waſh the parts, by preſſing the orifice of the prepuce together, ſo as to oblige the water to run back between the prepuce and glans; immediately after this the patient ſhould uſe the mercurial applications, otherways this operation of waſhing may do harm, as it will be waſhing away the former application of mercury; but in many caſes the parts are ſo ſore as not to allow of this practice.

A poultice of linſeed meal alone, or of equal parts of this and bread, ſhould be applied. This poultice is to be made with water, to which one-eighth of laudanum has been added. But previous to this, and immediately after the cleaning, it would be very proper to let the penis hang over the ſteam of hot water, with a little vinegar and ſpirits of wine in it, which is the neateſt way of applying fomentations.

The oftner this is practiſed the better, as it is keeping a mercurial application in contact with the diſeaſed parts a greater number of the hours out of the twenty-four, than otherways could be were the matter allowed to lie on the parts.

When to the abovementioned ſymptoms a bleeding of the chancre is added, I do not know a more troubleſome complaint, becauſe here the cells or veins have no great diſpoſition for contraction.* Oil of turpentine gives the

* I ſuſpect that where chancres bleed profuſely, the blood comes either from the glans, when there are chancres there, or from the ſpongy ſubſtance of the urethra where the chancre has begun

the beſt ſtimulus for the contraction of veſſels of all kinds; but where bleeding ariſes from an irritable action of the veſſels, which is ſometimes the caſe, then ſedatives, ſuch as opium, are the beſt applications. Whatever is uſed in ſuch a ſtate of the prepuce muſt be injected into the part.

When in conſequence of the treatment the inflammation begins to go off, and the chancres to heal, it will be neceſſary to move the prepuce upon the glans as much as they will allow of, to prevent adheſions which ſometimes happen when there have been chancres on both ſurfaces oppoſite to each other. Indeed the practice here recommended is ſuch as will in general prevent ſuch conſequences.

If this has not been properly attended to, and the parts have grown together, the conſequences may not be bad; but it muſt be very diſagreeable to the patient, and a reflection upon the ſurgeon.

I have ſeen the opening into the prepuce ſo much contracted from all theſe internal ulcers healing and uniting that there was hardly any paſſage for the water. If the paſſage in the prepuce ſo contracted be in a direct line with the orifice of the urethra, then a bougie may be readily paſſed; but this is not always the caſe: it often happens that they are not in a direct line, therefore an operation becomes neceſſary. The operation conſiſts in either ſlitting up part of the prepuce, or removing part of it; but as theſe parts have become very indiſtinct from the adheſions, either the ſlitting it up, or removing part of it, becomes a difficult operation. Whenever the urethra is diſcovered, or can be found out by a bougie, that is to be introduced, and it's application repeated till the paſſage becomes free and has got into the habit of keeping ſo.

I obſerved formerly that this tumefaction ſometimes produced a confinement of the matter formed by the chancre, and that while this effect laſted no ſubſiding of the inflammation or tumefaction could take place; that therefore thoſe diſeaſes continued to exiſt, and that the part thus circumſtanced came under our definition of an abſceſs; that is, the formation of matter in a ſtate of confinement. Although it never has been conſidered

begun about the frænum, for we ſeldom ſee profuſe bleedings from the prepuce when it's inſide is the ſeat of the chancre and can be expoſed; but indeed in ſuch caſes the inflammation is not violent.

in

in this light, yet the necessary treatment shows it to be such. This consists in laying it open from the external orifice to the bottom where the matter lies, as in a sinus, or fistola, so as to discharge it. However the intention annexed to this practice was not to allow of the discharge of the matter of the sore, but to admit of the application of dressings to it, for it has been recommended and practised, where there was no particular confinement of matter, which I have not found to be necessary, merely for that purpose, as we are in possession of an internal remedy; and if the opening produces no other good, but the allowing of the application of dressings it is not so material, because the sores may be washed with an injection through a syringe.

IV. OF THE COMMON OPERATION FOR THE PHYMOSIS PRODUCED BY CHANCRES.

THE common operation for the phymosis is slitting the prepuce nearly it's whole length, in the direction of the penis; but even this is sometimes thought not sufficient, and it is directed to cut the prepuce in two different places, nearly opposite to one another. When it was thought proper to be done in this way, it was imagined that it was seldom necessary to cut the whole length of the prepuce. It will in some degree depend on circumstances, which practice is to be followed. If it is a natural phymosis without tumefaction, and the chancre is near the orifice of the prepuce, which in such cases it most probably will be, as the glans is not denuded in coition so as to have chancres deeper seated, then it may be necessary only to go as far as the chancres extend.

From the common situation of the chancre, this disease of the phymosis arises more commonly from the tumefaction of the parts; and from the idea I have endeavoured to give of the inconveniences arising from this phymosis, where the chancres are placed behind the corona, producing a confinement of the matter behind the glans, slitting open the prepuce a little way cannot be sufficient, for in such cases it must be exposed to the bottom, or no good can arise from the operation.

Although

Although this operation will not take off the tumefaction of the prepuce so as to allow it to be brought back, yet it will allow of a free discharge of the matter, and also in some cases it will allow of dressings being applied to the sores; but not in all, for the tumefaction will not now allow more of an inversion of the prepuce than before, and in such the sores cannot have dressings applied to them.

In many cases it will be found that so violent an operation is improper; for it often happens that while the inflammation is so very considerable there is danger of increasing it by this additional violence, of which mortification may be the consequence; while on the other hand there are cases where a freedom given to the parts would prevent mortification, so that the surgeon must be guided by the appearances, and other circumstances. Besides these reasons for and against the operation arising from the disease itself, it will not always be consented to by the patients themselves, for some have such a dread of operations that they will not submit to cutting instruments; however in those cases where the matter is confined, it will be absolutely necessary to have an opening somewhere for the discharge of it. This is often produced by the ulcerative process going on on the inside, which makes an opening directly through the skin, laterally, which affords a direction for the surgeon; therefore the opening may be made directly into the cavity of the prepuce, through the skin, on the side of the penis, by a lancet; or a small caustic may be applied there, for which the lapis septicus is the most convenient.

The opening will allow of the discharge of the matter, and also admit any proper wash to be thrown in. But this opening should not be a large one, as in many cases the consequence of this lateral opening proves very troublesome; for from the tumefaction of the prepuce, the glans is squeezed on all sides, and rather more backwards upon the body of the penis than in any other direction, by which means it is often forced through this opening, whereby the glans is directed to one side, and the prepuce to the opposite, having a forked appearance. Besides this state of the parts tightens the skin of the penis round the root of the glans, acting there somewhat like a paraphymosis, and sometimes makes the whole prepuce mortify and drop off, which is often a lucky circumstance; but if this is not the consequence, then

then amputation of the prepuce becomes neceſſary; however this ſhould not be done till all inflammation is gone off, and the chancres are cured, when probably the tumefaction of the prepuce will have conſiderably ſubſided.

A mortification of the prepuce is ſometimes a conſequence of chancres when attended with violent inflammation, even without any previous operation; and I have ſeen caſes where the glans and part of the penis have mortified, while the prepuce has kept it's ground. But I ſhould ſuſpect in all ſuch caſes, that there is ſome fault in the conſtitution, and that the inflammation is of the eriſypelatous, not of the true ſuppurative kind.

I have ſeen the mortification go ſo far as to remove the whole of the diſeaſed prepuce, and the parts have taken on ſo favourable an appearance that I have treated it as a common ſore, and no bad conſequences have happened; in this caſe the diſeaſe performed what is often recommended in other diſeaſes of this part, that is circumciſion; but this is not always to be truſted to, for if abſorption of the venereal matter has taken place previous to the mortification, a lues venerea will be the conſequence, although the parts heal very readily.

V. OF THE CONSTITUTIONAL TREATMENT OF PHYMOSIS.

In thoſe caſes where violent inflammation has attacked the ſeat of a chancre, producing phymoſis, as before deſcribed, and often ſo as to threaten mortification, a queſtion naturally occurs, what is to be done? Is mercury to be given freely to get rid of the firſt cauſe? Or does that medicine increaſe the effect while it deſtroys the cauſe? Nothing but experience can determine this.

But I ſhould incline to believe that it is neceſſary that mercury ſhould be given, for I am afraid our powers to correct ſuch a conſtitution while the firſt cauſe ſubſiſts are weak. However on the other hand I believe the mercury ſhould be given ſparingly; for if it aſſiſts in diſpoſing the conſtitution to ſuch ſymptoms, we are gaining nothing, but may loſe by it's uſe. I therefore do ſuppoſe that ſuch medicines as may be thought neceſſary for the conſtitution ſhould be given liberally, as well as the ſpecific. Bark is the medicine that probably will be of moſt general uſe; opium in moſt caſes of this kind will alſo be of ſingular ſervice.

The bark ſhould be given in large quantities, and along with it mercury, while the virus is ſtill ſuppoſed to exiſt. Or if the inflammation has ariſen early in the diſeaſe, they may be then given together ſo as to counteract both diſeaſes, and not allow the inflammation to come to ſo great a height as it would otherways do if mercury was given at firſt alone.

This inflammation may be ſo great in many caſes, or be ſo predominant, that mercury may increaſe the diſpoſition and therefore become hurtful. Where this may be ſuppoſed to be the caſe, bark muſt be given alone.

VI. OF THE TREATMENT OF THE PARAPHYMOSIS FROM CHANCRES.

A prepuce in the ſtate of inflammation and tumefaction, and which has been either kept back upon the body of the penis while inflaming, or pulled back when inflamed, ſeldom can be again brought forwards while in this ſtate, therefore becomes alſo the ſubject of an operation, which conſiſts in dividing the ſame part, as in the phymoſis, only in a different way, ariſing from it's difference of ſituation; the intention of which operation is to bring the prepuce, when brought forwards, to the ſtate of a phymoſis that has been operated upon. This operation becomes more neceſſary in many caſes under this diſeaſe than under the phymoſis, becauſe it's conſequences are generally worſe; ſince, beſides the real diſeaſe, viz. Inflammation, tumefaction, ulceration, &c. there is a mechanical cauſe producing it's effects, by graſping the penis, which can of itſelf produce inflammation where the prepuce is naturally tight, as has been obſerved. From whatever cauſe it ariſes it often produces mortification in the parts between the ſtricture and the glans if it is not removed. This removal ſometimes happens naturally by the ulceration of the ſtrictured part; but an operation is generally neceſſary; and it is more troubleſome than in the former caſe, becauſe the ſwelling on each ſide of the ſtricture covers or cloſes in upon the tight part and makes it difficult to be got at.

The beſt way appears to be to ſeparate the two ſwellings as much as poſſible where you mean to cut, ſo as to expoſe the neck, then take a crooked biſtory which is pointed, and paſſing it under the ſkin at the neck divide it; no part of the two ſwellings on the ſides need be divided, for it is the looſeneſs of the ſkin in theſe parts which admits of their ſwelling. When this is done the prepuce may be brought forwards over the glans; but as this diſeaſe aroſe from chancres which may require being dreſſed, and as the ſtate of a phymoſis is a very bad one for ſuch treatment, it may be better now that the ſtricture is removed, to let it remain in the ſame ſituation till the whole is well.

If the paraphymoſis has ariſen from a natural tightneſs of the prepuce, and it's being forced back from accident, then no particular treatment after the operation is neceſſary, but to go on with the cure as recommended in chancres. It is indeed probable that in conſequence of the violence produced by the poſition of the prepuce, as alſo by the operation, a conſiderable inflammation may enſue; but as this will be an inflammation in conſequence of violence only, local treatment for the inflammation will be ſufficient, ſuch as fomentations, poultices, &c.

But if it is a paraphymoſis in conſequence of a diſeaſed phymoſis, then the ſame mode of treatment becomes equally neceſſary as was recommended in the phymoſis attended with conſiderable inflammation; and probably rather more attention is neceſſary here, as violence has been added to the former diſeaſe.

VII. OF THE CURE OF CHANCRES BY MERCURY GIVEN INTERNALLY.

While chancres are under local treatment, as before deſcribed, it is neceſſary to give mercurials internally, both for the cure of a chancre and the prevention of a lues venerea; and we may reaſonably venture to affirm, that the venereal diſpoſition of chancre will hardly ever withſtand both local and internal mercurials.

In

In cases of chancres where local applications cannot easily be made, as in cases of phymosis, internal mercurials become absolutely necessary; and more so than if they could be conveniently and freely applied externally. However, even in such cases internal mercurials will in the end effect a cure; so that we need seldom or ever be under any apprehension of not curing such a disease.

In every case of a chancre, let it be ever so slight, mercury should be given internally; even in those cases where they were destroyed on their first appearance. It should in all cases be given the whole time of the cure, and continue for some time after the chancres are healed; for as there are perhaps few chancres without absorption of the matter, it becomes absolutely necessary to give mercury to act internally, in order to hinder the venereal disposition from forming.

How much mercury should be thrown into the constitution in the cure of a chancre for the prevention of that constitutional affection is not easily ascertained, as there is in such cases no disease actually formed so as to be a guide, it must be uncertain what quantity should be given internally. It must in general be according to the size, number, and duration of the chancres. If large we may suppose that the absorption will be proportioned to the surface, and if long continued, the absorption will be according to the time; and if they have been many, large, and continued long, then the greatest quantity is necessary.

The circumstances therefore attending the chancre must be the guide for the safety of the constitution, especially in those cases where some stress in the cure is laid upon the external remedy.

The mercury given to act internally must be thrown in either by the skin or stomach, according to circumstances.

The quantity in either way should be such as may in common affect the mouth slightly; which method of giving mercury will be considered hereafter.

When the sore has put on a healthy look, when the hard basis has become soft, and it has skinned over kindly, it may be looked upon as cured.

But in very large chancres it may not always be necessary to continue the application of mercury either for external or internal action till the sore is healed;

healed; for the venereal action is just as soon destroyed in a large chancre as it is in a small one; for every part of the chancre being equally affected by the mercury, is equally easily cured. But the skinning is different; for a large sore is longer in skinning than a small one. A large chancre therefore may be deprived of it's venereal action long before it is skinned over; but a small one may probably skin over before the venereal action is entirely subdued. In the latter case, both on account of the chancre and constitution, it will be erring on the safe side to continue the medicine a little longer, which will most certainly in the end effect a cure: for we may reasonably suppose that the quantity of mercury capable of curing a local effect, although assisted by local applications, or of producing in the constitution a mercurial irritation sufficient to hinder the venereal irritation from forming, will be nearly as much as will cure a slight lues venerea.

I have formerly laid it down as a principle, that no new action will take place in another part of the body, however contaminated, whilst the body is under the beneficial operation of mercury; but there are now and then appearances which occur under the cure that will at first embarrass the practitioner. I have suspected that the mercury flying to the mouth and throat has sometimes produced sloughs in the tonsils, and these have been taken for venereal; the following cases in some degree explain this.

A young gentleman had a chancre on the prepuce, with a slight pain in a gland of one groin, for which I ordered mercurial ointment to be rubbed into the legs and thighs, especially on the side where the gland was swelled, and the chancre to be dressed with mercurial ointment. While he was pursuing this course the chancre became cleaner, the hardness at the base went off, and the pain in the groin was entirely removed. About three weeks after the first appearance of the disease he was attacked with a sore throat, and on looking into the mouth I found the right tonsil with a white slough which appeared to be in it's substance, with only one point yet exposed. From my mind being warped by the opinion that these complaints proceeded from the chancre, I immediately suspected that it was venereal; and the only way I could account for this seeming contradiction in one part healing while another was breaking out, was, that the healing sore

 was

was treated locally as well as conſtitutionally, while the tonſil, or the conſtitution at large, was only treated conſtitutionally, which was inſufficient.

Soon after this another gentleman was under my care for venereal ſcurfs, or eruptions on his ſkin, for which he uſed mercurial friction till his mouth became ſore; and in this ſtate he continued for three weeks, in which time the eruptions were all gone, diſcolourations being left only where the eruptions had been, yet at the end of three weeks a ſlough formed in one of the tonſils, exactly as in the former caſe. This made me doubtful how far ſuch caſes were venereal. I ordered the friction to be left off, to ſee what courſe the ulcers would take; the ſlough came out and left a foul ſore: I waited ſtill longer, and in a day or two it became clean and healed up.

The firſt mentioned caſe I did not ſee to an end; but I learned that the patient continued the mercury and got well; and the ulcer in the throat was ſuppoſed to be venereal; but from the circumſtances of the other caſe I now very much doubt of that.

It is more than probable that theſe effects of mercury only take place in conſtitutions that have a tendency to ſuch complaints in the throat. I know this to be the caſe with the laſt mentioned gentleman; and it is alſo probable that there may be an increaſed diſpoſition at the time, either in conſequence of the mercury, or ſome accidental cauſe. I have reaſon to ſuppoſe that mercury in ſome degree increaſes this diſpoſition, which will be further taken notice of when treating of the cure of the lues venerea.

In the cure of chancres I have ſometimes ſeen when the original chancre has been doing well, and probably nearly cured, that new ones have broken out upon the prepuce, near to the firſt, and have put on all the appearance of a chancre; but ſuch I have always treated as not venereal. They may be ſimilar to ſome conſequences of chancres, which will be taken notice of hereafter.

As ſwellings of the abſorbent glands take place in conſequence of other abſorptions beſides poiſons, we ſhould be careful in all caſes to aſcertain the cauſe, as has been already deſcribed; and here it may not be improper ſtill to obſerve further, that in the cure of chancres, ſwellings of the glands ſhall ariſe, even when the conſtitution is ſo much loaded with mercury as to be be sufficient for the cure of the sores; but then the mercury has been thrown into the constitution by the lower extremity; and therefore there is great room for suspicion that such swellings are not venereal, but arise from the mercury: for a real buboe, from absorption of venereal matter, if not come to suppuration, will give way to mercury rubbed into the leg and thigh. In such cases I have always desisted from giving the mercury in this way when I could give it by the mouth.

CHAPTER IV.

OF THE CURE OF CHANCRES IN WOMEN.

THE parts generally affected with chancres in this ſex, are more ſimple than in men, by which means the treatment in general is alſo more ſimple; but in moſt caſes they require nearly the ſame, both in the local application of mercury, and in throwing it into the conſtitution. It may be ſuppoſed however, that it will be neceſſary in many caſes to throw into the conſtitution more mercury than in men; becauſe in general there are more chancres, and the ſurface of abſorption of courſe larger.

As it is difficult to keep dreſſings on the female parts, it is proper they ſhould be waſhed often with ſolutions of mercury; perhaps corroſive ſublimate is one of the beſt, as it will act as a ſpecific, and alſo as a ſtimulant when that is wanted; but in chancres that are very irritable, the ſame mode of treatment as was recommended in men is to be put in practice. Afterwards the parts may be beſmeared with a mercurial application, either oily or watry, to be frequently repeated according to the circumſtances of the caſe.

If the ulcers ſhould have ſpread, or run up the vagina, great attention ſhould be paid to the healing of them; for it ſometimes happens that the granulations contract conſiderably ſo as to draw the vagina into a ſmall canal; at other times the granulations will unite into one another and cloſe the vagina up altogether; therefore in ſuch caſes it will be neceſſary to keep ſome ſubſtance in the vagina till the ſores are ſkinned, for which purpoſe probably lint may be ſufficient.

CHAPTER V.

OF SOME OF THE CONSEQUENCES OF CHANCRES —AND THEIR TREATMENT.

AFTER the chancres have been cured and all venereal taint removed, it ſometimes happens that the prepuce ſtill retains a conſiderable degree of tumefaction, which keeps up the elongation and tightneſs it acquired from the diſeaſe, ſo that it cannot be brought back upon the penis to expoſe the glans.

For this perhaps there is in many caſes no cure; however it is neceſſary to try every poſſible means. The ſteam of warm water is often of ſingular ſervice in theſe caſes; fomentations with hemlock, and alſo fumigations with cinnabar.

But if the parts ſtill retain their ſize and form, it may be very proper to remove part of the overgrown prepuce; how much muſt be left to the diſcretion of the ſurgeon; however I ſhould ſuppoſe that all that part which projects beyond the glans penis may be cut away.

The beſt way of removing it is by the knife, but great care ſhould be taken to diſtinguiſh firſt the projecting prepuce from the glans. When this is perfectly aſcertained, an inciſion may be made on the upper ſurface, the penis being held horizontally and followed down carefully; becauſe if the inciſion ſhould be too near the glans there may be danger of cutting it.

The parts may be allowed to heal with any common dreſſings, as it is to be conſidered as a freſh wound; however it will not heal ſo readily as a freſh wound made in an entirely ſound part, becauſe the operation conſiſts in taking away only a ſuperfluous part of a diſeaſed whole, and what is left is diſeaſed, but not ſo as to produce any future miſchief.

Some care may be neceſſary in the healing of the parts; for it is very poſſible that the cicatrix may contract, and ſtill form a phymoſis. This will be beſt prevented by the patient himſelf bringing the prepuce often back upon the penis; but it ſhould not be attempted till the part is nearly healed; and it is to be performed with great care, and ſlowly.

I. OF DISPOSITIONS TO NEW DISEASES TAKING PLACE DURING THE CURE OF CHANCRES.

CHANCRES both in men and women often acquire new diſpoſitions and modes of action in the time of the cure, which are of various kinds, ſome of which retard the cure, as deſcribed, and when the parts are cured leave them tumefied and indolent, as in the enlarged prepuce. In others a new diſpoſition takes place which prevents the cure or healing of the parts, and often produces a much worſe diſeaſe than that from which it aroſe. They alſo become the cauſe of the formation of tumors on theſe parts, which will be taken notice of hereafter.

Such new diſpoſitions take place oftner in men than in women, probably from the nature of the parts themſelves. They ſeldom or never happen but when the inflammation has been violent, which violence ariſes more from the nature of the parts than the diſeaſe, and therefore belongs more to the nature of the parts or conſtitution than to the diſeaſe; however I can conceive it may alſo take place where the inflammation has not been violent; although I can hardly ſay I have ever ſeen it.

In general they are ſuppoſed to be cancerous, but I believe they ſeldom are; although it is not impoſſible ſome may be ſo.

Of this kind may be reckoned thoſe continued and often increaſed inflammations, ſuppurations, and ulcerations, becoming diffuſed through the whole prepuce, as alſo all along the common ſkin of the penis, which becomes of a purple hue; the cellular membrane every where on the penis is very much thickened ſo as to increaſe the ſize of the whole conſiderably.

The ulceration on the inſide of the prepuce will ſometimes increaſe and run between the ſkin and the body of the penis, and eat holes through in different places till the whole is reduced to a numbers of ragged ſores. The glans often ſhares the ſame fate till more or leſs of it is gone; frequently the urethra

urethra at this part is wholly ulcerated away, and the urine comes out ſome way further back. If a ſtop is not put to the progreſs of the diſeaſe, the ulceration will continue till the parts are entirely deſtroyed. I ſuſpect that ſome of theſe caſes are ſcrofulous.

As this is an acute caſe immediate relief ſhould be given if poſſible; but as it may ariſe from various peculiarities in the conſtitution, and as theſe peculiarities are not at firſt known, no rational method can be here determined. The ſarſaparilla is often of ſervice in ſuch caſes, but requires to be given in large quantities.

The German diet-drink* has been of ſingular ſervice; I knew a caſe of this kind cured by it, after every known remedy had been tried.

The extract of hemlock is ſometimes of ſervice. I have known ſea-bathing cure theſe complaints entirely.

A gentleman came from Ireland with a complaint of this kind, and after trying every common, and known method, without effect, as ſarſaparilla, hemlock, German diet-drink; and after having uſed a great variety of dreſſings, which were all at laſt laid aſide, and opium only retained to quiet the pain, he went afterwards and bathed in the ſea, and got well.

It may be ſometimes neceſſary to paſs a bougie, to hinder the orifice of the urethra from cloſing or becoming too ſmall in the time of healing in ſuch caſes.

II. OF ULCERATIONS RESEMBLING CHANCRES.

It often happens that after chancres are healed, and all the virus gone, the cicatrices ulcerate again, and break out in the form of chancres.

* The following formulæ have been much recommended as diet-drinks. Take of crude antimony pulverized tied up in a bit of rag; pumice ſtone pulverized tied up in the ſame, of each one ounce; China-root ſliced; ſarſaparilla-root ſliced and bruiſed, of each half an ounce; ten walnuts with their rinds bruiſed; ſpring water four pints; boiled to half that quantity; filter it, and let it be drank daily in divided doſes.

Take ſarſaparilla, Sanders-wood, white and red, of each three ounces; liquorice and mezereon, of each half an ounce; lign. rhodii, guaic, ſaſſafras, of each one ounce; crude antimony, two ounces; mix them and infuſe them in boiling water, ten pints, for twenty-four hours; and afterwards boil them to five pints, of which let the doſe be from a pint and an half to four pints a day.

Although

Although this is moſt common in the ſeat of the former chancres, yet it is not always confined to them, for ſores often break out on other parts of the prepuce; but ſtill they appear to be a conſequence of a venereal complaint having been there, as they ſeldom attack thoſe who never had gonorrhœa or chancres. They often have ſo much the appearance of chancres, that I am perſuaded many are treated as venereal that are really not ſuch: they differ from a chancre in general by not ſpreading ſo faſt, nor ſo far; they are not ſo painful, nor ſo much inflamed, and have not thoſe hard baſis that the venereal ſores have, nor do they produce buboes. Yet a malignant kind of them, when they attack a bad conſtitution, may be taken for a mild kind of chancre, or a chancre in a good conſtitution. I have ſeen ſeveral that have puzzled me extremely.

Some ſtreſs is to be laid upon the account that the patient gives of himſelf; but when there is any doubt, a little time will clear it up. I have ſeen the ſame appearances after a gonorrhœa; but that more rarely happens. It would appear that the venereal poiſon could leave a diſpoſition for ulceration of a different kind from what is peculiar to itſelf. I knew one caſe where they broke out regularly every two months, exactly to a day.

As they are not venereal their treatment becomes difficult; for the cure conſiſts more in preventing a return, than in the healing up of the preſent ſores.

They require particular attention; for although they are not dangerous, they are often troubleſome, keeping the mind in ſuſpence for months.

I have tried a great variety of means, but with little ſucceſs, yet they have in general got well in the end. In the following caſe, the lixivium ſaponarium produced a ſpeedy cure.

A gentleman had three ſores broke out on the prepuce, which had very much the appearance of mild chancres. As I was doubtful of their nature, I waited ſome time, and only ordered them to be kept clean. As they did not get well, ſeveral things were tried. Mercurial dreſſings were applied, but they always produced conſiderable irritation, and it was neceſſary to leave them off. The mercurius calcinatus was given by way of trial, and to ſecure the conſtitution, but the ſores continued the ſame. They were eat down with the lunar cauſtic, which appeared to have a better effect than any

any other thing tried; but still they were not healed at the end of five months. I ordered forty drops of the lixivium tartari to be taken every evening and morning in a bason of broth. After using it three days he observed a considerable alteration in the sores, and in six they were perfectly skinned over. He had formerly had such sores often, which had always been treated as venereal; but he began to doubt whether they really were so from their getting so soon well in the present instance by the lixivium.

I knew a gentleman who had these sores breaking out and healing again for years, and by bathing in the sea for a month or two they healed up and never afterwards appeared.

III. OF A THICKENING AND HARDENING OF THE PARTS.

In some cases the parts do not ulcerate, but appear to thicken and become hard or firm; both the glans and prepuce seem to swell, forming a tumor or excrescence from the end of the penis, in form a good deal like a cauliflower, and when cut into showing radii running from it's base, or origin, towards the external surface, becoming extremely indolent in all it's operations. This gives more the idea of a cancer than the first, being principally a new formed substance. However it is not always a consequence of the venereal disease, I have known it to arise spontaneously.

This disease appears to be a tumor of so indolent a kind, that I do not know any medicine that stands the least chance of performing a cure. I have amputated them, and have also seen the same thing done by others, from the idea of their being cancerous, and the remaining part of the penis has healed kindly.

In most of these cases a considerable part of the penis must be removed. Immediately after the amputation, a suitable catheter should be introduced into the urethra; for if no such precaution is made use of, the consequences must be troublesome; for the first dressings become cemented to the orifice by the extravasated blood, and prevent the patient's making water, which must be attended with obvious inconveniences; this was the case with a patient whose penis I amputated.

IV. OF WARTS.

ANOTHER diſpoſition which theſe parts acquire from the venereal poiſon is the diſpoſition to form excreſcences, or cutaneous tumors, called warts. This diſpoſition is ſtrongeſt where the chancres were; and indeed chancres often heal into warts; but perhaps the parts acquire this diſpoſition from the venereal matter having been long in contact with their ſurfaces; for it often happens after gonorrhœas where there had been no chancres; and probably it is only in thoſe caſes where the venereal matter had produced the venereal ſtimulus upon the glans and prepuce, forming there what may be called an inſenſible gonorrhœa.

A wart appears to be an excreſcence from the cutis, or a tumor forming upon it, by which means it becomes covered with a cuticle, which like all other cuticles, is either ſtrong and hard, or thin and ſoft, juſt as the cuticle is which covers the parts from whence they ariſe. They are radiated from their baſis to the circumference, the radii appearing at the ſurface pointed or granulated, much like granulations that are healthy, except that they are harder, and riſe above the ſurface. It would appear that the ſurface on which each is formed has only the diſpoſition to form one, becauſe the ſurrounding and connecting ſurface does not go into the like ſubſtance; thus a wart once begun does not increaſe in it's baſis, but riſes higher and higher. They have an increaſing power within themſelves; for after riſing above the ſurface of the ſkin, on which they are not allowed to increaſe in breadth at the baſis, they ſwell out into a round thick ſubſtance which becomes rougher and rougher.

This ſtructure often makes them liable to be hurt by bodies rubbing againſt them; and often from ſuch a cauſe they bleed very profuſely, and are very painful.

Theſe excreſcences are conſidered by many not as ſimply a conſequence of the venereal poiſon, but as poſſeſſed of it's ſpecific diſpoſition, and therefore they have recourſe to mercury for the cure of them; and it is aſſerted that ſuch treatment often removes them. Such an effect of mercury I have never ſeen;

ſeen, although given in ſuch a quantity as to cure in the ſame perſon recent chancres, and ſometimes a pox.

As theſe ſubſtances are excreſcences from the body, they are not to be conſidered as truly a part of the animal, not being endowed with the common or natural animal powers, by which means the cure becomes eaſier. They are ſo little of the true animal, and ſo much of a diſeaſe, that many trifling circumſtances make them decay; an inflammation in the natural and ſound parts round the wart will give it a diſpoſition to decay; many ſtimuli applied to the ſurface will often make them die. Electricity will produce action in them which they are not able to ſupport; an inflammation is excited round them, and they drop off.

From this view of them, the knife and eſcharotics muſt appear not always neceſſary, although theſe modes will act more quickly than any other in many caſes, eſpecially if the neck is ſmall. In ſuch formed warts perhaps a pair of ſciſſars is the beſt inſtrument; but where cutting inſtruments of any kind are horrible to the patient, a ſilk thread tied round it's neck will do very well; but in whichſoever way it is ſeparated it will be in general neceſſary to touch the baſe with cauſtic.

Eſcharotics act upon warts in two different ways, one by deadening part and ſtimulating the remainder, ſo that by applying eſcharotic after eſcharotic, the whole decays tolerably faſt; and it is ſeldom neceſſary to eat them down to the very root, as the baſis or root often ſeparates and is thrown off. This however is not always the caſe, for we find that the root does not always ſeparate, and that it will grow again; therefore in ſuch caſes it is neceſſary to eat down lower than the general ſurface to remove the root.

Any of the cauſtics, ſuch as the lapis ſepticus, as alſo the metallic ſalts, ſuch as the lunar cauſtic, blue vitriol, &c. have this power. Merely as ſtimulants, the ruſt of copper and ſavine leaves mixed is one of the beſt.

After they have been to appearance ſufficiently deſtroyed they often riſe anew, not from any part being left, but from the ſurface of the cutis having the ſame diſpoſition as before; this requires a repetition of the ſame practice, ſo as to take off that ſurface of the cutis.

V. OF

V. OF EXCORIATIONS OF THE GLANS AND PREPUCE.

It very often happens that the ſurface of the glans and inſide of the prepuce excoriate, becoming extremely tender, and then a matter oozes out. The prepuce in ſuch caſes often becomes a little thickened, and ſometimes contracts in it's orifice, both of which render the inverſion of it difficult and painful. Whether this complaint ever ariſes from a venereal cauſe is not certain, as it often takes place where there never has been any venereal taint.

This diſeaſe is in the cutis; and under ſuch a diſpoſition it has no power of forming a good cuticle. It is very ſimilar to a gonorrhœa in this part, but is not venereal.

Drawing the prepuce back, and ſteeping the parts in a ſolution of lead, often takes off the irritation, and a ſound cuticle is formed. Spirits diluted often produce the ſame effect; the unguentum citrinum of the Edinburgh Diſpenſatory, lowered by mixing with it equal parts of hogs lard, is often of ſingular ſervice in ſuch caſes; but there are caſes which bid defiance to all our applications, in which I have ſucceeded by deſiring the perſon to leave the glans uncovered, which produced the ſtimulus of neceſſity for the formation of a natural cuticle.

PART

PART V.

CHAPTER I.

OF BUBO.

A Knowledge of the abſorbing ſyſtem, as it is now eſtabliſhed, gives us conſiderable information reſpecting many of the effects of poiſons, and illuſtrates ſeveral ſymptoms of the venereal diſeaſe, in particular the formation of buboes. Prior to this knowledge we find writers at a loſs how to give a true and conſiſtent explanation of many of the ſymptoms of this diſeaſe. The diſcovery of the lymphatics being a ſyſtem of abſorbents has thrown more light on many diſeaſes than the diſcovery of the circulation of the blood; it leads in many caſes directly to the cauſe of the diſeaſe.

The immediate conſequence of the local diſeaſes gonorrhœa and chancre, which is called bubo, as alſo the remote or lues venerea, ariſe from the abſorption of recent venereal matter from ſome ſurface where it has either been applied or formed. Although this muſt have been allowed in general ever ſince the knowledge of the diſeaſe and of abſorption, yet a true ſolution of the formation of bubo could not be given till we had acquired the knowledge of the lymphatics being the only abſorbents. Upon the old opinion of abſorption being performed by the veins, the lues venerea could have eaſily been accounted for, becauſe it could as readily be produced by the abſorbing power of the veins, if they had ſuch, as by the lymphatics; but the difficulty was to ſay how the bubo was formed. There they ſeemed to be at a loſs to account for this diſeaſe, yet they ſometimes expreſſed themſelves as if they had ſome idea of it, although at the ſame time they could have no clear notions of what they advanced; nor could they demonſtrate what they ſaid from the knowledge of the parts and their uſes.

Buboes are by ſome imputed to the ſtopping of a gonorrhœa, or as they expreſſed it, driving it to the glands of the groin, conformably to the idea they had of the cauſe of the ſwelling of the teſticle. But this is not juſt, for we know of no ſuch power as repulſion; and if it was driven there it could not be by ſtopping the formation of matter, but by increaſing the abſorption, of which they had no idea.

When we examine the opinions of authors concerning the formation of bubo, prior to the knowledge of the power of abſorption in the lymphatics, we ſhall find them making uſe of terms which they could not poſſibly underſtand. For inſtance, Heiſter ſays, "They are of two kinds, one venereal, and the other not;" but he does not ſay that the venereal ariſes only from impure coition.

Aſtruc ſays, page 326, that ſome buboes ariſe immediately from impure coition, and theſe he calls eſſential; others from ſuppreſſed gonorrhœa, or a ſmall diſcharge, or from chancres of the penis, and theſe he calls ſymptomatic; laſtly, that they ariſe ſpontaneouſly without any immediate previous coition, and are a pathognomonic ſign of a hidden pox.

In page 327 he ſhows the impoſſibility of this laſt happening from what we now call or underſtand by a lues venerea; but in page 328 he explains what he calls a latent lues venerea, which is local affections produced as he ſuppoſes from a lues venerea; but which moſt probably never yet happened; and if ever they had ariſen from ſuch a cauſe, even the abſorption of their matter could not produce a venereal bubo, as will be explained. In ſhort, from not knowing the true abſorbing ſyſtem, his ideas are become now unintelligible.*

We find Cowper, Drake, and Boerhaave, as well as Aſtruc, ſpeaking of the vitiated lymph not paſſing the glands, therefore inflaming them; alſo of the inſpiſſated lymph paſſing either by the circulation of the blood, that is, from the conſtitution to theſe glands, (an opinion held by ſome to this day) or by a ſhorter courſe, viz. The lymphatic veſſels which go to the inguinal glands. They alſo ſpeak of the ſwelling of the inguinal glands, or venereal buboes, from the contagion being communicated by the reſorbent lymphatics.

* The above extracts are from the Engliſh edition, publiſhed in the year 1754, page 326.

tics.

tici. Drake even speaks more pointedly, and if we considered him no further, he would almost make us believe that he knew that the lymphatics were the absorbents; but as he has no such ideas when treating of those vessels expressly, we are not to give him credit for it. His words are, "The venereal bubo may very likely take it's rise from some parts of the contagious matter of claps sucked up by the lymphatics of the penis, and thence imported to the inguinal glands where they deposit their liquor; and thence it well behoves the surgeon to be as early as may be in the opening of such tumors, before by the exporting vessels of that class the poison is carried further into the blood, which very probably may be the case where such tumor ariseth immediately upon the stopping of a gonorrhœa, as does the hernia humoralis; but when the same appears some months after that was removed, we are to suppose as in cases of other poisons laying hold of the blood, by the strength of nature it is thrown forth, either by means of the lymphatics of the blood vessels themselves, if not spewed out of the nervous tubes, as Wharton surmised, and deposited in these emunctories."

Here he compares it to the formation of a hernia humoralis, which plainly shows that he understood neither of them.

Even so late as the year 1748, we do not find any new ideas on this subject: Freke says, "By sealing up the mouths of the glands of the urethra, the poison is thence by the ducts leading to the inguinal glands conveyed to them."

In the year 1754, eight years after Dr. Hunter having publicly taught his opinion of the lymphatics being a system of absorbents, we find a treatise on this disease by Mr. Gataker, where as little new is advanced on this subject, as in any of the former.

When we come so low down as the year 1770, in an abridgement of Astruc by Dr. Chapman, (second edition) in which he introduces his own knowledge and ideas, we find the absorbing power of the lymphatics brought in as a cause of the formation of buboes; but by this time the knowledge of the lymphatics being the system of absorbents was in this country generally diffused.

The doctrine of absorption being now perfectly understood, we have only to explain the different modes in which it may take place.

The

The venereal matter is taken up by the abſorbents of the part in which it is placed; and although the abſorption of the matter and the effects after abſorption are the ſame, whether from the matter of the gonorrhœa or chancre, yet I ſhall divide the abſorption into three kinds, according to the three different ſurfaces from which the matter may be abſorbed, beginning with the leaſt frequent.

The firſt and moſt ſimple is where the matter either of a gonorrhœa or chancre has only been applied to ſome ſound ſurface, without having produced any local effect on the part, but has been abſorbed immediately upon it's application. Inſtances of this I have ſeen in men, and ſuch are perhaps the only inſtances that can be depended upon; for it is uncertain in many caſes, whether a woman has a gonorrhœa or not. I think however I may venture to affirm that I have ſeen it in women, or at leaſt there was every reaſon to believe that they had neither chancre, nor gonorrhœa preceding, as there was no local appearance of it, nor did they communicate it to others who had connection with them.

It muſt be allowed that this mode of abſorption is very rare; and if we were to examine the parts very carefully, or inquire of the patient very ſtrictly, probably a ſmall chancre might be diſcovered to have been the cauſe, which I have more than once ſeen. For when we conſider how rarely it happens from a gonorrhœa, in which the mode of abſorption is ſimilar, we can hardly ſuppoſe it probable that it ſhould here ariſe from ſimple contact, the time of the application of the venereal matter being commonly ſo very ſhort. We might indeed ſuppoſe the frequency to make up for the length of time, which we can hardly allow, for the ſame frequency ſhould give the chance of producing it locally. Therefore very particular attention ſhould be paid to all the circumſtances attending ſuch caſes.

There is however no great reaſon why it ſhould not happen, and the poſſibility of it leſſens the faith that is to be put in the ſuppoſition, that the diſeaſe may be years in the conſtitution before it appears; for whenever it does appear in a lues venerea, it's date is always carried back to the laſt local affection, whether gonorrhœa or chancre, and the latter connections are never regarded.

The

The ſecond mode of abſorption of this matter is more frequent than the former, and it is when the matter applied has produced a gonorrhœa; and it may happen while the complaint is going on, either under a cure or not. Some of the matter ſecreted by the inflamed ſurfaces having been abſorbed and carried into the circulation, produces the ſame complaints as in the former caſe, by which means a perſon gives himſelf the lues venerea.

The third mode is the abſorption of the matter from an ulcer, which may either be a chancre, or a bubo. This mode is by much the moſt frequent; which with many other proofs would ſhow that a ſore, or ulcer, is the ſurface moſt favourable for abſorption. Whether ulcers in every part of the body have an equal power of abſorption I have not been able to determine; but I ſuſpect that an ulcer on the glans, is not ſo good a ſurface for abſorption as one on the prepuce, although I have ſeen both buboes and the lues venerea ariſe from the former, but not ſo often as from the latter.

To theſe three methods may be added a fourth, abſorption from a wound; which I have already remarked is perhaps not ſo frequent as any of the former.

As the venereal poiſon has the power of contaminating whatever part of the body it comes in contact with, it contaminates the abſorbent ſyſtem, producing in it local venereal complaints. It is hardly neceſſary to obſerve, that what is now commonly underſtood by a bubo, is a ſwelling taking place in the abſorbing ſyſtem, eſpecially in the glands, ariſing from the abſorption of ſome poiſon, or other irritating matter; and when ſuch ſwellings take place in the groin, they are called buboes, whether from abſorption or not, but are moſt commonly ſuppoſed to be venereal, even although there has been no viſible preceding cauſe. This has been ſo much the caſe, that all ſwellings in this part have been ſuſpected to be of this nature; femoral ruptures, and aneuriſms of the femoral artery have been miſtaken for venereal buboes.

I ſhall call every abſceſs in the abſorbing ſyſtem, whether in the veſſels or the glands, ariſing in conſequence of the abſorption of venereal matter, a bubo.

This matter when abſorbed from either of the four different ſurfaces, which are common ſurfaces, wounds, inflamed ſurfaces, and ulcers, is carried along the abſorbent veſſels to the common circulation, and in it's paſſage often produces the ſpecific inflammation in theſe veſſels; the conſequence of which is the formation of buboes, which are venereal abſceſſes, exactly ſimilar in their nature and effects to a chancre; the only difference being in ſize. As the abſorbents with the glands are immediately irritated by the ſame ſpecific matter which has undergone no change in it's paſſage, the conſequent inflammation muſt therefore have the ſame ſpecific quality, and the matter ſecreted in them be venereal.*

As this ſyſtem of veſſels may be divided into two claſſes, the veſſels themſelves, and their ramifications and convolutions, called the lymphatic glands, I ſhall follow the ſame diviſion in treating of their inflammations.

Inflammation of the veſſels is not nearly ſo frequent as that of the glands. In men ſuch inflammations in conſequence of chancres upon the glans or prepuce generally appear like a chord leading along the back of the penis from the chancres. Sometimes they ariſe from the thickening of the prepuce in gonorrhœas, that part in ſuch caſes being generally in a ſtate of excoriation, as was deſcribed when on that form of the diſeaſe. Theſe chords often terminate inſenſibly on the penis, near it's root, or near the pubes; at other times they extend further, paſſing to a lymphatic gland in the groin: this chord can be eaſily pinched up between the finger and thumb, and it often gives a thickneſs to the prepuce, making it ſo ſtiff at this part as to make the inverſion of it difficult, if not impoſſible, producing a kind of phymoſis.

I think I have obſerved this appearance to ariſe as frequently from the gonorrhœa, when attended with the before mentioned inflammation and tumefaction of the prepuce, as from chancres; which if my obſervation is juſt, is not eaſily accounted for. I have obſerved that abſorption is more common to ulcers than inflamed ſurfaces; or at leaſt the formation of a bubo in the gland, and it's effects in the conſtitution, are more common from an ulcer; but it may be remarked, that the inſide of the prepuce, from whence this chord appears to ariſe, is in an excoriated ſtate. It is poſſible that this

* I do not know how far this reaſoning will hold good in all caſes of poiſons, for I very much ſuſpect that the bubo that is ſometimes formed in conſequence of inoculation of the ſmallpox does not produce variolus matter; the natural poiſons in producing buboes certainly do not form a poiſon ſimilar to themſelves.

effect

effect may arise from the lymphatics sympathising with the inflammation of the urethra; but I believe the affection is truly venereal; or it is possible that even the absorption of the coagulable lymph which was produced from the venereal inflammation, and which is the cause of the tumefaction, may have the power of contamination, as appears to be the case in the cancer.

The thickening, or the formation of this hard chord, probably arises from the thickening of the coats of the absorbents, joined with the extravasation of coagulable lymph, thrown in upon it's inner surface, as in inflamed veins.

This chord often inflames so much as to suppurate, and sometimes in more places than one, forming one, two, or three buboes, or small abscesses in the body of the penis. When this is going on, we find in some parts of this chord a circumscribed hardness, then suppuration takes place in the centre, the skin begins to inflame, the matter comes nearer to it, and the abscess opens like any other abscess.

I have seen a chain of these buboes, or little abscesses along the upper part of the penis through it's whole length.

This may be supposed to be exactly similar to the inflammation and suppuration of a vein after being wounded and exposed.

Inflammation of the glands is much more frequent than the former, and arises from the venereal matter being carried on to the lymphatic glands; the structure of which appears to be no more than the ramifications and reunion of the absorbent vessels, by which means they form these bodies.

From this structure we may reasonably suppose that the fluid absorbed is in some measure detained in these bodies, and thereby has a greater opportunity of communicating the disease to them than to the distinct vessels, where it's course is perhaps more rapid; which may account for the glands being more frequently contaminated.

Swellings of these glands are common to other diseases, and should be carefully distinguished from those that arise from the venereal poison. The first inquiry should be into the cause, to see if there is any venereal complaint at some greater distance from the heart, as chancres on the penis, or any preceding disease on the penis; to learn if mercurial ointment has been at all applied to the legs and thighs of that side; for mercury applied to those parts for the cure of a chancre will sometimes tumefy the glands, which has been

been supposed to be venereal. We should further observe, if there be no preceding disease in the constitution, such as a cold, fever, &c. the progress of the swelling with regard to quickness is also to be attended to, as also to distinguish it from a rupture, lumbar abscess, or aneurism of the crural artery.

Perhaps these bodies are more irritable, or more susceptible of stimuli than the vessels, they are certainly more susceptible of sympathy; however we are not yet sufficiently acquainted with the use of these glands to be able to account satisfactorily for this difference.

It would appear in some cases, that it is some time after the absorption of the venereal matter before it produces it's effects upon the glands; in some it has been six days at least. This could only be known by the chancres being healed six days before the bubo began to appear; and in such cases it is more than probable that the matter had been absorbed a much longer time before, for the last matter of a chancre most probably is not venereal; and indeed it is natural to suppose that the poison may be as long before it produces an action on the parts, when applied in this way, as it is either in the urethra, or in forming a chancre; which I have shown to be sometimes six or seven weeks.

The glands nearest to the origin of the disease are in general the only ones that are attacked, as those in the groin, when the matter has been taken up from the penis in men. In the groin, between the labia and thigh, and the round ligaments, when absorbed from the vulva, in women.

I think there is commonly but one gland at a time that is affected by the absorption of venereal matter, which if so becomes in some sort a distinguishing mark between venereal buboes and other diseases of these bodies.

We never find the lymphatic vessels, or glands, that are second in order, affected; as those along the iliac vessels, or back; and I have also seen when the disease has been contracted by a sore, or cut upon the finger, the bubo come on a little above the bend of the arm, upon the inside of the biceps muscle; and in such where the bubo has come in that part none have formed in the arm-pit, which is the most common place for the glands to be affected by absorption.

But

But this is not universal, although common, for I was informed by a gentleman who contracted the disease in the before mentioned way, that he had buboes both on the inside of the biceps muscle, and in the arm-pit. Another case of this kind I have heard of since; why it is not more common is perhaps not easily explained.

It might be supposed that the matter was weakened, or much diluted by the absorptions from other parts by the time it gets through these nearest ramifications, and therefore has not power to contaminate those which are beyond them; but it is most probable that there are other reasons for this. I once suspected that the nature of the poison was altered in these glands as it passed through them, which was the reason why it did not contaminate the second or third series of glands; and also why it did not affect the constitution in the same way as it did the parts to which it was first applied; but this explanation will not account for the next order of glands to suppurating buboes not being affected by the absorption of venereal matter. It appears to me that the internal situation of the other glands prevents the venereal irritation from taking place in them; and this opinion is strengthened by observing when one of these external glands suppurates and forms a bubo, which is to be considered as a large venereal sore or chancre, that the absorption from it, which must be great, does not contaminate the lymphatics or glands next in order, by the venereal matter going directly through them.

If this be true, then the skin would seem to be the cause of the susceptibility of the absorbents to receive the irritation. Whether the skin has the power inherent in itself, or acquires it from some other circumstance, as air, cold, or sense of touch, is not easily ascertained, but whichever it be, it shows that the venereal matter of itself is not capable of irritating, and that it requires a second principle to compleat it's full effect, that is, a combination of the nature of the poison and the influence of the skin, and that influence must be by sympathy, and therefore weaker than if acting in the same part, that is, the skin itself; which perhaps is the reason why the venereal matter does not always affect those vessels and glands, while it always does the skin, if inserted into it.

The ſituation of buboes ariſing from the venereal diſeaſe in the penis, are in men, in the abſorbent glands of the groin: if a gonorrhœa is the cauſe of a bubo, one groin is not exempted more than the other, both may be affected; but if a bubo ariſes in conſequence of a chancre, then the groin may be generally determined by the ſeat of the chancre; for if the chancre is on one ſide of the penis then the bubo will commonly be on that ſide; however this is not univerſally the caſe, for I have known inſtances, although but few, where a chancre on one ſide of the prepuce, or penis, has been the cauſe of a bubo on the oppoſite ſide, which if ariſing from that chancre is a proof that the abſorbents either anaſtomoſe, or decuſſate each other. If the chancre be on the frænum, or on the middle of the penis, between the two ſides, then it is uncertain which ſide will be affected.

The ſituation of the glands of the groin is not always the ſame, and therefore the courſe of the abſorbent veſſels will vary accordingly. I have ſeen a venereal bubo which aroſe from a chancre on the penis, a conſiderable way down the thigh; on the contrary I have ſeen it often as high as the lower part of the belly, before Poupart's ligament, and ſometimes near the pubis, all of which three ſituations may lead to ſome variations in the method of cure, therefore it may be proper to attend to them.

As the diſeaſe moſt commonly ariſes from copulation, the ſituations of buboes are generally in the groin; but as no part of the body under certain circumſtances is exempt from this diſeaſe, we find the neareſt external glands between the part of abſorption, and the heart, every where in the body ſhare the ſame fate with thoſe of the groin, eſpecially if external.

CHAPTER

CHAPTER II.

OF BUBOES IN WOMEN.

THE same diseases in the absorbents in consequence of the absorption of the venereal matter, take place in this sex as well as in men. I never saw but one case where the absorbent vessels were diseased; but this is nearly in the same proportion as those I have seen in men, when I consider the proportion the number of the one sex bears to that of the other who apply to me for a cure of the venereal disease in any form. The case was a gonorrhœa with violent itching and soreness when the patient sat or walked; but she had very little pain in making water. When I examined the parts I could see no difference between them and sound parts, excepting that the left labium was swelled, or fuller than the other, and a hard chord passed from the centre of that labium upwards to the os pubis, and passed on to the groin of the same side, and was lost in a gland as high as Poupart's ligament. It was not to be felt but by pressing the parts with some force, and it gave considerable pain upon pressure.

The swelling of the labium appeared to be somewhat similar to the swelling of the prepuce in similar cases in men, so that they would appear to arise from the same cause.

One would naturally suppose that what has been said of this complaint in the lymphatic glands in men, would be wholly applicable to women; and also that nothing peculiar to women could take place; but the seat of absorption is more extensive in this sex, and the course of some of the absorbents is also different, from whence there are three situations of buboes in women, two of which are totally different from those in men, and these I suspect to be in the absorbents.

The third situation of buboes in this sex is similar to that in men, and therefore they may be divided into three, as in men.

When

When buboes arise in women where there is no chancre, it is more difficult to know whether they are venereal or not than in men; for when they arise in men without any local complaint, it is known that no such complaint exists, and therefore the bubo cannot be venereal, excepting by immediate absorption; but in women it is often difficult to know whether there be any infection present or not; and therefore in order to ascertain the nature of the bubo, attention must be paid to it's manner of coming on, progress, and other circumstances.

When chancres are situated forwards, near to the meatus urinarius, nymphæ, clitoris, labia, or mons veneris, then we find that the matter absorbed is carried along one or both of the round ligaments, and the buboes are formed in those ligaments just before they enter the abdomen, without I believe ever going further. These buboes I suspect not to be glandular, but inflamed absorbents; and if so it strengthens the idea that it is only an external part that can be affected in this way.

When the chancres are situated far back, near the perinæum, or in it, the matter absorbed is carried forwards along the angle between the labium and the thigh to the glands in the groin, and often in this course there are formed small buboes in the absorbents, similar to those on the penis in men; and when the effects of the poison do not rest here it often produces a bubo in the groin as in men.

CHAPTER

CHAPTER III.

OF THE INFLAMMATION OF BUBOES, AND THE MARKS THAT DISTINGUISH THEM FROM OTHER SWELLINGS OF THE GLANDS.

THE bubo commonly begins with a ſenſe of pain which leads the patient to examine the part, where a ſmall hard tumor is to be felt.* This increaſes like every other inflammation that has a tendency to ſuppuration; and if not prevented, goes on to ſuppuration and ulceration, the matter coming faſt to the ſkin.

But we find caſes where they are ſlow in their progreſs, which I ſuſpect either ariſes from the inflammatory proceſs being kept back by mercury, or other means; or being retarded by a ſcrofulous tendency, ſuch a diſpoſition in the parts not ſo readily admitting the true venereal action.

At firſt the inflammation is confined to the gland, which is moveable in the cellular membrane; but as it increaſes in ſize, or as the inflammation, and more eſpecially the ſuppuration, advances, which in all caſes produce rather a common effect than a ſpecific, the ſpecific diſtance is exceeded, the ſurrounding cellular membrane becomes more inflamed, and the tumor is more diffuſed. Some become eriſypelatous, by which means they are rendered more diffuſed and œdematous, and do not readily ſuppurate, a circumſtance often attending the eriſypelatous inflammation.

To aſcertain what a diſeaſe is, is the firſt ſtep in the cure; and when two or more cauſes produce ſimilar effects, great attention is neceſſary to

* It muſt be remarked here, that whenever a perſon has either a gonorrhœa or a chancre, he becomes apprehenſive of a bubo; and as there are in the gonorrhœa, and ſometimes in the chancre, ſympathetic ſenſations in or near the groin, they are ſuſpected by the patient to be beginning buboes, and the hand is immediately applied to the part; and if he feels one of the glands, although not in the leaſt increaſed, the ſuſpicions are confirmed from a belief that he has no ſuch parts naturally.

diſtinguiſh one effect from another, ſo as to come at the true cauſe of each.

The glands of the groin from their ſituation are liable to ſuſpicion, for beſides being ſubject to the common diſeaſes, they become expoſed to others by allowing whatever is abſorbed to paſs through them; and as the rout of the venereal poiſon to the conſtitution is principally through them, and being oftner ill from this cauſe than any other, they often are ſuſpected of this diſeaſe without foundation.

To diſtinguiſh with certainty the true venereal bubo from ſwellings of thoſe glands ariſing from other cauſes may be very difficult. We muſt however examine all circumſtances to aſcertain in what the bubo differs from the common diſeaſes of thoſe glands, whether in the groin or elſewhere; in which examination the apparent cauſes are not to be neglected. I have already given the character of the venereal bubo in general terms; but I ſhall now be more particular, as the two are to be contraſted.

The true venereal bubo in conſequence of a chancre is moſt commonly confined to one gland. It keeps nearly it's ſpecific diſtance till ſuppuration has taken place, and then becomes more diffuſed.* It is rapid in it's progreſs from inflammation to ſuppuration and ulceration. The ſuppuration is commonly large for the ſize of the gland, and but one abſceſs. The pain is very acute. The colour of the ſkin where the inflammation attacks is of a florid red.

It may be obſerved, that the buboes in conſequence of the firſt mode of abſorption, viz. where no local diſeaſe had been produced, will always be attended with a greater uncertainty of the nature of the diſeaſe than thoſe attended or preceded by a diſeaſe in the penis; becauſe a ſimple inflammation and ſuppuration of theſe glands is not ſufficient to mark it to be venereal; but as we always have this diſeaſe in view when ſuch parts as the glands of the groin are the ſeat of the diſeaſe, the patient runs but little riſk of not being cured if it ſhould be venereal; but I am afraid that patients have often undergone a mercurial courſe when there has been no occaſion for it.

* It may be obſerved here, that the glands and ſurrounding parts being diſſimilar, inflammation does not ſo readily become diffuſed as when it takes place in a common part.

It

It will perhaps be difficult to find out the ſpecific difference in the diſeaſes themſelves; but I think that ſuch buboes as ariſe without any viſible cauſe are of two kinds, one ſimilar to thoſe ariſing from chancres or gonorrhœa; that is, inflaming and ſuppurating briſkly. Theſe I have always ſuſpected to be venereal; for although there is no proof of there being ſo, yet from theſe circumſtances it is a ſtrong preſumption that they are.

The ſecond are generally preceded and attended with ſlight fever, or the common ſymptoms of a cold, and they are generally indolent and ſlow in their progreſs. If they ſhould be more quick than ordinary, they become more diffuſed than the venereal, and may not be confined to one gland. When very ſlow they give but little ſenſation; but when more quick the ſenſation is more acute, though not ſo ſharp as in thoſe that are venereal; and moſt commonly they do not ſuppurate, but often become ſtationary. When they do ſuppurate it is ſlowly, and often in more glands than one, the inflammation being more diffuſed, and commonly ſmall in proportion to the ſwelling. The matter comes ſlowly to the ſkin, not attended with much pain, and the colour is different from that of the other, being more of the purple. Sometimes the ſuppurations are very conſiderable but not painful.

Now let us ſee what other cauſes there are for the ſwelling of theſe glands beſides venereal infection, to which I have aſcribed one of the modes of ſwelling; for there muſt be other cauſes to account for the other modes of it.

The firſt thing to be attended to is, whether or not there are any venereal complaints; and if not, this becomes a ſtrong preſumptive proof that they may not be venereal, but proceed from ſome unknown cauſe. If the ſwelling is only in one gland, very ſlow in it's progreſs, and gives but little or no pain, it is probably merely ſcrofulous; but if the ſwelling is conſiderable, diffuſed and attended with ſome inflammation and pain, then it is moſt probable that there is a conſtitutional action conſiſting in ſlight fever, the ſymptoms of which are laſſitude, loſs of appetite, want of ſleep, ſmall quick pulſe, and an appearance of approaching hectic. Such ſwellings are ſlow in their cure, and do not ſeem to be affected by mercury, even when very early applied.

A gentleman

A gentleman had all the ſymptoms of a ſlight fever; the pulſe a little quick and hard, loſs of appetite, and of courſe loſs of fleſh; a liſtleſſneſs and a ſallow look. While in this ſtate a ſwelling took place in the glands of one of the groins. He immediately ſent for me becauſe he imagined it to be venereal. From the hiſtory of the caſe I gave it as my firm opinion it was not; in this he had not much faith. The ſwellings were not very painful, and after having acquired a conſiderable ſize they became ſtationary. To pleaſe him I gave him a box of mercurial ointment to be rubbed on the leg and thigh only, of the ſide affected, that it might have a ſufficient local effect, and as little go into the conſtitution as poſſible; but it did not appear to be of any ſervice to the ſwellings in the groin, they remaining ſtationary, and almoſt without pain. His friends became uneaſy, and ſent their ſurgeons to him, who without knowing he was my patient, and of courſe without knowing my opinion, imagined that the diſeaſe was venereal, as they talked of giving mercury. With reſpect to the cure, I thought he ſhould go to the ſea and bathe.

Allowing the chance of the diſeaſe being venereal or not venereal, to be equal, I reaſoned upon that ground. His preſent want of health could not be ſuppoſed to ariſe from any venereal cauſe as it was prior to the ſwelling in the groin, and therefore though the ſwelling was venereal, he was not at preſent in a condition to take mercury, as a ſufficient quantity of that medicine for the cure would kill him; and if it ſhould not be venereal, that ſtill a greater quantity of mercury muſt be given than what was neceſſary if it was venereal; becauſe it's not giving way readily would naturally make the ſurgeon puſh the mercury further; and beſides this diſagreeable circumſtance, the diſeaſe in the groin might be rendered more difficult of cure. But if he went to the ſea his conſtitution would be reſtored; and if the diſeaſe in the groin proved to be venereal, he would be in a proper condition to go through a mercurial courſe, and by that means get rid of both diſeaſes by the two methods. But if I ſhould be right in my opinion, that there was nothing venereal in the caſe, then he would get well by the ſea-bathing alone.

Theſe arguments had the deſired effect, he went directly to the ſea, and began to recover almoſt immediately. About a fortnight after a ſmall ſup-

puration

puration took place in one of the glands, I directed a poultice should be made with sea-water and applied, and if it broke that it should not be further opened, but poulticed till healed. In six weeks he came back perfectly recovered in every respect.

The above appearance, with the constitutional affections, I have seen take place when there were chancres, and I have been puzzled to determine whether it was sympathetic, from a derangement of the constitution, or from the absorption of matter.

I have long suspected a mixed case, and I am now certain that such exists. I have seen cases where the venereal matter, like a cold or fever, has only irritated the glands to disease, producing in them scrofula, to which they were predisposed.

In such cases the swellings commonly arise slowly, give but little pain, and seem to be rather hastened in their progress if mercury is given to destroy the venereal disposition. Some come to suppuration while under this resolving course; and others which probably had a venereal taint at first, become so indolent that mercury has no effect upon them, and in the end get well either of themselves or by other means, which I imagine may have induced some to think that buboes are never venereal. Such cases require great attention to be able to determine them properly; and I believe this requires in many cases so nice a judgment that we shall be often liable to mistakes.

Buboes are undoubtedly local complaints, as has been explained.

How far the lymphatic glands are to be considered as guards against the further progress of this or any other disease caught by absorption is not easily determined; we must however allow that they cannot prevent the poison from getting into the constitution in cases where it produces buboes; for whenever it affects these glands in it's course it produces the same disease in them which is capable of furnishing the constitution with an increased quantity of the same kind of poison.

CHAPTER IV.

GENERAL REFLECTIONS ON THE CURE OF BUBOES.

FROM what has been ſaid upon the hiſtory of buboes it will be needleſs here to enter into a diſcuſſion of the opinion of their being a depoſit from the conſtitution, and of the concluſion drawn from this opinion, that they ought not to be diſperſed; for according to this theory, to diſperſe them would be to throw the venereal matter upon the conſtitution. But if this were really the caſe then there would be no occaſion for the uſe of mercury, provided that the bubo be allowed to proceed, as it would prove it's own cure; but even thoſe who were of this opinion were not ſatisfied with the cure which they ſuppoſed nature had pointed out, but gave mercury and in very large quantities. From the ſame hiſtory of a bubo I have alſo endeavoured to ſhow that there are ſeveral buboes which are not in the leaſt venereal, but ſcroſulous; and that there are alſo buboes which appear to be only in part venereal; or perhaps only a gland diſpoſed to ſcrofula brought into action by the venereal irritation, ſimilar to what happens often from the matter of the ſmallpox in inoculation. Therefore prior to the method of cure the true venereal bubo is to be diſtinguiſhed from the others if poſſible. When it is well aſcertained to be venereal, reſolution is certainly to be attempted if the bubo be in a ſtate of inflammation only. The propriety of the attempt depends upon the progreſs the diſeaſe has made. If it be very large, and ſuppuration appears to be near at hand, it is probable that reſolution cannot be effected; and if ſuppuration has taken place, I ſhould very much doubt the probability of ſucceſs, and an attempt might now poſſibly only retard the ſuppuration, and protract the cure.

The reſolution of thoſe inflammations depends principally upon mercury, and almoſt abſolutely upon the quantity that can be made to paſs through them;

them; and the cure of them, if allowed to come to suppuration, depends upon the same circumstances. The quantity of mercury that can be made to pass through a bubo, depends principally upon the quantity of external surface for absorption beyond the bubo.

Mercury is to be applied in the most advantageous manner, that is, to those surfaces by an absorption from which it may pass through the diseased gland; for by destroying the disease there the constitution has less chance of being contaminated. The powers of mercury may often be increased from the manner in which it is applied. In the cure of buboes it should always be made to pass into the constitution by the same way through which the habit received the poison; and therefore to effect this, it must be applied to the mouths of those lymphatics which pass through the diseased part, and which will always be placed on a surface beyond the disease.

But the situation of many buboes is such as not to have much surface beyond them, and thereby not to allow of a sufficient quantity of mercury being taken in in this way; as for instance, those buboes on the body of the penis arising from chancres on the glans or prepuce.

These two surfaces are not sufficient to take in the necessary quantity to cure those buboes in it's passage through them; therefore whenever the first symptoms of a bubo appear, it's situation is well to be considered, with a view to determine if there be a sufficient surface to effect a cure, without having recourse to other means. It is first to be observed, whether the absorbent vessels on the body of the penis are affected, or the glands in the groin. If the disease be in the groin, it must be observed in which of the three situations of the bubo before taken notice of, it is; whether on the upper part of the thigh and groin, on the lower part of the belly before Poupart's ligament, or near to the pubes. If they are on the body of the penis this shows that the absorbents leading directly from the surface of absorption are themselves diseased. If in the groin, and on the upper part of the thigh, or perhaps a little lower down than what is commonly called the groin, then we may suppose it is in the glands common to the penis and thigh. If high up, or on the lower part of the belly, before Poupart's ligament, then it is to be supposed that those absorbents that arise from about the groin, lower part of the belly and pubes, pass through the bubo; and if far forwards,

forwards, then it is most probable that only the absorbents of the penis and skin about the pubes pass that way. The knowledge of these situations is very necessary for the application of mercury for the cure by resolution, and for the cure after suppuration has taken place.

The propriety of this prctice must appear at once, when we consider that the medicine cannot pass to the common circulation without going through the diseased parts; and it must promote the cure in it's passage through them; while at the same time it prevents the matter which has already passed, and is still continuing to pass into the constitution from acting there, so that the bubo is cured and the constitution preserved.

But this practice alone is not always sufficient, there are many cases which mercury by itself cannot cure. Mercury can only cure the specific disposition of the inflammation; and we know that this disease is often attended with other kinds of inflammation besides the venereal.

Sometimes the common inflammation is carried to a great height, at other times the inflammation is erisypelatous, and I suspect often scrofulous. We must therefore have recourse to other methods.

Where the inflammation rises very high, bleeding, purging, and fomenting, are generally recommended. These will certainly lessen the active power of the vessels, and render the inflammation more languid, but they can never lessen the specific effects of this poison, which were the first cause, and are still in some degree the support of the inflammation. Their effects are only secondary; and if they reduce the inflammation within the bounds of the specific, it is all the service they can perform. If the Inflammation be of the erisypelatous kind, perhaps bark is the best medicine that can be given; or if it be suspected to be scrofulous, hemlock, and poultices made with sea-water may be of service.

Vomits have been of service in resolving buboes, even after matter has been formed in them, and after they have been nearly ready to burst; this acts upon the principle of one irritation destroying another; and the act of sickness and vomiting perhaps gives a disposition for absorption. A remarkable instance of this kind happened in an officer who had a bubo at Lisbon. It came to fair suppuration, and was almost ready to burst. The skin was thin and inflamed, and a plain fluctuation felt. I intended opening it, but as he was going on board a ſhip for England on the day following, I thought it better to defer it till then. When he went on board, he ſet ſail immediately, and the wind blew ſo very hard that nothing could be done for ſome days, all which time he was very ſick, and vomited a good deal; when the ſickneſs went off, he found the bubo was entirely gone, and it never afterwards appeared. When he came to England, he went through a regular courſe of mercury.

I. OF RESOLUTION OF THE INFLAMMATION OF THE ABSORBENTS ON THE PENIS.

THE ſurface beyond the ſeat of the diſeaſe in this caſe, that is all that part of the penis before the bubo, is not large enough to take in a quantity of mercury ſufficient to prevent the effects of abſorption, and therefore recourſe is to be had to other means; yet this application ſhould by no means be neglected, and this ſurface, ſmall as it is, ſhould be conſtantly covered with mercurial ointment, which will aſſiſt in the cure of the local diſeaſe. It may be diſputed whether any medicine can paſs through diſeaſed lymphatics, ſo as to have any effect upon them, but from experience it certainly can. As this ſurface is too ſmall, and as it is neceſſary that a larger quantity ſhould be taken in, it becomes proper to give it either by the mouth, or by friction on ſome larger ſurface; this is neceſſary to prevent the lues venerea, as well as to cure the parts themſelves. The quantity cannot be determined, that muſt be left to the ſurgeon, who muſt be directed by the appearances of the original complaint, and the readineſs with which they give way.

The ſame method is to be followed in women; but as there is a larger ſurface in this ſex, more mercury may poſſibly be abſorbed; and there ſhould be a conſtant application of ointment to the inſide, and outſide of the labia.

II. OF THE RESOLUTION OF BUBOES IN THE GROIN.

The inflammation of the glands is to be treated exactly upon the ſame principle with the other; but we have in general a larger ſurface of abſorption, ſo that we can make a greater quantity of mercury paſs through the diſeaſed parts.

It will be proper to apply the mercury according to the ſituation of the inflamed gland. If the bubo be in the groin, according to our firſt ſituation, then it is neceſſary to rub the mercurial ointment upon the thigh. This ſurface will in general abſorb as much mercury as will be ſufficient to reſolve the bubo, and to preſerve the conſtitution from being contaminated by the poiſon that may get into it; but if reſolution does not readily take place, then the ſurface of friction may be increaſed, by rubbing the ointment upon the leg.

But if the bubo be on the lower part of the belly, that is, in the ſecond ſituation, then the ointment ſhould be rubbed alſo upon the penis, ſcrotum, and belly; and the ſame, if the bubo ſhould be ſtill further forwards; for probably thoſe glands receive the lymphatics from all the ſurfaces mentioned, as well as from the thigh and leg.

The length of time the frictions ſhould be continued, muſt be according to circumſtances. If the bubo gives way, they muſt be continued till it has entirely ſubſided, and perhaps longer, on account of the cauſe of it, a chancre, which may not yield ſo ſoon as the bubo. If it ſtill goes on to ſuppuration, the frictions may, or may not be continued; for I do not know for certain if any thing is to be gained by their continuance in this ſtate.

The quantity here recommended may affect the mouth, and it muſt alſo be regulated accordingly.

III. OF

III. OF THE RESOLUTION OF BUBOES IN WOMEN.

When on the seat of buboes in women I observed that of the different situations when arising from the parts of generation in this sex, two were peculiar to them, the others similar to those in men.

In the treatment of buboes in women some attention should be paid to their situation, for on that depends in some degree the method of resolution and cure when they suppurate. The first was in the round ligament, the second between the labium and thigh, and the third in the groin.

In the first and second situations the surface of absorption beyond the bubo is by much too small to be depended upon for throwing in a sufficient quantity of mercury to produce resolution, especially in the first situation; but in the second, that is, between the labia and thigh, the mercury may be rubbed in all about the anus and buttock, as all the absorbents of those parts probably pass that way; we know at least that they do not pass into the pelvis by the anus, but go by the groin. Other means of introducing mercury must be recurred to, as is recommended in men; but still it will be proper to rub in on these surfaces as much as possible.

In the situations common to both sexes, we have a larger field, yet as they are divisible into three, the same observations hold good, and a similar mode of practice is to be followed in women as in men.

IV. OF BUBOES IN OTHER PARTS.

As venereal buboes arise from other modes of application of the poison besides coition, they are to be found in different parts of the body; but the hands appear to be the next in order of frequency. They arise in the armpit from wounds in the hands or fingers being contaminated by venereal matter, and reduced to a chancre. In such cases it becomes necessary that the ointment should be rubbed on the arm and fore-arm; but this surface may

may not be sufficient, therefore we must apply it in another way, or to other parts, to produce it's effects upon the constitution.

I have seen a true venereal chancre on the middle of the lower lip produce a bubo on each side of the neck under the lower jaw, just upon the maxillary gland. By applying strong mercurial ointment to the under lip, chin, and swellings, they were resolved.

V. OF THE QUANTITY OF MERCURY NECESSARY FOR THE RESOLUTION OF A BUBO.

THE quantity of mercury necessary for the resolution of a bubo must be proportioned to the obstinacy of the bubo, stopping short of certain effects upon the constitution. If it be in the first situation, and yields readily upon rubbing in half a dram of mercurial ointment made of equal parts of quicksilver and hogs lard every night, and the mouth does not become sore, or at most only tender, then pursuing this course till the gland is reduced to it's natural size will be sufficient, and probably will be a good security for the constitution, provided the chancre, which may have been the cause of the bubo, heals at the same time. If the mouth is not affected in six or eight days, and the gland does not readily resolve, then two scruples, or a dram, may be rubbed in every night; and if there be no amendment, then more must be rubbed in; in short, if the reduction is obstinate the mercury must be pushed as far as can be done without producing a salivation.

If there be a bubo on each side, then there cannot be so much mercury applied locally to each; for the constitution most probably could not bear double the quantity which is necessary for the resolution of one. But in such cases we must not so much mind the soreness of the mouth as when there is but one; however the buboes must be allowed to go on to suppuration, rather than affect the constitution too much by the quantity of mercury; and therefore when there are two they are more likely to suppurate then where there is only one.

In the second and third situation of buboes, if we find that most probably a sufficient quantity of mercury does not pass through them for their resolution,

lution, it may be continued to be thrown in by the leg and thigh to act upon the constitution, as has been already observed. The quantity taken in in this way must be greater than what would be necessary if the whole could be made to pass through the bubo. The mouth must be affected, and that in proportion to the state and progress of the bubo.

This method of resolving buboes occurred to me at Bellisle, in the year 1761, where I had good opportunities of trying it upon the soldiers; and I can say with truth, that only three buboes have suppurated under my care since that time, and two of these were in one person, where a small quantity of mercury had considerable effects on the constitution, and therefore a sufficient quantity could not be sent through the two groins for their resolution; but in both cases the suppurations were small in comparison to what they threatened to be, which I imputed to the mode of treatment.

Many buboes after every attempt remain swelled without either coming to resolution or suppuration, but rather become harder and scirrhous. Such I apprehend were either scrofulous at first, or became so when the venereal disposition was removed. The cure of them should be attempted by hemlock, sea-water poultices, and sea-bathing, as will be further taken notice of.

VI. OF THE TREATMENT OF BUBOES WHEN THEY SUPPURATE.

After every known method has been used, buboes cannot in all cases be resolved, but come to suppuration. They then become more an object of surgery, and are to be treated in some respects like any other abscess. If it be thought proper to open a bubo, it should be allowed to go on thinning the parts as much as possible. The great advantage arising from this is, that these parts having become very thin, lose the disposition to heal, which gives the bottom of the abscess a better chance of healing along with the superficial parts; by this means too, a large opening is avoided, and the different modes made use of for keeping the skin from healing till the bottom is healed, become unnecessary.

 It

It may admit of diſpute, whether the application of mercury ſhould be continued or not through the whole ſuppuration. I ſhould be inclined to continue it, but in a ſmaller quantity; for although the parts cannot ſet about a cure till opened, yet I do imagine that they may be better diſpoſed to it; and I think that I have ſeen caſes where ſuppuration took place although under the above practice, that were very large in their inflammation, but very ſmall in their ſuppuration, which I imputed to their having taken mercury in the before mentioned way, both before and while ſuppuration was going on.

It has been diſputed more in this kind of abſceſs than in others, whether it ſhould be opened or allowed to burſt of itſelf; and likewiſe whether the opening ſhould be made by inciſion or cauſtic.

There appears to be nothing in a venereal abſceſs different from any other to recommend one practice more than another. The ſurgeon ſhould in ſome degree be guided by the patient.

Some patients are afraid of cauſtics, others have a horror of cutting inſtruments; but when it is left wholly to the ſurgeon, and the bubo but ſmall, I ſuppoſe a ſlit with a lancet will be ſufficient; in this way no ſkin is loſt.

But when a bubo is very large, in which caſe there is a large quantity of looſe ſkin, perhaps the cauſtic will anſwer better, both on account of it's deſtroying ſome ſkin, and becauſe the deſtruction is attended with leſs inflammation than what attends inciſion. If done by a cauſtic the lapis ſepticus is the beſt*; but it is not neceſſary to open every bubo, and perhaps it may be difficult to point out thoſe where opening would be of ſervice or neceſſary.

The bubo is to be dreſſed afterwards according to the nature of the diſeaſe, which I have already obſerved is often ſo complicated as to baffle all

* I once opened two buboes in the ſame perſon, one immediately after the other. The firſt was with the lapis infernalis, which gave him conſiderable pain, and therefore he would have the other opened with a lancet, as the pain would only be momentary. But it was ſo great, and the ſoreneſs continued ſo long, while there was no pain in the other deadened by the cauſtic, after it had done it's buſineſs; that next day he ſaid if he was ever obliged to have one opened again it ſhould be with cauſtic.

our ſkill. The conſtitution at the ſame time is to be attacked with mercury, either by applying it internally or externally; if the mercury is applied externally, it ſhould be applied to that ſide, and beyond where the bubo is, as before directed in treating of the reſolution of buboes, as it may have ſome influence on the diſeaſe in it's paſſing through the part.

Giving mercury in theſe caſes anſwers two purpoſes, it aſſiſts the external applications to cure the buboes, and it prevents the effects of the conſtant abſorption of the venereal matter from the ſore.

How far it is neceſſary to purſue the mercurial courſe with a view to prevention it is not poſſible to determine, but it may be ſuppoſed that it is neceſſary to give the ſame quantity to prevent a diſeaſe that would cure one that has already taken place. It will be neceſſary to continue the courſe till the bubo is healed, or till it has for ſome time loſt it's venereal appearance; but it may be difficult to aſcertain this laſt fact; therefore we muſt have recourſe to experience, not theory, and continue the courſe in general till the whole is healed, and even longer, eſpecially if the bubo heals very readily; for we find in many caſes that the conſtitution ſhall be ſtill tainted after all; however ſome reſtrictions are to be made here, for I have already obſerved, that it often happens that buboes aſſume other diſpoſitions beſides the venereal, which mercury cannot cure, but will even make worſe. It is therefore very neceſſary to aſcertain the diſtinction; which will be taken notice of.

The treatment of buboes in women, when they ſuppurate, is the ſame with thoſe of men.

CHAPTER

CHAPTER V.

OF SOME OF THE CONSEQUENCES OF BUBOES.

I Formerly obferved that the venereal difeafe was capable of bringing latent difpofitions or fufceptibilities into action. This is remarkably the cafe with buboes, and I believe the difpofition is more of the fcrofulous kind than any other; whether this arifes from the buboes being formed in lymphatic glands, or not, is probably not eafily determined.

It fometimes happens that thefe fores when lofing, or entirely deprived of the venereal difpofition, form into a fore of another kind, and moft probably of various kinds. How far it is a difeafe arifing from a venereal taint, and the effects of a mercurial courfe jointly, is not certain, but moft probably thefe two have fome fhare in forming the difeafe. If this idea of it were juft, it would become a fpecific difeafe and be reduceable to one method of cure; but I fhould fufpect that either the conftitution or the part hath fome, if not the principal fhare in it; that is, the parts fall into a peculiar difeafe independent of the conftitutional difeafe or method of cure; for if it arofe out of the two firft entirely, we might expect to meet with it oftner. So far as the conftitution or the part has a fhare in forming this difeafe, it becomes more uncertain what the difeafe is, becaufe it muft in fome degree partake of the conftitution or nature of the part. I am apt to fufpect fomething fcrofulous in them, efpecially as they are difeafes of the lymphatic glands.

Such difeafes make the cure of the venereal much more uncertain, becaufe when the fore becomes ftationary, or the mercury begins to difagree, we are ready to fufpect that the virus is gone, but this is not always the cafe; the virus is perhaps only lefs powerful than the new formed difeafe, and as it were lies dormant, or ceafes to act, and when the other becomes weaker, the venereal begins to fhow itfelf again.

The

The treatment in ſuch caſes is to attack the predominant diſeaſe, but ſtill the difficulty is to find out the diſeaſe, and when it is or is not venereal. The following caſe explains this difficulty very well.

A gentleman had a very large venereal bubo: it was opened; he took a great deal of mercury for about two months, but I ſuſpect not in ſufficient doſes, which produced a mercurial habit; the bubo had no diſpoſition to heal, and he came to me. From the account he gave me, I ſuſpected that he had then too much of a mercurial habit to receive at this time any further good from that medicine, I therefore adviſed him to uſe a good nouriſhing diet for near a month; after that I put him upon a briſk mercurial courſe by friction, and the parts put on a better appearance. This courſe he continued for near two months, and then the ſore, although much mended, began to be ſtationary. I did now conceive that the venereal action was deſtroyed, and therefore immediately left off the mercurial courſe and put him upon a milk diet, and ſent him into the country. But not gaining much ground, he had a ſtrong decoction of the ſarſaparilla with mezereon given him, which although continued for above a month produced little or no effect. I alſo gave him the cicuta as much as he could bear, with the bark almoſt the whole time, without effect; new ſinuſes formed which were opened, and the ſore became extremely irritable, with thickened lips. The dreſſings were poultices made with the juice of hemlock, ſea-water, opium, and a gentle ſolution of lunar cauſtic; but nothing ſeemed to affect it. I ſuſpected ſomething ſcrofulous, therefore propoſed he ſhould go and bathe in the ſea, but this then could not be done. Theſe different treatments after mercury had been left off took up about four months without the leaſt benefit. Being doubtful whether there might not be ſtill ſomething venereal in the ſore, eſpecially as appearances were growing worſe, and it was now four months ſince he had taken any mercury, I was inclined to try it once more, and ſent him two portions of ointment, half an ounce each, to rub in in two nights. He had caught a little cold, and therefore did not rub in the mercury the two evenings as ordered; and called upon me the third day and told me he was much better; the ſore now became eaſy, the watry or tranſparent inflammation began to ſubſide, the lips became flatter and thinner, and the edges of the ſore began to heal.

4 C I then

I then desired him not to rub in the ointment, but wait a little. In eight or ten days the sore had contracted to three quarters of it's former size, and had all the appearance of a healing sore.

Quere: What conclusions should we draw from this case? I think the following; that the virus may be gone although the sore has no disposition to heal, therefore we are not to look upon the not healing of a bubo as a sign of the presence of the original disease. Secondly; that the sarsaparilla, mezereon, cicuta, and the bark, will not do in all such cases; and thirdly, that some of these diseases are capable of wearing out the unhealthy disposition of themselves, and that we should not be too ready to attribute cures to our treatment; for if the mercury had been rubbed in, and the same effects had still taken place, I should then have certainly pursued the mercury with vigor, and attributed the cure to it; but I should not have rested here, I should have related the case as an instance of the disease continuing after repeated courses of mercury, and that it was necessary in such cases where the mercury appeared to lose it's power, and even do harm, to wait, and season the constitution to strength and the loss of the mercurial habit; and that even four months was sometimes necessary for this purpose, after which we must begin again to give mercury.

A gentleman had a common gonorrhoea which was severe, I gave him an injection of a grain of corrosive sublimate in eight ounces of water, with a few mercurial pills. After having continued the injection for ten, or twelve days without any visible benefit, I gave it as my opinion that it would be of no service to continue it any longer, and therefore desired he would be quiet for a little time. About this time a swelling in each groin took place, and supposing them to be venereal, I ordered mercurial ointment to be rubbed into both the legs and thighs to resolve them if possible. He appeared to be less uneasy about the buboes than he was about the gonorrhoea; but I told him that the cure of that complaint would be insensibly involved in the resolution of the buboes. I spoke too confidently of my powers of the resolution of the buboes, for they both suppurated; although the suppuration was small in comparison to the magnitude of the buboes when they first inflamed. The frictions were left off.

While

While we were attempting to refolve the buboes he got well of the gonorrhœa. The fkin covering the buboes became thin, they were both opened, one with a cauftic, the other with a lancet; when opened, he was ordered to rub in mercury again on the thighs and legs for their cure. They began foon to look well, and to clofe faft, but when about half healed they became ftationary. I fufpected that a new difeafe was forming. On continuing the frictions a little longer they began to inflame and fwell anew, and a fuppuration took place about half an inch above each of the firft fuppurations, which broke into the firft. I left off the mercury immediately upon their inflaming, and faid that now a new difeafe had formed. I ordered poultices made with fea-water to be applied, and alfo a decoction of farfaparilla to be taken, but this appeared not to be fufficient for the cure of this new difeafe. I then ordered him to the fea, and to go into the tepid fea-bath every evening, the heat of the water to be about ninety degrees. By the time he had been in the bath four times, the inflammation and fwelling had very much abated, and the firft fores, or original buboes, were beginning to heal. He went on with the bathing every evening for about three weeks, when the fores rather began to look worfe; I then fufpected that the venereal difpofition was become predominant, and I ordered him to rub in as before, which he did, and in about a fortnight the firft buboes healed, but the fecond fuppurations were not yet healed; then I fuppofed it to be entirely the new formed difeafe, and he went into the country, where I defired he might go into the open fea every day, as he then could have an opportunity, which he did, and got perfectly well, and has continued fo.

This cafe plainly fhows that there was another difpofition formed befides the venereal, and which was put into action by the venereal irritation, which I fufpect was of a fcrofulous kind, and probably not truly fuch.

I have feen fome buboes moft exceedingly painful and tender to almoft every thing that touched them, and the more mild the dreffings that were applied, the more painful the parts became.

In fome the fkin feems only to take on the difeafe. Ulceration going on in the furrounding fkin, while a new fkin forms in the centre and keeps pace with the ulceration, forming an irregular fore like a worm-eaten groove all round. This like the erifypelatous inflammation, as alfo fome others, appears

pears to have only the power of contaminating the parts that have not yet come into action; and those that have already taken it seem to lose the diseased disposition, and heal readily.

In some they spread to an amazing extent, as the following case shows, the circumstances of which are very remarkable.

A young gentleman, aged eighteen years, in consequence of a venereal infection had two buboes, which were both opened. They were treated in the usual manner, and at first put on a favourable appearance; but when they were nearly healed they began to ulcerate at their edges and spread in all directions, rising above the pubes almost to the navel, and descending upon each thigh. His nights became restless, and his general health was affected. A great variety of medicines were tried, particularly mercury in different forms, with little or no effect. Extract of hemlock did more good than any thing else, and was taken in unusual quantities. An ounce was swallowed in the course of the day for some time, which was afterwards increased to an ounce and an half, two ounces, and even two ounces and an half. It produced indistinct vision and blindness, loss of the voice, falling of the lower jaw, a temporary palsy of the extremities, and once or twice a loss of sensation; and notwithstanding he was almost every night in a state, as it were, of complete intoxication from the hemlock; his general health did not suffer, but on the contrary kept pace in it's improvement with the ulcers. They could not however be healed by the hemlock; and among many other things, Æthiops mineral, and Plummer's pill were liberally given, seemingly with advantage. Recourse was had to the hemlock from time to time. A great many different kinds of dressings were made trial of, none of which were found to exceed dry lint. The ulcers were nearly all healed, after having tormented him upwards of three years, when committing some irregularities in diet, and the sores getting worse, he returned to the extract of hemlock, which he had for some time laid aside, and of himself swallowed in the course of the morning ten drams. This quantity was only the half of what he had formerly taken in twenty-four hours, but his constitution had been at that time gradually habituated to the medicine. The ten drams produced great restlessness and anxiety; he dropt insensible from his chair, fell into convulsions, and expired in two hours.

To

To return to the cure of buboes; where they only become ſtationary and appear to have but little diſpoſition to ſpread, which is moſt common; and perhaps a ſinus or two may be found running into them from ſome other gland. I have often ſeen them give way to hemlock, and ſooner than to any thing I am acquainted with, eſpecially if joined to the bark. If the hemlock is applied both internally and externally it anſwers better.

Sarſaparilla is often of ſingular ſervice here, as well as in other caſes ariſing ſeemingly from the ſame cauſe; and I have ſeen ſea-bathing of great ſervice, as alſo ſea-water poultice.

At the Lock Hoſpital they uſe goldrefiners water as an application, which is of ſervice in ſome caſes. Dr. Fordyce recommends the juice of oranges to be drank in large quantities, which I have ſeen good effects from in ſome caſes. The mezereon is in ſome inſtances of ſingular uſe.

PART VI.

CHAPTER I.

OF THE LUES VENEREA.

THE lues venerea, I have already observed, arises in consequence of the poisonous matter being absorbed and carried into the common circulation. This form of the disease, which I have called the constitutional,* would appear to be much more complicated, both in the different ways in which it may be caught, and in it's effects when caught, than either a gonorrhœa or chancre. It generally arises from the local complaints before taken notice of, by the matter being absorbed from them and carried into the constitution. The matter however appears to be capable of being taken into the constitution by simple application, without first having produced either of the before mentioned local effects, as was taken notice of in treating of the formation of the bubo; but this seems to be only when applied to some particular parts of our body, such as may be called a half internal surface, as the glans penis. I think it is probable that it is not capable of being taken in by the absorbents of the sound skin, at least I know of no instance of it; however this is only opinion.

* The term constitutional is perhaps not strictly a proper term; for by constitutional disease strictly, I would understand that in which every part of the body is acting in one way, as in fevers of all kinds, either sympathetic or original; but the venereal poison appears to be only diffused through the circulating fluids, and as it were, to force certain parts of the body to assume the venereal action, which action is perfectly local, and takes place in different parts in regular succession of susceptibilities; there are but few parts therefore acting at the same time; and a person may be constitutionally affected in this way, and yet almost every function going on well.

It

It is likewiſe capable of being taken into the conſtitution by being applied to common ulcers, although not neceſſarily rendering theſe ulcers themſelves venereal; alſo by wounds, as has been obſerved; but I believe always previouſly producing ulceration in the wound.

Many other modes of infection have been ſuppoſed, but I believe erroneouſly; ſuch ſuppoſitions moſt probably having taken their riſe from ignorance or deceit, two great ſources of error in this diſeaſe.

It is moſt likely that contamination takes place about the beginning of the local complaints, eſpecially when from a chancre; for there is in moſt caſes leſs chance of it's happening afterwards, becauſe the patient commonly flies to medicine, which generally becomes a prevention of contamination. For if it could take place through the whole time of the cure, we ſhould have the parts contaminated at different periods, coming into action at different times, each according to it's ſtated time, although in ſimilar parts both in their nature and other circumſtances; but as theſe ſimilar parts do not vary much in their times of coming into action, it is reaſonable to ſuppoſe they were contaminated at or near the ſame time, and therefore that no contamination was taking place in the time of the cure, although we may ſuppoſe abſorption to be going on equally then as at any other time.

In caſes of contamination from a gonorrhœa where no mercury has been taken, we might expect this irregularity in ſimilar ſtructures; but as contamination ſo ſeldom takes place in this way, we have not a chance of great variety from ſuch; however it would be worth while to aſcertain the matter, which from a great many caſes might be done.

Without being very exact in aſcertaining the different proportions in thoſe who have the lues venerea that originates from the three ſeveral modes above deſcribed, I think one may venture to ſay from general practice or experience, that where one contracts it from the firſt cauſe, that is, where no local effects have been produced, an hundred have it from the ſecond, or gonorrhœa; and where one has it from the ſecond, an hundred have it from the third, or chancre; and perhaps not one in five hundred who have connection with venereal women, have it in the firſt way, and not one in an hundred have it from the ſecond; while not one in an hundred would

eſcape

escape having it from the third, if the means of prevention were not made use of in the common method of cure of the chancre.

I. OF THE NATURE OF THE SORES OR ULCERS PROCEEDING FROM THE LUES VENEREA.

In consequence of the blood being contaminated with real venereal pus, it might naturally be supposed that the local effects arising therefrom would be the same with the original which produced them; but from observation and experiment I have reason to believe that they are not.

In considering this subject we may first observe, that local effects from the constitution are all of one species, that is ulcers, let the surface upon which they appear be what it will, whether the throat or common skin, which is not the case in the local application of the matter in gonorrhœa and chancre; for there I observed that it produced effects according to the nature of the surfaces. Now if the matter when in the constitution were to act upon the same specific principles with that which is applied, we should have gonorrhœas when it attacked a canal; sores or chancres when it attacked other surfaces; but it has never been yet known to produce a gonorrhœa from the constitution, though this has indeed been suspected. For some gonorrhœas in which it has not been clear how they were contracted, and which did not easily give way to the common methods of cure, have been supposed to have arisen from the constitution. Whenever the disease affects the mouth and nose, it has always been looked upon as producing a true chancre; yet even here I find that such ulcers in their first appearance are very different from chancres. The true chancre, I observed, produces considerable inflammation, which of course brings on quickly suppuration, attended often with a great deal of pain; but the local effects from the constitution are slow in their progress attended with little inflammation, and are seldom or ever painful, except in particular parts. However this sluggishness in the effects of the poison is more or less according to the nature of the parts which become diseased; for when the tonsils, uvula, or nose are affected, it's progress is rapid, and the sores have more of the chancre in their appearance than when it affects the ſkin; yet I do not think that the inflammation is ſo great in them as in chancres that are ulcerating equally faſt.

It has been ſuppoſed that even all the ſecretions from the contaminated blood could be affected ſo as to produce a like poiſon in them; and as the parts of generation are thrown in the way of receiving it, when freſh contracted, ſo they ſtill lie under the cenſure of having it returned upon them from the conſtitution. Hence it has been ſuppoſed that the teſticles and veſiculæ ſeminales may be affected with the diſeaſe; the ſemen may become venereal, may communicate the diſeaſe to others, and after impregnation may even grow into a pocky child: but all this is without foundation; otherways when a perſon has the lues venerea no ſecreting ſurface could be free from the ſtate of a gonorrhœa, nor could any ſore be other than venereal. Contrary to all which the ſecretions are the ſame as before; and if a ſore is produced by any other means in a ſound part, that ſore is not venereal, nor the matter poiſonous, although formed from the ſame blood.

The ſaliva in the caſe of a mad dog being a natural ſecretion rendered poiſonous, may be brought as an argument in contradiction to this theory; yet it is eaſily accounted for, and might be produced rather as an argument in ſupport of it. In the dog there is an irritation peculiar to the hydrophobia in the ſalivary glands; but the other and natural ſecretions of the ſame dog, are not capable of giving this infection, becauſe they are not ſuſceptible of the hydrophobiacal irritation, and therefore have it not.

The breath and ſweat are ſuppoſed to carry along with them contagion. The milk of the breaſt is ſuppoſed to be capable of containing venereal poiſon, and of affecting the child who ſucks it; but there are ſeveral reaſons which overturn theſe opinions. Firſt, we find that no ſecretion is affected by this poiſon, excepting where the ſecreting organs have been previouſly affected with venereal inflammation or irritation, or it's ſpecific mode of action. Again, if they were contaminated ſo as to produce matter ſimilar to that of an ulcer in the throat, ſuch matter would not be poiſonous, nor poſſeſs a power of communicating the diſeaſe, as will be explained more fully hereafter. Further, true venereal matter, even when taken into the ſtomach, does not affect either the ſtomach or conſtitution, but is digeſted; as was evident in the two following caſes.

A gentleman

A gentleman who had chancres which discharged largely, used to wash the parts with milk in a tea-cup with some lint, and generally let the lint lie in the cup in the milk. A little boy in the house stole the milk and drank it, but whether or not he swallowed the lint was not known. No notice was taken of this by the gentleman either to the family or the boy; and attention unknown to the family was paid to the boy even for years, but nothing happened that could give the least suspicion of it's having affected him either locally in the stomach or constitutionally.

A gentleman had a most violent gonorrhœa in which both the inflammation and the discharge were remarkably great. He had also a chordee which was very troublesome at night when in bed. In order to cool the parts and keep them clean he had a small bason of milk by the bed side, in which, when the chordee was troublesome, he got up and dipped or washed the penis. This operation he frequently repeated in the night. Under such complaints he allowed a young lady to sleep with him. Her custom was to have by the bed side a bason of tea to drink in the morning before she got up; but unfortunately for the lady, she drank one morning the milk instead of the tea. This was not known till she got up, which was five or six hours after. I was sent for directly, and in the mean time she endeavoured to vomit, but could not. When I came I ordered ipecacuanha, which was to be sent for, and which is slow in it's operation. She vomited, but it was more than eight hours after drinking the milk and water, and what came up was nothing but slime, mucus, or water, the milk being digested. I was attentive to what might follow, but nothing uncommon happened, at least for many months.

It is also supposed, that a fœtus in the womb of a pocky mother may be infected and have the disease from her, as it were naturally interwoven with it. This I should doubt very much, both from what may be observed of the secretions, and from finding that even the matter from such constitutional inflammation is not capable of communicating the disease as before mentioned. However, one can conceive the bare possibility of a child being affected in the womb of a pocky mother, not indeed from the disease of the mother, but from a part of the same matter which contaminated the mother and was absorbed by her; and whether irritating her solids to action

or

or not may poſſibly be conveyed to the child, pure as abſorbed; and if ſo it may affect the child exactly in the ſame way it did or might have done the mother. This idea has been carried ſtill further; for it has been ſuppoſed that ſuch a contaminated child could contaminate the breaſts of a clean woman by ſucking her, the poſſibility of which will be conſidered preſently. We may obſerve, that even the blood of a pocky perſon has no power of contaminating, and is not capable of giving the diſeaſe to another even by inoculation; for if it were capable of irritating a ſound ſore to a venereal inflammation, no perſon that had this matter circulating, or had the lues venerea, could eſcape having a venereal ſore whenever he is bled or receives a ſcratch with a pin, the part ſo wounded turning into a chancre. For if venereal matter had been on the point of the lancet, or on the point of the pin, the punctures would have become chancres.

II. OF THE MATTER FROM SORES IN THE LUES VENEREA COMPARED WITH THAT FROM CHANCRES AND BUBOES.

When the matter has got into the conſtitution it from thence produces many local effects on different parts of the body, which are in general a kind of inflammation, or at leaſt an increaſed action occaſioning a ſuppuration of it's own kind; it is ſuppoſed that the matter produced in conſequence of theſe inflammations, ſimilar to the matter from a gonorrhœa or chancre, is alſo venereal and poiſonous. This I believe till now has never been denied; and upon the firſt view of the ſubject one would be inclined to ſuppoſe that it really ſhould be venereal: for firſt the venereal matter is the cauſe; and again the ſame treatment cures both diſeaſes; thus mercury cures both a chancre and a lues venerea; however this is no deciſive proof, as mercury cures many diſeaſes beſides the venereal. On the other hand there are many ſtrong reaſons for believing that the matter is not venereal. There is one curious fact which ſhows it is either not venereal, or if it be, that it is not capable of acting in ſome reſpects on the ſame body or ſame ſtate of conſtitution as that matter does which is produced from a chancre

or

or gonorrhœa. The pus from these latter when absorbed generally produces a bubo, as has been described; but we never find a bubo from the absorption of matter from a pocky sore; for instance, when there is a venereal ulcer in the throat, we have no buboes in the glands of the neck; when there are venereal sores on the arms, or even suppurating nodes on the ulna, there are no swellings of the glands of the arm-pit; although such will take place if fresh venereal matter is applied to a common sore on the arm, hand, or fingers. No swelling takes place in the glands of the groin from either nodes or blotches on the legs and thighs. It may be supposed that there is no absorption going on from such sores; but I think we have no grounds for such supposition. It's mode of irritation, or the action of the parts affected is very different from what happens in the chancre, gonorrhœa or bubo, being hardly attended with inflammation, which in them is generally violent.

It might be supposed that a constitution truly and universally pocky, is not to be affected locally by the same species of matter; but from the following experiments it would appear that matter from a gonorrhœa or chancre is capable of affecting a man locally that is already poxed; and that matter from pocky sores, arising from the constitution, has not that power.

A man had been affected with the venereal disease a long time, and had been several times salivated, but the disease still broke out anew. He was taken into St. George's Hospital, affected with a number of pocky sores; and before I put him under a mercurial course I made the following experiment: I took some matter from one of the sores upon the point of a lancet, and made three small wounds upon the back where the skin was smooth and sound, deep enough to draw blood. I made a wound similar to the other three, with a clean lancet, the four wounds making a quadrangle; but all the wounds healed up and none of them ever appeared after.

This experiment I have repeated more than once, and with the same result; it shows that a pocky person cannot be affected locally with the matter proceeding from the sores produced by the lues venerea. But to see how far real venereal matter was capable of producing chancres on a pocky person, I made the following experiment.

A man who had venereal blotches on many parts of his ſkin, was inoculated in ſound parts with matter from a chancre, and alſo with matter from his own ſores. The wounds impregnated with the matter from the chancres became chancres, but the others healed up. Here then was a venereal conſtitution capable of being affected locally with freſh venereal matter. This experiment I have likewiſe repeated more than once, and always with the ſame effect.

I ordered a perſon at St. George's Hoſpital to be inoculated with the matter taken from a well marked venereal ulcer on the tonſil, and alſo with matter from a gonorrhoea, which produced the ſame effects as in the preceding experiment; that is, the matter from the gonorrhoea produced a chancre, but that from the tonſil had no effect.

A woman, aged twenty-five, came into St. George's Hoſpital, Auguſt 21, 1782, with ſores on her legs, and blotches over her body. Her huſband was a ſoldier. He gave her the venereal diſeaſe, December 1781. Her ſymptoms then were a diſcharge from the vagina, and a ſmall ſwelling of the glands of the groin, which were painful. She had taken ſome pills, ſuppoſed to be mercurial, to the number of thirty. February 1782, about three months after being infected, the diſcharge ſtopped, but the ſwelling, which had been gradually increaſing ever ſince it's firſt appearance, had now ſuppurated. She applied ſome ointment to it which was brought her by her huſband, and in two months it got well, that is, in April 1782. After the bubo got well, a diſcharge from the vagina came on, for which ſhe took more of the ſame pills ſhe had taken before, to the number of thirty. After this time blotches came out over her whole body; ſome of which about her legs, under her arms, and upon her nipples, ulcerated.

Twins, which ſhe bore at eight months, in March 1782, at the time the bubo was healing, had blotches upon them at their birth, and died ſoon after.

Another girl, about two years old, whom ſhe ſuckled, was alſo covered with blotches when ſhe came to the hoſpital.

To aſcertain whether her ſecondary ulcers were infectious, that is, whether the matter of them would have the ſpecific effects of venereal matter, ſhe

was

was inoculated with ſome matter from one of her own ulcers, and with ſome matter from a bubo of another perſon where mercury had not been uſed. This was done, September 18, 1782. September 19, the puncture where ſhe was inoculated with her own matter gave her pain three hours from the time of inoculation, and the day following it inflamed a little. The other had not then inflamed at all.

September 20, both the punctures had ſuppurated and had the appearance of a ſmallpox puſtule; they ſpread conſiderably, and were attended with a good deal of inflammation. That from her own matter healed with common poultices, and ointments without mercury; but the other, although treated in a ſimilar way, continued in the ſame ſtate, attended with much pain and inflammation.

September 22, the child was inoculated with ſome matter from one of it's own ulcers, and with ſome common pus. The punctures both inflamed in a ſmall degree, but neither of them ſuppurated.

The mother and the child went into the ſalivation ward, October 21, 1782; the child took no mercury. It was ſuppoſed that it's gums became a little ſore; and the blotches got well.

During the time that the mother was uſing mercury, the ulcer from inoculation began to get well, and all her venereal ſymptoms diſappeared. What ſhall we ſay to this caſe? Were the blotches venereal? There was every leading circumſtance to make us think ſo, which was ſtrengthened by the method of cure. If they were venereal it ſtrengthens my opinion that the conſtitutional appearances of the diſeaſe do not produce matter of the ſame ſpecies that produced them. If it was not venereal, then it ſhows we have no abſolute rule by which to judge in ſuch caſes.

It has been ſuppoſed and aſſerted from obſervation, that ulcers in the mouths of children from a conſtitutional diſeaſe, which conſtitutional diſeaſe was ſuppoſed to be derived from the parent, produced the ſame diſeaſe upon the nipples of women who had been ſucked by them, giving it as it were at the third hand; that is, the children were contaminated either by their mothers or fathers having the diſeaſe in form of a lues venerea (of which I have endeavoured to ſhow the impoſſibility); the child was the ſecond, and

and the nurfe was the third. If however it were poffible to contaminate once in this way it would be poffible to contaminate for ever.

How far the obfervations upon which the before mentioned opinion is founded have been made with fufficient accuracy to overturn thofe which I made with a view to afcertain the truth, I know not. But from a more accurate inveftigation of fome of thofe cafes which were by moft of the faculty called venereal, they appeared evidently not to be fuch: to fay what they were would lead us into the confideration of other difeafes. The following cafe may leffen our faith in the hiftories of fuch as have been fuppofed to be venereal.

Before I defcribe the cafe I fhall firft mention fome of the circumftances leading to it.

A child was fuppofed to infect it's nurfe with the venereal difeafe. The parents had been married above twelve years when this child was born. The father was a very fond hufband, and the mother one of the mildeft and moft affectionate women that could poffibly exift. The father had a venereal gonorrhœa two years before he married, that is, fourteen years before the birth of the child. About nine months after marriage they had a child, and afterwards a fecond, both of which were extremely healthy at birth, and ftill continue fo. The mother fell into a weakly ftate of health and mifcarried of her third child at the end of five months. The fourth child came at feven months, but was puny, weak, and had hardly any cuticle when born. It was immediately after birth attacked with a violent diforder in the bowels fo as to purge blood. It died in a few days and was opened by me. The whole fkin was almoft one excoriated furface. The inteftines were violently inflamed and thickened.

With her fifth child, from great care, fhe went eighth months, and it was now hoped that fhe might go the full time, and alfo that this child might be more healthy than the former. When fhe was delivered, the child was very thin, but free from any vifible complaint.

Some days after birth it became bliftered in a vaft number of places on it's body, which blifters were filled with a kind of matter, and when they broke they difcharged a thinnifh pus. The infide of the mouth was in the fame condition. Bark was given to the nurfe. Dark in milk was given

to

to the child by the mouth, and it was fomented with decoction of bark; but in about three weeks after birth it died.

Some weeks after the death of the child the nurse's nipple, and the ring round the nipple, inflamed, and sores or ulcers were formed with a circumscribed base.* They were poulticed, but without benefit. She also complained of a sore throat, but the sensation she complained of was so low in the throat that nothing diseased could be seen. A swelling took place in the glands of the arm-pit, but they did not suppurate. She applied to a physician, and from the account she gave he pronounced her disease to be venereal, and that she had given suck to a *foul* child; and ordered ten boxes of mercurial ointment to be rubbed in on her legs and thighs, eight of which had been used when I saw her, and then her mouth was become extremely sore.

These circumstances came to the ears of the family, and an alarm took place. The husband went from surgeon to surgeon, and from physician to physician, to know if it was possible for him to have the disease for fourteen years, and never to have perceived a single symptom of it in all that time: or if it was possible he could get children with the disease now, when the two first were healthy. He also wanted to know, if it was possible for his wife to have caught the disease from him under such circumstances; and also, if she could breed children with this disease, although she herself never had a single symptom of it. If we take all the above mentioned circumstances as facts, it was impossible there could be any thing venereal in the case; but as they could not be absolutely proved to be facts, there remained a doubt in the mind, a something still to be proved.

Now let us see what the result of the case itself says. The nurse's mouth was become extremely sore from the mercury when I first saw her. I desired that Mr. Pott might see her along with me; and it was the opinion of us both, that the sores on the nipple and round it were not venereal; but it was alledged, that as she had taken mercury their not having a venereal appearance now was owing to that cause. The bark was given, as also the sarsaparilla, but the sores did not heal, nor did they get worse; nor did the mouth get better by leaving off the mercury; they both as it were become

* She had but one breast that gave milk.

ſtationary. I ordered the hemlock, but that appeared to have no effect. While this was going on eruptions broke out on the ſkin. The ſkin of the hands and fingers peeled off; the nails of both fingers and toes ſeparated, and ſores formed about their roots, which were all ſuppoſed (by many) to be venereal. But ſome of them appearing while the conſtitution was full of mercury, and others diſappearing without any further uſe of that medicine, I was clear they were not. We ſuſpected that her mode of living was ſuch as contributed greatly to the continuance of her firſt complaint, and gave riſe to the new ones; ſhe looked dejected and ſallow. She was deſired to go into an hoſpital; which ſhe did. As ſoon as ſhe got into a warm bed, and had good wholeſome food ſhe began to mend, and in about five or ſix weeks ſhe had got fat and almoſt well, the ſore only about the root of the nail of the great toe had not healed; but that appeared now to be owing to the root of the nail being detached, therefore acting as an extraneous body. She came out of the hoſpital before this toe had got well, and by returning to her old poor mode of living the ſoreneſs in the mouth returned; however ſhe mended in the end without the uſe of more mercury.

This caſe I ſhall further conſider when on diſeaſes reſembling the venereal.

The following caſe will further prove that we often ſuſpect complaints to be venereal when they really are not.

A gentleman had for ſome time blotches on his ſkin. The face, arms, legs and thighs, were in many places covered with them, and they were in their different ſtages of violence. In this ſituation he applied to me; and I muſt own they had a very ſuſpicious appearance. I aſked him what he ſuppoſed theſe blotches were; he ſaid he ſuppoſed them to be venereal. I aſked him when he had a recent venereal complaint; he told me not for above twelve months. I then aſked him how long he had had the blotches; and the anſwer was, above ſix months. As this was a ſufficient time for making obſervations upon them that might aſcertain better than the mere appearance what they were, I aſked him if any of the blotches that came firſt had diſappeared in that time; and he ſaid many; I deſired to ſee where thoſe had been; and on examining I found only a diſcoloured ſkin, common to the healing of ſuperficial ſores. I then declared to him that they were not venereal, for none would have diſappeared if they had. He now informed

formed me, that he had been taking mercury; and this information obliged me to have recourse to further inquiries; and I therefore asked him, whether while he was taking mercury many of the first got well? The answer was, yes. And was the cure of those imputed to the mercury? The answer was again, yes. I then asked him, if while he was taking the mercury, which appeared to have cured some, did those that now remain, arise? Yes. My next question was, how long had he taken mercury? He said for six months. I then declared they were not venereal, nor ever had been venereal. I asked him, what was now the opinion of his surgeon? He said that his opinion still was, that they were venereal and that he should go on with the mercury. I advised him to take no medicines whatever; to live well, avoiding excess, and to come to me in three weeks; which he did, and then he was perfectly well, only the skin was stained where the blotches had been. He now asked me, what he was next to do? I told him he might go to the sea and bathe for a month. This he did, and returned well and healthy, and has continued so.

III. OF THE LOCAL EFFECTS ARISING FROM THE CONSTITUTION CONSIDERED AS CRITICAL—SYMPTOMATIC FEVER.

How far the eruptions or local effects of this disease arising from the constitution are an effort of nature to clear herself of this disease, is not certain. I observed, that a gonorrhœa might be produced by a general law in the animal œconomy by which it endeavours to relieve itself of the irritation by producing a discharge; and that in chancres a breach is made in the solids for the same purpose, although this purpose is not answered in either; nature not having a provision against this poison. But how far a similar attempt takes place in a lues venerea I do not know; and if it was upon the same principle, the same reason might be expected to be given, why the constitution is not capable of relieving itself in the present instance that was given when treating of the primary affections, because in this as it was in the other, the matter formed might be supposed to be venereal; and therefore

therefore by being absorbed by the very surface which produced it as in a chancre, it might keep up the constitutional disease. If this were really the case it would be very different from many other specific diseases; for the reason why many specific diseases cure themselves, is that the irritation cannot last beyond a stated time; and also that in many, the patient is never susceptible of the same disease a second time, as in the smallpox. If this was not the case, a person once having the smallpox would always have them; for according to one supposition, that absorption of it's own pus keeps up the disease; and according to another, that the irritation never wears itself out, the patient would either never be free, or have them repeated for ever; for his own matter would give the disease a second time, a third time and so on.* But the venereal matter when taken into the constitution produces an irritation which is capable of being continued independent of a continuance of absorption; and the constitution has no power of relief, therefore a lues venerea continues to encrease. This circumstance is perhaps one of the best distinguishing marks of the lues venerea, for in it's ulcers and blotches it is often imitated by other diseases, which not having this property will therefore heal and break out again in some other part; diseases in which this happens show themselves not to be venereal; however we are not to conclude, because they do not heal of themselves and give way only to mercury that therefore they are venereal, although this circumstance joined to others gives a strong presumption of their being such.

When the parts contaminated assume the venereal action, we commonly find fever, restlessness or want of sleep, and often headach; but I believe that these symptoms are rather peculiar to the disease when the second order of parts, the periosteum and bones, come into action, although they are sometimes found of the first. Do these symptoms arise from the local irritations affecting the constitution? And are they merely sympathetic? Whatever the immediate cause may be, they never go off till the local irritations are removed. This fever at first has much the appearance of the rheumatic

* This circumstance alone is a strong proof that people cannot have the smallpox twice, at least at any distance of time between, if they had fair eruptions the first time; for if the constitution was not so altered as not to be susceptible of this irritation a second time, a person would have them immediately upon the going off of the first.

fever;

fever, and after a time it partakes a good deal of the nature of the hectic.

These symptoms often take place independent of or unattended by any local action, and when that is the case it becomes very uncertain what the disease is; for we may observe that in the proof of any point which cannot be made out directly it is the concurrence of circumstances that becomes the proof. Many of these symptoms give way to mercury, which is probably the only concurring circumstance attending this complaint that is a proof of it's being venereal.* It rather however appears to be against this idea that for the most part a much smaller quantity is sufficient for the cure of such symptoms than what is necessary for the cure of local complaints. But if mercury always cured them it would not be very material what they were called. It is worth consideration however, how far the venereal poison when in the constitution does or does not always produce local effects, that it in general does we are certain; but whether it is ever a cause of constitutional symptoms, simply, such as loss of appetite, wasting, debility, want of sleep, and fever, at last becoming hectic, is uncertain; and it is also uncertain if it is ever capable of producing local actions from irritations only without an alteration of the structure of the parts irritated, as cough, secretion from the lungs, purging, headachs, sickness, pains in different parts of the body like rheumatic pains, but not from an alteration of the structure of the part taking place, as beginning nodes. If such effects take place, we must in such a case rely entirely on the history of the disease, and pronounce according to probability. Such complaints come oftner under the management of the physician than the surgeon, to whom I would recommend a particular attention to this.

The fever in consequence of the venereal irritation, like most other fevers, deranges the constitution which thereupon assumes such actions as it has the greatest tendency to. It is capable of producing glandular swellings in many parts of the body, and probably many of the nodes

* Here it is to be understood, that having had the disease in the form of gonorrhœa or chancre is not to be considered as strong evidence.

that arise in the time of this fever may proceed from the fever, and similar to every such effect from whatever cause it does not partake of the disease which produced it, for it is not venereal: it only takes place in constitutions very susceptible of such action where the predisposing cause is strong and probably at seasons most fitted to produce it, only waiting the immediate cause to put them into action, such will and do go away of themselves when the predisposing cause ceases, such as season.

IV. OF THE LOCAL AND CONSTITUTIONAL FORMS OF THE DISEASE NEVER INTERFERING WITH ONE ANOTHER.

I observed when treating of the gonorrhœa and chancre, that they do not interfere when occurring in the same person, the one neither increasing the symptoms, nor retarding the cure of the other. And it may also be observed, that the chancre or gonorrhœa and the constitutional form of the disease meeting in the same person do not interfere with each other, either in their symptoms or cure; therefore a man may have any one of the kinds, and then get another without increasing the first, or having the last increased by the first.

To explain these effects more fully, let me observe, that if a man has a gonorrhœa, and a chancre appears some days after, the chancre does not either increase or diminish the gonorrhœa. Again, if a man has either a gonorrhœa, a chancre, or both, and a lues venerea ensue in consequence of either of these, neither the gonorrhœa nor chancre is affected by it. If a man has a lues venerea and gets either a gonorrhœa, or chancre, or both, neither of them affects the lues venerea, nor are their symptoms the worse. Nor is the cure of either singly, retarded by the presence of the other; for a gonorrhœa is as easily cured when there are chancres, as when there are none, even although the chancres are not attempted to be cured; and a chancre may be cured locally independent of the gonorrhœa. Further, a gonorrhœa, chancre, or both, may be as easily cured, when the constitution is poxed either by them, or previous to their appearance, as when the person is in perfect

perfect health; but the chancre has this advantage, that the constitution cannot be cured without it's being likewise cured.

The gonorrhœa and chancre indeed so far influence one another, as the one can be in some degree a cause of prevention of the other, as has been already observed; but I believe that this circumstance does not assist in the cure of either, yet I could conceive it might, each acting as a derivator to the other, without increasing it's own specific mode of action.

V. OF THE SUPPOSED TERMINATION OF THE LUES VENEREA IN OTHER DISEASES.

THIS disease seldom or ever interferes with other disorders, or runs into, or terminates in any other, although it has been very much accused of doing so; for a termination of one disease in another, as I understand the expression, must always be a cure of the one terminated; but the venereal disease never terminates till the proper remedy is applied, and therefore never can run into any other disease.

That venereal complaints may be the cause of others I think is very probable. I have seen a chancre the immediate cause of an erisypelatous inflammation, but the venereal did not terminate in the erisypelatous inflammation, for if it had the chancre would have been cured; nor was the erisypelatous inflammmation venereal; the chancre only acted here as a common irritator, independent of the specific quality of the disease as a cause. I have known a venereal bubo become a scrofulous sore as soon as the venereal action was destroyed by mercury; this was not a venereal terminating in a scrofulous affection, for in such a view the scrofula must have cured the venereal. The venereal disease would seem only to partake of the nature of such disorders as the constitution was previously disposed to, and may push into action the causes of these disorders. The same observation and mode of reasoning holds equally good with respect to other diseases. The common symptoms however of the lues venerea, though in some degree according to the constitution, are not so much so as either in the chancre, or the gonorrhœa; for the lues venerea is attended with very little

little inflammation, which in general partakes much more of the nature of the constitution than any other diseased action.

VI. OF THE SPECIFIC DISTANCE OF THE VENEREAL INFLAMMATION.

I have already observed, that many specific diseases, as also those arising from poison, have their local effects confined to certain distances, which I have called their local specific distance; and it would appear from observation, that the venereal irritation and inflammation, of whatever kind it may be, is guided by this principle; for it seldom extends far beyond the surface that receives it; the neighbouring part not having a tendency to sympathise, or run easily into this kind of inflammation. This is the reason why we find a gonorrhœa for weeks confined to one spot in the urethra in men, and for months to the vagina in women, not extending farther in either. In chancres also the inflammation is confined to the seat of the sore without becoming so diffused as when from common accidents. As a further proof of this fact, we find it is also confined to the glands of the groin in cases of buboes till matter is formed in them; which matter acts as a common irritator and the specific is in some degree lost, and then the inflammation becomes somewhat more diffused, as happens in common inflammation. We also see that the same thing happens in venereal ulcers when they arise from the constitution; their size is at first but small and they are merely local, but as the disease increases, the size increases, but still they remain circumscribed, not becoming diffused. Perhaps all poisons and specific diseases agree in this property of having their inflammation limited and circumscribed in a manner peculiar to themselves, for we find that the inflammation of the smallpox, measles and chickenpox, is each circumscribed in it's own way. From hence it must appear, that the human body in general is not so susceptible of specific irritations as it is of the common, or what may be called the natural. But we must also consider, that the common inflammation in very healthy constitutions has it's specific distance, although not so determined or circumscribed as is that of the specific in such constitutions, therefore we may reasonably

reasonably suppose, that such healthy constitutions are the furthest in disposition from the inflammatory action; and we may also suppose still more so from the specific. What would appear to strengthen this idea is, that when the constitution is such as readily goes into inflammation, the more readily does the inflammation spread, every part being susceptible of such action; and we find that in many the specific also spreads, although not in so great a degree, from which we may suppose that the specific is always a more confined mode of action. I have suspected that when the body was disposed to increase the inflammation beyond the specific distance, it was of the erisypelatous kind, as was mentioned before, and which is to be attended to in the cure.

VII. OF THE PARTS MOST SUSCEPTIBLE OF THE LUES VENEREA—OF THE TIME AND MANNER IN WHICH THEY ARE AFFECTED—WHAT IS MEANT BY CONTAMINATION, DISPOSITION AND ACTION—SUMMARY OF THE DOCTRINE.

WHEN I assigned the causes for so great a difference in the effects of the same poison upon two different surfaces, as forming the gonorrhœa and chancre, I then said I did not know whether similar surfaces in every part of the body were equally susceptible of this irritation, having but few comparative trials of the direct application of the poison to other parts besides those of generation. But it would appear that some parts of the body are much less susceptible of the lues venerea than others; and not only so, but many parts, so far as we know, are not susceptible of it at all. For we have not yet had every part of the body affected; we have not seen the brain affected, the heart, stomach, liver, kidneys, nor other viscera; although such cases are described in authors. But as there are different orders of parts respecting the times of the disease appearing, and as the person commonly flies to relief upon the first or second appearances, it may be supposed that the whole disease in the parts actually affected is cured before the other parts have had time to come into action, which will therefore be cured under the ſtate of a diſpoſition only, if we can conceive that a cure can take place before parts have come into action. But if the parts viſibly affected are cured while thoſe only diſpoſed are not, and afterwards come into action, they would form a ſecond order reſpecting time; and if theſe again are cured, and other parts under a diſpoſition ſhould come into action, ſuch would form a third order of parts reſpecting time. The lungs have been believed to have been affected with the venereal diſeaſe, both from the circumſtances preceding the complaint, and from the complaint itſelf being cured by mercury; and their being affected when the other viſcera are not, may ariſe from their being in ſome degree an external ſurface, as will be explained hereafter.

It is this form of the diſeaſe therefore that gives us the comparative ſuſceptibility of parts both for diſpoſition and action. For we muſt ſuppoſe that all parts are equally and at once expoſed to the action of the poiſon; but though there may be various degrees of ſuſceptibility, it will be ſufficient for practice to divide them into two, under the following appellations of *firſt in order*, and *ſecond in order*, to which we may add the intermediate.

Whether the parts that are really firſt affected are naturally more eaſily affected by this kind of irritation, or that ſome other circumſtance which belongs to theſe parts is the cauſe, cannot be abſolutely determined; but from conſidering the matter attentively it would appear to be owing to ſomething foreign to the conſtitution, and alſo not depending on the nature of the parts themſelves; for if we take a view of all the parts that are firſt affected by this diſeaſe when ariſing from the conſtitution, which I ſhall ſuppoſe are the parts moſt ſuſceptible of it, we ſhall ſee that in the recent ſtate of the diſeaſe theſe parts are ſubject to one general affection, while there are ſimilar parts of the body not affected by this diſeaſe, and not ſubject to this general affection. Probably the parts ſecond in order may naturally be as ſuſceptible of the irritation as thoſe firſt in order; but not being under the influence of an irritating cauſe they are later in coming into action; and there are alſo probably other cauſes in the nature of the parts themſelves, ſuch as being indolent in all their actions, and of courſe indolent in this, therefore later in coming into action. However it is not univerſally the caſe that the parts which I have called firſt in order are always ſo; on the

the contrary, we find that this order is inverted in fome cafes, although but rarely. We cannot fuppofe that this difference arifes from any active power in the poifon, nor any particular direction of it, but from properties in the parts themfelves; for it may be allowed us to fuppofe, that when this matter has got into the circulation, it acts on all parts of the body with equal force; that is, it is not determined to any one part more than another by any general or particular power in the animal machine; nor is the nature of the poifon fuch as will fall more readily on one part of the body than another, when they are all in fimilar circumftances. That fome parts therefore are more readily affected by it than others, owing to circumftances which are no part of the animal principle, nor of the poifon; and alfo that fome parts of the body have a greater tendency to be irritated by it than others, muft be allowed.

The parts that are affected by this form of the difeafe when in it's early ftage or appearance, which I have called firft in order, are the fkin, tonfils, nofe, throat, infide of the mouth, and fometimes the tongue.* When in it's later ftate, the periofteum, fafciæ, and bones come into action, and thefe I call *fecond in order of parts*. Perhaps the bones come into action from the membrane being affected.

That we may be able to account in fome meafure for thefe fimilar effects as to time in diffimilar parts, fuch as the fkin and the tonfils, two very different kinds of parts, let us confider in what circumftance they agree, and why they are more fufceptible of this irritation than thofe parts that probably are naturally as much fo, although they do not take it on fo readily, fuch as the periofteum, fafciæ, and bones.

The moft remarkable circumftance perhaps to which the external furface is expofed, and to which the internal is not, is cold, or a fucceffion of different degrees of cold. For we may obferve in general, that the atmofphere

* The tongue is very fubject to have ulcers formed on it, efpecially on it's edges. They are feldom very large, nor are they often either very foul or have a hard bafis: thefe are commonly fuppofed to be venereal; but I believe they feldom are. I do not know whether I am, or not, acquainted with the diftinguifhing marks. I never faw but one that I fufpected to be either venereal or cancerous from it's foul look and it's hard bafis. It gave way readily to mercury, therefore I fuppofed it to be venereal.

in

in which we live is colder than the human body* in it's usual temperature, therefore the skin, &c. is continually exposed to a cold greater than what the internal parts are; and we find that all those parts which are most exposed to this, admit of being much more easily affected, or come more readily into action in this disease than the others.

It is certain that cold has very powerful effects on the animal œconomy. It would at least appear to have great powers of disposing the body for receiving the venereal irritation, and going readily on with it.

From this idea we may account for several circumstances respecting this disease; why the mouth, nose and skin are the most frequently affected by it, because they are most susceptible of it from the causes before mentioned, and for the same reason they come more readily into action. If this is a true solution, it also accounts for those second in order; for if the poison has contaminated both the order of parts as to the susceptibility and time of coming into action, it is natural to suppose that those parts that are as it were predisposed by the common causes, and therefore most easily affected, viz. the surfaces that are most exposed shall come first into action; the parts exposed to cold in the next degree, forming the second in order, come next into action, such as bones, periosteum, &c. but even in them it is not in every bone alike, or every part alike in any one bone; for it appears first in those that are in some measure within the power of being affected by sympathy from application of cold to the skin: we find that when the deeper seated parts, or the parts second in order come into action, such as the periosteum or bones, it is first in these that are nearest the external surface of the body, such as the periosteum or bones of the head, the tibia, ulna, bones of the nose, &c. nor does it affect these bones on all sides equally, but first on that side next the external surface. However, it would appear that in the bones there is another cause besides the vicissitudes of weather, why this disease should attack them; for the periosteum of bones, or bones themselves, are not liable to be diseased on all parts in propor-

* It is to be understood that this cannot hold good as an universal principle; it can only take place in the temperate and frigid zone; for in the torrid the heat of the surrounding atmosphere is sometimes greater than that of the human body.

tion to the diſtance from the ſkin, the perioſteum which covers the ankles, or many of the joints being as near the external ſurface as many other parts of the perioſteum or bones that are affected. The nature of the bones themſelves which are covered by that perioſteum are ſomewhat different, they are ſofter in their texture, therefore they would ſeem to be affected in proportion to their nearneſs to the ſkin and hardneſs of the bones jointly; which would incline us to believe that the bones are more eaſily affected, and rather have ſome influence upon the perioſteum in this diſeaſe, than the perioſteum upon them; and this ſuſceptibility in the hard bones would appear to be in proportion to their quantity of earth and expoſure to cold combined.

It may be objected to this theory, that the fore part of the tibia, &c. cannot be really colder than the back part; but then it may be ſuppoſed, that it is not neceſſary that the part ſhould be actually cold, but only within the power of ſympathy. For a part that is not actually cold is capable of being affected from it's ſympathiſing with a cold part in the ſame manner as if actually cold; although perhaps not in ſo great a degree, and therefore requires a longer time to come into action than if it were actually cold. We find for example, that when the ſkin is actually cold, the muſcles underneath are thrown into alternate action, ſo that we tremble, or our teeth chatter with cold, and yet it is poſſible that theſe muſcles may not be colder at this time than any other; although it is moſt probable that they are really colder,* which will aſſiſt the power of ſympathy. So far as cold can affect the actions of parts, ſo far alſo will the ſympathiſing part be affected in proportion as it is nearer to the parts actually cold; therefore the deeper ſeated parts in the venereal diſeaſe are later in coming into action.

The actual cold parts come firſt into action, then thoſe that are leſs ſo, and next thoſe that are neareſt in ſympathy, and ſo on, except the parts firſt in order of ſuſceptibility have been only partially cured, and then their recurrence may correſpond with the action of thoſe that are ſecond in order of ſuſceptibility, and all the parts will come into action together. What would ſeem to ſtrengthen this opinion is, the different effects that ariſe from different climates: in warm climates the diſeaſe ſeldom or ever ariſes to ſuch

* Vide Philoſophical Tranſactions, vol. 68, part I, page 7.

a height as in cold climates; it is more flow in it's progrefs and much more eafy to cure, at leaft if we may give credit to the accounts we have received of the difeafe in fuch climates.

Whether the difference in the time of appearance between the fuperficial and deeper feated parts in warm climates is the fame as in cold ones, I do not know; but from the above theory it fhould not be fo great in the warm as in the cold climates.

Befides the caufes already mentioned, it would appear that there are others by which the lues venerea may be brought fooner into action than it otherways would be if left entirely to the nature of the conftitution; for I think I have feen cafes where fever has brought it into action when the difpofition had been previoufly formed. Like moft other difeafes to which there is a fufceptibility or difpofition, we find that any difturbance in the conftitution fhall call it forth: fcrofula, gout, and rheumatifm are often called forth in this way.

Having faid that the deeper feated parts of the body come into action later than thofe that are fuperficial, I fhall now obferve, that when the lues venerea has been cured fo far as only to remove the firft actions, but not to eradicate the difpofition in the deeper feated parts, as has been explained, under fuch circumftances of the difeafe it never attacks again the external, or the parts that were firft affected, but only the deeper feated parts which are fecond in order of time. The reafon is, that the deeper feated parts had not affumed the action at the time of the cure of the firft. The following cafes, felected from a great number of fimilar ones, will illuftrate the doctrines we have laid down.

In January 1781, A. B. had connection with a woman, and two days after perceived an itching in the glans: at the end of four days he found chancres upon the prepuce. He took about twenty grains of calomel, and then applied to a furgeon, under whofe care he remained three months, that is, till April. He thought himfelf nearly well, and went into the country, taking a few pills with him, and at the end of another month believed himfelf perfectly cured. Three months after, that is in Auguft, by lying in damp fheets he caught cold, and had confiderable fever, for which James's powders were given. Soon after taking that medicine, fpots of a

copper

copper colour appeared upon his legs, and he had violent pains in his shin bones. By the order of a country surgeon he rubbed in about an ounce of mercurial ointment, and had a slight spitting; the pain ceased, the spots disappeared, and in a month he again conceived himself to be well; this was in October 1781. In June 1782, he had the influenza: about a fortnight afterwards his left eye inflamed, and he had a pain in the head, and a noise in his ears. Five days afterwards his throat became sore. Three weeks after the inflammation of his eye several pustules made their appearance near the anus. These symptoms remained till the 21st of August, when he came into St. George's Hospital. He rubbed in strong mercurial ointment till his mouth became sore; he sweated very much; the pain in his head remained, but the complaint in his eye, and about the anus, together with the sore throat, were totally removed.

It would appear that in this case it required some additional power acting upon the body to dispose it more readily to assume the venereal action. That cold has a strong power of this kind we have allowed, which appears in this case to have been the first immediate cause; but a fever appears to have been equally effectual in producing the second return of the symptoms.

Here was the venereal disposition in the constitution from April 1781, the time he was cured of the local complaint, till June 1782, fourteen months after; and then it reappeared eleven months after that, which periods might have been longer if it had not been called forth by the two circumstances of cold and fever.

Let us consider how far this case corresponds with the opinion of the action being easier of cure than the disposition. The first action, that is, the chancres, were perfectly cured by the quantity of mercury he took at first, for they never recurred; but the venereal matter had produced the disposition in the constitution, which was not cured by the same quantity of mercury, for blotches appeared three months after; but all the parts that had taken on the disposition at that time had not then come into action; therefore only the parts which had come into action were cured by the second course of mercury; and the other parts which had not yet taken on the action, went on with the disposition till the influenza (which happened eleven months after) brought them into action. The first class of pocky appearances were perfectly

perfectly cured by the ſecond courſe of mercury, as the local had been cured by the firſt; for they never reappeared, not even with the ſecond. The ſecond ſet of pocky ſymptoms, we have obſerved, appeared to be perfectly cured by the third courſe of mercury. How far there may be a third ſet of pocky ſymptoms to come forth, time can only tell.

This caſe further proves that ſometimes the ſecond ſet of ſymptoms appear firſt, and the firſt ſecond; and alſo ſhews the difference in times between the firſt pocky appearances after the healing of the local, and between the ſecond appearance of the ſymptoms after the healing of the firſt.

A gentleman had a chancre in May 1781: in the ſame month next year, 1782, he had a gonorrhœa; and in May 1783 he had a ſore throat. He had no connection with any woman from September 1782, till May 1783, which was about a fortnight before his throat became ſore, and had had no immediate local complaints.

When I ſaw the throat firſt, I ſaid it was not venereal; and he being rather of a hectic habit, was deſired to go to Briſtol. When at Briſtol, an ulcer appeared at the root of the uvula, which made him immediately come back to London. When I ſaw this ulcer I ſaid it was venereal. He now went through what I ſuppoſed was a ſufficient courſe of mercury, and all the venereal ſymptoms appeared to be cured.[a] He went into the country about the month of Auguſt; and about the beginning of January 1784, viz. four months after the ſuppoſed cure, he felt a pain, together with a ſwelling, in his ſhin bones, for which he went through a courſe of mercury which removed both the pain and the ſwelling.

In this caſe we have every reaſon to ſuppoſe that the diſpoſition had taken place in the bones, or their coverings, from the ſame cauſe that affected the uvula; but the uvula came firſt into action, being of the firſt order of parts. Whether this was really the caſe or not, we muſt allow that in the parts ſecond in order, the diſpoſition, and not the action, did exiſt at the time when the diſeaſe in the uvula came into action, as alſo at the time when he went through a courſe of mercury ſufficient to cure the uvula;

[a] I may remark here, that only the venereal ulcer got well by the mercury, for the former excoriation of the throat continued, but was afterwards cured by bark and ſarſaparilla.

we

we muſt alſo allow that the diſpoſition was not removed by the quantity of mercury which was capable of removing the diſeaſe in the uvula. From all which I would draw the following inferences in confirmation of the preceding doctrine: firſt, that the parts about the throat are capable of aſſuming the action ſooner than the bones. Secondly, it is probable that mercury can cure the action only, and not the diſpoſition; and thirdly, that the venereal pus is not preſent in the circulation while the ſecondary actions take place; for if it were, the parts firſt in order would ſtand an equal chance of being again contaminated, and of coming into action a ſecond time; ſuppoſing the venereal matter ſtill to exiſt in the conſtitution after the parts firſt thrown into action are abſolutely cured, ſo as to contaminate the parts that are ſecond in order of action, we ſhould certainly have the parts firſt in order take on the diſeaſe a ſecond and even a third time, and ſo on, while the ſecond or third in order would be going on and only coming into their firſt action; and therefore we might have thoſe that are firſt in order and thoſe that are ſecond in order in action at the ſame time. This might be carried ſtill further, for as it is poſſible for the parts firſt in order of ſuſceptibility to have the diſeaſe a ſecond time, while the parts ſecond in order are under the influence of the firſt infection, thoſe firſt in order may be contaminated a ſecond time from a new or freſh infection, which would be a lues venerea upon a lues venerea, a caſe which certainly may happen. If the matter does really continue in the conſtitution it would be natural to ſuppoſe that the parts moſt eaſily affected by it would remain ſo as long as the poiſon remained. It may indeed be alledged, that parts which have already been accuſtomed to this irritation and cured, are rendered by that means leſs ſuſceptible of it.

If the poiſon were ſtill capable of circulating after it's viſible effects were cured, then giving mercury in the time of a chancre can be of little ſervice, as it can only aſſiſt in the cure of the chancre, but cannot preſerve the conſtitution from infection, which does not agree with experience; for practice informs us, that not one in fifty would eſcape the lues venerea if the chancre were only cured locally; ſo that mercury has the power of preventing a diſpoſition from forming, and therefore neceſſary to be given while we ſuppoſe abſorption going on, or while there is matter that may be abſorbed.

4 L Mercury,

Mercury, prior to the action, will not remove the disposition, and of course will not hinder the action coming on afterwards; however, it is possible, and most probable, that the medicine while it is present will hinder the action taking place; so that no venereal complaints will take place while under the course of mercury, although the parts may be contaminated.

This is not peculiar to the venereal disease, but common to many others, and in some it may be reversed, for there are diseases whose disposition can be cured, and therefore the action prevented by such medicines as would rather increase the action if given in the time of it.

The parts first affected are more easily cured, according to our present method, than the parts second in order. A part once perfectly cured is never irritated again by the same stock of infection, though probably some other parts in the constitution are still under the venereal irritation. If the facts stated be just, the circumstance of the disease appearing to leave the parts first attacked and attacking the secondary parts is easily accounted for. It is no more than the first parts being cured while the secondary are not, and of course going on with the disease, the first remaining well.

If this mode of accounting for these circumstances be just, it proves two things; first a former assertion, that this disease in the form of lues venerea has not the power of contaminating parts, not already under it's influence, even in the same constitution; secondly, that the venereal poison is not circulating in the blood all the time the disease is going on in the constitution; so that most probably the poison only irritates when just absorbed, and is soon expelled or thrown out in some of the secretions.

The above account of the lues venerea may be reduced to the following heads.

First, that most parts, if not all, that are affected in the lues venerea are affected with the venereal irritation at the same time.

Secondly, the parts exposed to cold are the first that take on the venereal action; then the deeper seated parts, according to their susceptibility for such action.

Thirdly, the venereal disposition when once formed in a part must necessarily go on to form the venereal action.

Fourthly,

Fourthly, that all parts of the body under ſuch diſpoſition do not run into action equally faſt, ſome requiring ſix or eight weeks, others as many months.

Fifthly, in the parts that come firſt into action the diſeaſe goes on increaſing without wearing itſelf out, while thoſe that are ſecond in time follow the ſame courſe.

Sixthly, mercury hinders a diſpoſition from forming, or in other words, prevents contamination.

Seventhly, mercury does not deſtroy a diſpoſition already formed.

Eighthly, mercury hinders the action from taking place although the diſpoſition be formed; and

Ninthly, mercury cures the action.

Theſe principles being eſtabliſhed, the facts reſpecting the cure are eaſily accounted for.

CHAPTER II.

OF THE SYMPTOMS OF THE LUES VENEREA.

WHEN the venereal matter has got into the conſtitution in any of the ways before mentioned, it has the whole body to work upon, and ſhews itſelf in a variety of ſhapes; many of which putting on the appearance of a different diſeaſe we are often obliged to have recourſe to the preceding hiſtory of the caſe before we can form any judgment of it. Probably the varieties in the appearances may be refered to the three following circumſtances; the different kinds of conſtitutions; the different kinds of ſolids affected; and the different diſpoſitions the ſolids are in at the time; for I can eaſily conceive that a peculiarity of conſtitution may make a very material difference in the appearance of the ſame ſpecific complaint; and I am certain that the ſolids according to their different natures produce a very different appearance when attacked with this diſeaſe; and I can alſo eaſily conceive that a different diſpoſition from the common in the ſolids at the time, may make a conſiderable difference in the appearances.

The difference of conſtitution, and of the ſame parts at different times, may have conſiderable effects in the diſeaſe appearing ſooner, or later; this I am certain of, that the different parts of the body produce a very conſiderable difference in the times of appearance of this diſeaſe. That it appears much ſooner in ſome parts than in others is beſt ſeen where different parts are affected in the ſame perſon; for I have already endeavoured to ſhow that it is moſt probable all the parts affected are contaminated nearly at the ſame time. This difference in the times is either owing to ſome parts being naturally put into action more eaſily by the poiſon than others, or that they are naturally more active in themſelves, and therefore probably will take on more quickly the action of every diſeaſe that is capable of affecting them.

When on the general hiſtory of the lues venerea, I divided the parts into two orders, according to the time of their appearance; I alſo obſerved that the

the first were commonly the external parts, as the skin, nose, tonsils; and that the second were more internal, as the bones, periosteum, fasciæ, and tendons.

The time necessary for it's appearance, or for producing it's local effects in the several parts of the body most readily affected after it has got into the constitution is uncertain; but in general it is about six weeks; in many cases however it is much later, and in others much sooner. In some cases it appears to produce it's local effects within a fortnight after the possibility of the absorption of the matter. In one case a gentleman had a chancre, and a swelling in the groin came on, and within the before mentioned time he had venereal eruptions all over the body. He could not impute this to any former complaint, yet there is a possibility of it's having arisen from the first mode of catching the disease, by simple contact, at the time he got the local or chancre, which might extend the time to a week or more, although this is not probable. In another case, three weeks after the healing of a chancre, eruptions broke out all over the body, and this happened only a fortnight after leaving off the course of mercury that cured the chancre. The effects on other parts of the body that are less susceptible of this irritation, or are slower in their action, are of course much later in appearing; and in those cases where both orders of parts are contaminated, it is in general not till after the first has made it's appearance for a considerable time, and even perhaps after it has been cured; for while the parts first in order of action were contaminated and under cure, the second in order are only in a state of contamination, and go on with the disease afterwards, although it may never again appear in the first.

From this circumstance of the parts second in order coming later into action, we can plainly see the reason why it shall appear in them, although the first in order may have been cured; for if the external parts, or first in order, have been cured, and the internal, or second, have not been cured, such as the tendons, bones, periostrum, &c. then it becomes confined solely to these parts. The order of parts may sometimes be inverted, for I have seen cases where the periosteum, or bone, was affected prior to any other part; whether in the same case it might in the end have affected the skin, or throat, I will not pretend to say, as it was not allowed to go on; but it is possible the se-

 cond

cond order of parts may be affected without the first having ever been contaminated.

It's effects upon the deeper seated parts are not like those produced in the external, and the difference is so remarkable as to give the appearance of another disease; and a person accustomed to see it in the first parts only, would be entirely at a loss about the second.

The parts which come first into action go on with it, probably on the same principle, much quicker than what the others do; and this arises from the nature of the parts, as has already been observed.

Each succeeding part that becomes affected is slower and slower in it's progress, and more fixed in it's symptoms when produced; this arises also from the natural disposition of such parts, all their actions being slow, which indolent action may be assisted by the absence of the great disposing cause, that is cold. I should however suspect that warmth did not contribute much to their indolence of action, for if it did it would assist in the cure, which it appears not to do, these parts being as slow in their operations of restoration as they are in their actions of disease. We may also observe, that similar parts come sooner into action, and appear to go on more rapidly with it, as they are nearer the source of the circulation. It appears earlier on the face, head, shoulders, and breast, than on the legs, and the eruptions come sooner to suppuration in the before mentioned parts.*

The circumstance of it's being very late in appearing in some parts, when it had been only cured in it's first appearances, as mentioned, has made many suppose that the poison lurked somewhere in the solids; and others that it kept circulating in the blood for years.

It is not however easy to determine this point, but there can be no good reason for the first hypothesis, as the lurking disposition never takes place prior to it's first appearance; for instance, we never find that a man had a chancre a twelvemonth ago, and that it broke out after in venereal scurfs upon the skin, or ulcers in the throat.. The slowness of it's progress is only when the parts less susceptible of it's irritation have been affected by it.

* Vide Introduction.

I. OF

I. OF THE SYMPTOMS OF THE FIRST STAGE OF THE LUES VENEREA.

The first symptoms of the disease after absorption appear either on the skin, throat, or mouth; these differ from one another according to the nature of the parts affected, therefore I shall divide them into two kinds, although there appears to be no difference in the nature of the disease itself.

The appearance on the skin I shall call the first, although it is not always the first appearance; for that in the throat, is often as early a symptom as any. The appearances upon the skin generally show themselves in every part of the body, no part being more susceptible than another, first in discolourations, making the skin appear mottled, many of them disappearing, whilst others continue, and increase with the disease.*

In others it will come on in distinct blotches, often not observed till scurfs are forming; at other times they appear in small distinct inflammations, containing matter and resembling pimples, but not so pyramidal, nor so red at the base.

Venereal blotches at their first coming out are often attended with inflammation, which gives them a degree of transparency, which I think is generally greater in the summer, than in the winter, especially if the patient be kept warm. In a little time this inflammation disappears, and the cuticle peels off in the form of a scurf. This sometimes misleads the patient, and the surgeon, who look upon this dying away of the inflammation as a decay of the disease, till the succession of scurfs undeceive them.

These discolourations of the cuticle arise from the venereal irritation, and are seldom to be reckoned a true inflammation, for they seldom have any of it's characteristics, such as tumefaction and pain; but this is true only on those parts most exposed; for in parts well covered, and in parts constantly

* This is not peculiar to this disease, it often takes place in the smallpox. It appears as if the skin took on a general disposition for disease, but the specific taking place and remaining, the other eruptions disappear. If this is really the case in the lues venerea, it must be a consequence of fever.

in

in contact with other parts there is more of the true inflammatory appearance, especially about the anus.

The appearance of the parts themselves next begins to alter, forming a copper coloured dry inelastic cuticle, called a scurf; this is thrown off, and new ones are formed. These appearances spread to the breadth of a sixpence or shilling, but seldom broader, at least for a considerable time, every succeeding scurf becoming thicker and thicker, till at last it becomes a common scab, and the disposition for the formation of matter takes place in the cutis under the scab, so that at last it turns out a true ulcer; in which state it commonly spreads, although but slowly.

These appearances arise first from the gradual loss of the true sound cuticle; the diseased cutis having lost the disposition to form one; and as a kind of substitute for this want of cuticle, an exudation takes place forming a scale, and afterwards becoming thicker the matter acquiring more consistence it at last forms a scab; but before it has arrived at this stage the cutis has given way and ulcerated, which continues gradually to change the discharge more and more into a true matter or pus. When it attacks the palms of the hands and the soles of the feet, where the cuticle is thick, a separation of the cuticle takes place, and it peels off, a new one is immediately formed, which also separates, so that a series of new cuticles takes place from it's not so readily forming scurfs as on the common skin. If the disease is confined to those parts it becomes more difficult to determine whether or not it be venereal; for most diseases of the cutis of these parts produce a separation of the cuticle attended with the same appearances in all, and having nothing characteristic of the the venereal disease.

Such appearances are peculiar to that part of the common skin of the body which is usually exposed; but when the skin is opposed by another skin which keeps it in some degree more moist, as between the nates, about the anus, or between the scrotum and the thigh, or in the angle between the two thighs, or upon the prolabium of the mouth, and in the arm-pits, the eruptions never acquire the above described appearances, and instead of scurfs or scabs we have the skin elevated, or as it were tumefied by the extravasated lymph into a white, soft, moist, flat surface, which discharges a white matter. This may perhaps arise from there being more warmth, more

more perſpiration, and leſs evaporation, as well as from the ſkin being thinner in ſuch places. What ſtrengthens this idea ſtill more is, that in many venereal patients I have ſeen an approach towards ſuch appearances on the common ſkin of the body; but then it was on ſuch parts as were covered with the cloaths; for on thoſe parts of the ſkin that were not covered there was only the flat ſcurf: theſe however were redder than the ab c deſcribed appearances, but hardly ſo high.

How far this is peculiar to the venereal diſeaſe I know not, as it may take place in moſt ſcurfy eruptions of the ſkin. From a ſuppoſition of this not being venereal, I have deſtroyed them at the ſide of the anus with cauſtic, and the patient has got well; however, from my idea of the diſeaſe, that every effect from the conſtitution is truly local, and therefore may be cured locally, this treatment having proved a cure does not determine the queſtion.

This diſeaſe on it's firſt appearance often attacks that part of the fingers upon which the nail is formed, making that ſurface red which is ſeen ſhining through the nail, and if allowed to continue a ſeparation of the nail takes place, ſimilar to the cuticle in the before deſcribed ſymptoms; but here there cannot be that regular ſucceſſion of nails as there is of cuticle.

It alſo attacks the ſuperficies of the body which is covered with hair, producing a ſeparation of the hair; a prevention of the growth of young hair is alſo the conſequence while the diſeaſe laſts.

The ſecond part in which it appears is moſt commonly the throat, ſometimes the mouth and tongue. In the throat, tonſils, and inſide of the mouth, the diſeaſe generally ſhows itſelf at once in the form of an ulcer without much previous tumefaction, ſo that the tonſils are not much enlarged; for when the venereal inflammation attacks theſe parts it appears to be always upon the ſurface, and it very ſoon terminates in an ulcer.

Theſe ulcers in the throat are to be well diſtinguiſhed from all others of the ſame parts. It is to be remarked, that this diſeaſe when it attacks the throat, always I believe produces an ulcer; although this is not commonly underſtood; for I have ſeen caſes where no ulceration had taken place, called by miſtake venereal; it is therefore only this ulcer that is to be diſtinguiſhed from other ulcers of theſe parts. This ſpecies of ulcer is generally tolerably well marked, yet it is perhaps in all caſes not to be

 diſtinguiſhed

diſtinguiſhed from others that attack this part, for ſome ſhall have the appearance of being venereal, and what are really venereal ſhall reſemble thoſe that are not. We have ſeveral diſeaſes of this part which do not produce ulceration on the ſurface, one of which is common inflammation of the tonſils, which often ſuppurates in the centre, forming an abſceſs, which burſts by a ſmall opening, but never looks like an ulcer began upon the ſurface as in the true venereal; and this caſe is always attended with too much inflammation, pain, and tumefaction of the parts to be venereal; and if it ſuppurates and burſts it ſubſides directly, and it is attended probably with other inflammatory ſymptoms in the conſtitution.

There is another diſeaſe of theſe parts which is an indolent tumefaction of the tonſils, and is peculiar to many people or conſtitutions, having ſomething of the ſcrofula in them, producing a thickneſs in the ſpeech. Sometimes the coagulable lymph is thrown out on the ſurface, and called by ſome ulcers, by others ſloughs, and ſuch are often called putrid ſore throats. Thoſe commonly ſwell to too large a ſize for the venereal; and this appearance is eaſily diſtinguiſhed from an ulcer or loſs of ſubſtance; however, where it is not plain at firſt ſight it will be right to endeavour to remove ſome of it; and if the ſurface of the tonſil is not ulcerated, then we may be ſure it is not venereal. I have ſeen a chink filled with this, appearing very much like an ulcer; but upon removing the coagulable lymph the tonſil has appeared perfectly ſound. I have ſeen caſes of a ſwelled tonſil where a ſlough formed in it's centre, and that ſlough has opened a paſſage out for itſelf; and when it has been as it were ſticking in this paſſage it has appeared like a foul ulcer.

The moſt puzzling ſtage of the complaint is when the ſlough is come out, for then it has moſt of the characters of the venereal ulcer; but when I have ſeen the diſeaſe in it's firſt ſtages, I have always treated it as of the eriſypelatous kind, or as ſomething of the nature of a carbuncle.

When I have ſeen them in their ſecond ſtage only I have been apt to ſuppoſe them venereal; however, no man will be ſo raſh as to pronounce what a diſeaſe is from the eye only, but will make inquiries into all the circumſtances before he forms a judgment. If there have been no preceding local ſymptoms within the proper date, he will ſuſpend his judgment and wait

wait a little to fee how far nature is able to relieve herfelf. If there has been any preceding fever it will be ftill lefs probable that it is venereal. However, I will not fay of what nature fuch cafes are, but only that they are not venereal, as they are often believed to be. I have feen a fore throat of this kind taken for venereal, and mercury given till it fhould affect the mouth, which when it did it brought on a mortification on all thofe parts concerned in the firft difeafe, fo that the tonfils and the uvula mortified and floughed away. It would therefore appear that this fpecies of the fore throat is aggravated by mercury.

There is another complaint of thofe parts which is often taken for venereal, which is an ulcerous excoriation, where the ulceration or excoriations run along the furface of the parts, becoming very broad and fometimes foul having a regular termination, but never going deep into the fubftance of the parts as the venereal do. There is no part of the infide of the mouth exempted from this ulcerous excoriation; but I think it is moft frequent about the root of the uvula, and fpreads forwards along the palatum molle. That fuch are not venereal is evident from their not giving way in general to mercury; and I have feen them continue for weeks without altering, and a true venereal ulcer appear upon the centre of the excoriated part.

The difference between the two is fo ftrong that there can be no miftake; the patients have gone through a courfe of mercury which has perfectly cured the venereal ulcers, but has had no effect upon the others, which were afterwards cured by bark.

The true venereal ulcer in the throat is perhaps the leaft liable to miftake of any of the forms of the difeafe. It is a fair lofs of fubftance, part being dug out as it were from the body of the tonfil, with a determined edge, and is commonly very foul, having thick white matter adhering to it like a flough, which cannot be wafhed away.

Ulcers in fuch fituations are always kept moift, the matter not being allowed to dry and form fcabs, as in thofe upon the fkin; the matter is carried off the ulcers by deglutition, or the motion of the parts, fo that no fucceffion of fcurfs or fcabs can take place, as on the fkin.

Their progrefs is alfo much more rapid than on the common fkin, ulceration taking place very faft.

Like

Like moſt other ſpreading ulcers they are generally very foul, and for the moſt part have thickened or bordered edges, which is very common to venereal or cancerous ſores, and indeed to moſt ſores which have no diſpoſition to heal, whatever the ſpecific diſeaſe may be.

When it attacks the tongue it ſometimes produces a thickening and hardneſs in the part; but this is not always the caſe, for it very often ulcerates as in the other parts of the mouth.

They are generally more painful than thoſe of the ſkin; although not ſo much ſo as common ſore throats ariſing from inflamed tonſils.

They oblige the perſon to ſpeak thick, or as if his tongue was too large for his mouth, with a ſmall degree of ſnuffling.

Theſe are the moſt common ſymptoms of this ſtage of the diſeaſe; but it is perhaps impoſſible to know all the ſymptoms this poiſon produces when in the conſtitution. I knew a gentleman who had a teaſing cough, which he imputed to it; for it came on with the ſymptomatic fever and continued with it, and by uſing mercury both diſappeared.

There are inflammations of the eyes which are ſuppoſed to be venereal; for after the uſual remedies againſt inflammation have been tried in vain, mercury has been given on the ſuppoſition of the caſe being venereal, and ſometimes with ſucceſs, which has tended to eſtabliſh this opinion. But if ſuch caſes are venereal, the diſeaſe is very different from what it is when attacking other parts, from the conſtitution, for the inflammation is more painful than in venereal inflammation proceeding from the conſtitution; and I have never ſeen ſuch caſes attended with ulceration, as in the mouth, throat, and tongue, which makes me doubt much of their being venereal.

II. EXPERIMENTS MADE TO ASCERTAIN THE PROGRESS AND EFFECTS OF THE VENEREAL POISON.

To aſcertain ſeveral facts relative to the venereal diſeaſe, the following experiments were made. They were begun in May 1767.

Two

Two punctures were made on the penis with a lancet dipped in venereal matter from a gonorrhœa; one puncture was on the glans, the other on the prepuce.

This was on a Friday; on the Sunday following there was a teasing itching in those parts which lasted till the Tuesday following. In the mean time these parts being often examined, there seemed to be a greater redness and moisture than usual, which was imputed to the parts being rubbed. Upon the Tuesday morning the parts of the prepuce where the puncture had been made were redder, thickened, and had formed a speck; by the Tuesday following the speck had increased and discharged some matter, and there seemed to be a little pouting of the lips of the urethra, also a sensation in it in making water, so that a discharge was expected from it; the speck was now touched with lunar caustic, and afterwards dressed with calomel ointment. On Saturday morning the slough came off, and it was again touched, and another slough came off on the Monday following. The preceding night the glans had itched a good deal, and on Tuesday a white speck was observed where the puncture had been made; this speck when examined was found to be a pimple full of yellowish matter. This was now touched with the caustic, and dressed as the former. On the Wednesday the sore on the prepuce was yellow, and therefore was again touched with caustic. On the Friday both sloughs came off, and the sore on the prepuce looked red, and it's basis not so hard; but on the Saturday it did not look quite so well, and was touched again; and when that went off it was allowed to heal up, as also the other, which left a dent in the glans. This dent on the glans filled up in some months, but for a considerable time it had a bluish cast.

Four months afterwards the chancre on the prepuce broke out again, and very stimulating applications were tried; but these seemed not to agree with it, and by letting it alone it healed up. This it did several times afterwards, but always healed up of itself. That on the glans never did break out, and herein also it differed from the other.

While the sores remained on the prepuce and glans, a swelling took place in one of the glands of the right groin. I had for some time conceived an idea that the most effectual way to put back a bubo was to rub in mercury on that leg and thigh, which would send a current of mercury

 through

through the inflamed gland; this afforded a good opportunity of making the experiment. I had often succeeded in this way, but now wanted to put it more critically to the test.* The sores upon the penis were healed before the reduction of the bubo was attempted. A few days after beginning the mercury in this method the gland subsided considerably, it was then left off; for the intention was not to cure it completely at present. The gland some time after began to swell again, and as much mercury was rubbed in as appeared to be sufficient for the entire reduction of the gland; but it was meant to do no more than to cure the gland locally, without giving enough to prevent the constitution from being contaminated.

About two months after the last attack of the bubo, a little sharp pricking pain was felt in one of the tonsils in swallowing any thing; and on inspection a small ulcer was found, which was allowed to go on till the nature of it was ascertained, and then recourse was had to mercury. The mercury was thrown in by the same leg and thigh as before, to secure the gland more effectually, although that was not now probably necessary.

As soon as the ulcer was skinned over the mercury was left off, it not being intended to destroy the poison, but to observe what parts it would next affect. About three months after, copper coloured blotches broke out on the skin, and the former ulcer returned in the tonsil. Mercury was now applied the second time for those effects of the poison from the constitution, but still only with a view to palliate.

It was left off a second time, and the attention was given to mark where it would break out next, but it returned again in the same parts. It not appearing that any further knowledge was to be procured by only palliating the disease a fourth time in the tonsil, and a third time in the skin, mercury was now taken in a sufficient quantity, and for a proper time, to complete the cure.

The time the experiments took up, from the first insertion to the complete cure, was about three years.

The above case is only uncommon in the mode of contracting the disease, and the particular views with which some parts of the treatment were di-

* The practice in 1767 was to apply a mercurial plaister on the part, or to rub in mercurial ointment on the part, which could hardly act by any other power than sympathy.

rected;

rected; but as it was meant to prove many things which though not uncommon are yet not attended to, attention was paid to all the circumstances. It proves many things, and opens a field for further conjectures.

It proves first, that matter from a gonorrhœa will produce chancres.

It makes it probable that the glans does not take on the venereal irritation so quickly as the prepuce. The chancre on the prepuce inflamed and suppurated in somewhat more than three days, and that on the glans in about ten; this is probably the reason why the glans did not throw off it's sloughs so soon.

It renders it highly probable that mercury applied to the legs and thighs, is the best method to resolve a bubo; and therefore also the best method of applying mercury to assist in the cure, even when the bubo suppurates.

It also shews that buboes may be resolved in this way and yet the constitution not safe; and therefore that more mercury should be thrown in, especially in cases of easy resolution, than what simply resolves the bubo.

It shews that parts may be contaminated, and not having taken on the action may have the poison kept dormant in them while under a course of mercury for other symptoms, but break out afterwards.

It also shews that the poison having orginally only contaminated certain parts, when not completely cured can break out again only in those parts.

III. OF THE SYMPTOMS OF THE SECOND STAGE OF THE LUES VENEREA.

THIS stage of the disease is not so well marked as the former, and as it is of more importance it requires all our discernment to determine what the disease is.

The parts less susceptible of this irritation are such as are more out of the way of the great exciting cause, which is the external air, as has been before related. And they begin to take on the venereal action whether it may or it may not have produced it's local effects upon the external or exposed surfaces; and they even go on with the action in many cases after these surfaces first affected have taken on the action and have been cured, as has been already observed.

obſerved. Theſe deeper ſeated parts are the perioſteum, tendons, faciæ, and ligaments; however what the parts affected may be when the diſeaſe is in this ſtage is not always certain; I have known it produce total deafneſs, and ſome of thoſe caſes to end in ſuppuration, attended with great pain in the ear, and ſide of the head; ſuch caſes are generally ſuppoſed to ariſe from ſome other cauſe; and nothing but ſome particular circumſtance in the hiſtory of the caſe, ſome ſymptom attending it, or a lucky idea ſtriking the ſurgeon, can lead to the nature of the complaint.

When theſe deeper ſeated parts become irritated by this poiſon, the progreſs is more gradual than in the firſt; they have very much the character of ſcrofulous ſwellings, or chronic rheumatiſm, only in this diſeaſe the joints are not ſo ſubject to it as they are in the rheumatiſm. We ſhall find a ſwelling come upon a bone when there has been no poſſible means of catching the infection for many months, and it will be of ſome ſize before it is taken notice of, from having given but little pain. On the other hand there ſhall be great pain, and probably no ſwelling to be obſerved till ſome time after. The ſame obſervations are applicable to the ſwelling of tendons, and faſciæ.

As theſe ſwellings increaſe by ſlow degrees, they ſhow but little ſigns of inflammation. When they attack the perioſteum, the ſwelling has all the appearance of a ſwelling of the bone, by being firm and cloſely connected with it.

The inflammation produced in theſe later ſtages of the diſeaſe can hardly get beyond the adheſive, in which ſtate it continues getting worſe and worſe, and when matter is formed it is not true pus, but a ſlimy matter. This may ariſe in ſome degree from the nature of the parts not being in themſelves eaſily made to ſuppurate; and when they do ſuppurate the ſame languidneſs ſtill continues, in ſo much that this matter is not capable of giving the extraneous ſtimulus, ſo as to excite true ſuppuration or ulceration, even after the conſtitution is cleared of the original cauſe, and then the diſeaſe is probably ſcrofulous. Some nodes either in the tendons, or bones, laſt for years before they form any matter at all; and in this caſe it is doubtful whether they are venereal or not, although commonly ſuppoſed to be ſo.

I have

I have already obſerved that the pain in the firſt ſtages of this diſeaſe is much leſs than might be expected, conſidering the effects produced by the poiſon. The diſeaſe being very ſlow and gradual in it's progreſs may account for it's giving little pain; an ulcer in the throat cauſes no great pain, and the ſame may be ſaid of blotches on the ſkin, even when they become large ſores.

When the perioſteum and bones become affected, the pain is ſometimes very conſiderable, and at other times there is hardly any; it is not perhaps eaſy to account for this; we know alſo that the tendinous parts when inflamed give in ſome caſes very conſiderable pain, and that of the heavy kind, while in others they will ſwell conſiderably without giving any pain.

Theſe pains are commonly periodical or have their exacerbations, being commonly worſt in the night; this is common to other aches or pains, eſpecially of the rheumatic kind, which the venereal pains reſemble very much.

When the pain is the firſt ſymptom it affords no diſtinguiſhing mark of the diſeaſe, it is therefore often taken for the rheumatiſm.

IV. OF THE EFFECTS OF THE POISON ON THE CONSTITUTION.

THE poiſonous matter ſimply as extraneous matter produces no change whatever upon the conſtitution, and whatever effects it has depend wholly upon it's ſpecific quality as a poiſon. The general effects of this poiſon on the conſtitution are ſimilar to other irritations, either local or conſtitutional. It produces fever, which is of the ſlow kind; and when it continues a conſiderable time it produces what is called a hectic diſpoſition, which is no more than an habitual ſlow fever ariſing from a cauſe the conſtitution cannot overcome. While this exiſts it is impoſſible that any thing ſalutary can go on in ſuch a conſtitution: the patient loſes his appetite, or even if his appetite is good, loſes his fleſh, becomes reſtleſs, loſes his ſleep, and looks ſallow.*

* This kind of look although ariſing entirely from a harraſſed conſtitution is always ſuppoſed to be peculiar to a venereal one; this idea however does not ariſe from the look only but from the leading ſymptoms.

4 P In

In the firſt ſtage of this diſeaſe before it begins to ſhow itſelf externally the patient has generally rigors, hot fits, headachs, and all the ſymptoms of an approaching fever.

Theſe ſymptoms continuing for ſome days, and often for weeks, ſhow that there is ſome irritating cauſe which works ſlowly upon the conſtitution; it is then ſuppoſed to be whatever the invention or ingenuity of the practitioner ſhall call it; but the venereal eruptions or nodes upon either the perioſteum, bones, tendons, or other parts, appearing, ſhow the cauſe, and in ſome degree carry off the ſymptoms of fever and relieve the conſtitution for a little time, but they ſoon recur.

Theſe conſtitutional complaints however are not always to be found, the poiſon ſtimulating ſo ſlowly as hardly to affect the conſtitution, unleſs the poiſon is allowed to remain in it a long time.

There are a number of local appearances mentioned by authors which I never ſaw, ſuch as the fiſſures about the anus, &c. There are alſo a number of diſeaſes deſcribed by authors as venereal, eſpecially by Aſtruc and his followers, which are almoſt endleſs; the cancer, ſcrofula, rheumatiſm, and gout, are conſidered as ariſing from it, which may be in ſome meaſure true, but they are with them the diſeaſe itſelf, and all their conſequences, as conſumption, waſting from want of nouriſhment, jaundice, and a thouſand other diſeaſes which happened many years before the exiſtance of the lues venerea, are all attributed to it.

There is even at this day hardly any diſeaſe the practitioner is puzzled about, but the venereal comes immediately into his mind; and if this became the cauſe of careful inveſtigation, it would be productive of good, but with many the idea alone ſatisfies the mind.

CHAPTER

CHAPTER III.

GENERAL OBSERVATIONS ON THE CURE OF THE LUES VENEREA.

IT has been obſerved before, that there are three forms of the venereal infection, gonorrhœa, chancre, and the lues venerea, which various forms I have endeavoured to account for. As they all three ariſe from the ſame poiſon, and as the two firſt depend only on a difference in the nature of the parts, and the lues venerea on another circumſtance which has been explained, it would be natural to ſuppoſe that one medicine, whatever it is, would cure all the forms of this diſeaſe. But we find from experience, that this does not hold good; for one medicine, that is mercury, cures only the chancre and the lues venerea, and the gonorrhœa is not in the leaſt affected by it; and what is ſtill more remarkable is, that the two which it cures are in no reſpect ſimilar, while the gonorrhœa which it does not cure is ſimilar in ſome reſpects to the chancre, which it does cure.

It may be remarked in general, that there is not only a difference in the form of the diſeaſe, but alſo in the modes of cure, and in the times neceſſary for the cure of the different forms of the diſeaſe, even when the ſame medicine cures. The gonorrhœa in it's cure is the moſt uncertain of the three, the chancre next, and the lues venerea the moſt certain, although cured by the ſame medicine which cures the chancre.

A gonorrhœa in ſome caſes ſhall be cured in ſix days, and in others require as many months; which in regard to time is about the proportion of thirty to one. A chancre may be ſometimes cured in two weeks, and often requires as many months; which is in the proportion of four to one. The lues venerea in general may be cured in one or two months; which is only two to one. This calculation ſhows the regularity and irregularity as to time in the cure of each form of the diſeaſe.

I have

I have formerly obſerved, that indiſpoſitions of the body often affect this diſeaſe very conſiderably, more eſpecially the gonorrhœa and the chancre.

When an increaſe of ſymptoms takes place in a gonorrhœa from an indiſpoſition of body, nothing ſhould be done for the gonorrhœa, the indiſpoſition of body being only to be attended to; becauſe we have no ſpecific for the gonorrhœa, and in time it cures itſelf. But this practice is perhaps not to be followed in a chancre, or lues venerea. It may be neceſſary in thoſe to continue the mercury, although perhaps more gently, for the mercury is a ſpecific that cannot be diſpenſed with, becauſe neither the chancre nor lues venerea get well of themſelves, but always increaſe.

This form of the venereal diſeaſe I have divided into two ſtages. When in the parts moſt ſuſceptible of the diſeaſe, which I have called the firſt order of parts, and which appear to be the ſuperficies only; the lues venerea is perhaps ſubject to leſs variety than either the gonorrhœa or chancre, and it's mode of cure is of courſe more uniform; although the diſeaſe be leſs eaſily aſcertained, at leaſt for ſome time. In the ſecond order of parts the lues venerea becomes more complicated, and it's cure ſtill leſs to be depended upon.

The cure of this form is much more difficultly aſcertained than either of the two former, they being always local, and their effects viſible, become more the object of our ſenſes, ſo that we are ſeldom or ever deceived in the cure; although at the ſame time the cure is often more tedious and difficult; for whenever the ſymptoms of the gonorrhœa or chancre have entirely diſappeared, in general the patient may look upon himſelf as cured of them; but this is not the caſe in the lues venerea.

A lues venerea is the effects of the poiſon having circulated in the blood till it has irritated parts ſo as to give them a venereal diſpoſition, which parts ſooner or later aſſume the venereal action, according to the order of their ſuſceptibility.

When the venereal matter is circulating, I have ſuppoſed that certain parts are irritated by it, and that a vaſt number of other parts eſcape, as is evidently the caſe with the chancre; for in the caſe of a chancre the whole glans, prepuce, and ſkin of the penis, have had the matter applied to them, yet only one or more parts are contaminated or irritated by it, all the others

eſcape;

escape; and we often see in the lues venerea, that when the parts contaminated assume the action, it is confined to them without affecting other parts, although the disease be allowed to go on for a considerable time without any attempt to a cure; and also if these parts are imperfectly cured the disease returns only in them; therefore these effects, although arising from the constitution, are in themselves entirely local, similar to the gonorrhœa and chancre, and like them may be cured locally; and the person may still continue to have the lues venerea, although not in these, yet in other parts, because there may be many other parts in the same body that are under the venereal disposition although they may not yet have assumed the venereal action. To cure the local and visible effects of the disease we must attack it through that medium by which it was communicated, that is, the blood, without however considering the blood itself as a diseased part, or containing the poison, but as the vehicle of our medicine which will be carried by it to every part of the body where the poison was carried, and in it's course it will act upon the diseased solids. This practice must be continued some time after all symptoms have disappeared; for the venereal action may to appearance be stopped, and symptoms disappear, and yet all return again, the venereal action not being completely destroyed. If the medicine were also a cure for the disposition in the parts second in order, and could prevent their coming into action, it would be necessary to continue it somewhat longer on their account; but this is not the case, for the visible effects, symptoms, or appearances, in the first order of parts give way to the treatment, while the parts that have only acquired the disposition, and are still inactive, afterwards assume the action and continue the disease. This deceives the surgeon and leaves the ground-work for a second set of local effects in the parts second in order; but I have asserted that what will cure an action will not cure a disposition; if so we should push our medicine no further than the cure of the visible effects of the poison, and allow whatever parts may be contaminated to come into action afterwards.

The parts that first assume the venereal action are easiest of cure; and I have suspected that those effects of the disease being external, were in some degree assisted in their cure by the local action of the medicine, which evidently passes off through those parts.

4 Q When

When the disease has attacked the parts second in order of susceptibility, it generally happens that they are more difficult of cure than the former; therefore when they appear at the same time with the former, and are cured, we may be sure that the first will be also cured. From hence as it would appear that the parts most susceptible of the disease are also easiest of cure, it follows that the parts least susceptible of the disease are also most difficult of cure; and I believe that this is seldom or ever reversed, therefore those second in order of susceptibility have this advantage, that we have the local complaints for our guide to judge of the whole; and in such we have only to continue the treatment till they all vanish, being certain that the cure of the first, if there are any, will be involved in those of the second.

As the second are attended with more tumefaction or swelling than the first, it becomes a question, whether the mercurial course should be continued till the whole has subsided. But I believe it is not necessary to continue the method of cure till the whole tumefaction disappears; for as those local complaints cannot contaminate the constitution by reabsorption, and as the venereal disposition and action from the constitution can be cured while the local effects still remain, even where the tumefaction forming nodes on the bones, fasciæ, &c. is carried the length of suppuration, there can be no occasion for continuing the course longer than the destruction of the venereal action. But this effect of our medicine is not easily known, therefore it will be necessary to pursue the method of cure till the appearances become stationary, and probably a little longer to destroy the whole action of the disease. From these circumstances it would appear that the venereal irritation when in this stage of the disease is easier of cure than the effects of that irritation, such as the tumefaction.

I. OF THE USE OF MERCURY IN THE CURE OF THE LUES VENEREA.

Mercury in the lues venerea, as in the chancre, is the great specific, and hardly any thing else is to be depended upon. It is necessary that we should always consider well the effects of this medicine, both on the constitution

tution at large, and the disease for which it is given. The effects of mercury on a constitution will always be as the quantity of mercury in that constitution; and when the same quantity affects one constitution more than another, it is in the proportion of the irritability of that constitution, to the powers of mercury, entirely independent of any particular preparation, or any particular mode of giving it.

With regard to the preparations of the medicine, and the modes of applying it, we are to consider two things. First, the preparation and mode that is attended with the least trouble or inconvenience to the patient; and second, the preparation and mode of administering it that most readily conveys the necessary quantity into the constitution.

Nothing can show more the ungrateful or unsettled mind of man, than his treatment of this medicine. If there is such a thing as a specific, mercury is one for the venereal disease in two of it's forms; yet mankind are in pursuit of other specifics for the disease, as if specifics were more common than diseases; while at the same time they are too often contented with the common mode of treating many other diseases for which they have no specific; and these prejudices are supported by the public, who have in their minds a dread of this medicine, arising from the want of knowledge of our predecessors in administering it; and many of the present age, who are equally ignorant, take advantage of this weakness.

Mercury in the constitution acts on all parts of the machine, cures those which are diseased, affecting but little those that are sound. Mercury is carried into the constitution in the same way as other substances, either externally by the skin, or internally by the mouth: it cannot however in all cases be taken into the constitution in both ways; for sometimes it happens that the absorbents on the skin will not readily receive it, at least no effect will be produced either on the disease or constitution from such application; when this is the case it is to be considered as a misfortune, for then it must be given internally by the mouth, although possibly this mode may be very improper in other respects, and often inconvenient. On the other hand it sometimes happens that the internal absorbents will not take up this medicine, or at least no effect is produced either upon the disease or constitution; in such cases it is right to try all the different preparations of the

the medicine; for it will sometimes happen that one preparation will succeed when another will not. I have never seen a case where neither external nor internal applications of mercury were not absorbed; such a case must be miserable indeed.

I may just observe here, that many surfaces appear to absorb this medicine better than others; and most probably all internal surfaces and sores are of this kind; for when we find that thirty grains of calomel rubbed in on the skin has no more effect than three or four taken by the mouth, it becomes a kind of proof that the bowels absorb it best; also, when dressing a small sore with red precipitate produces a salivation, it shows that sores are good absorbing surfaces, especially too when we know that the lues venerea generally arises from a chancre.

A patient with a stump which produced too much granulations, was dressed with ointment containing a large proportion of red precipitate; the sore was about the size of a crown piece, it very nearly brought on a salivation, and the patient was obliged to leave it off.

A mulatto woman had upon her leg a very bad ulcer which was about the breadth of two palms; it was dressed with red precipitate mixed with common ointment, which soon threw her into a violent salivation.

A lady, in the month of December 1782, was burnt over the whole breast, neck, and shoulders, as also between her shoulders, on which parts deep sloughs were formed. The sores at first healed nearly up, and tolerably well for burns; but they broke out anew and then became more obstinate. Seven months after the accident she came to London, with very large sores extending across the breast, and upon each side to the shoulders; they were extremely tender and painful. They continued to heal for some time after she came to London; but she became ill, having been affected with extreme irritability, loss of appetite, sickness, and throwing up of her food and medicines. At this time the sores again began to spread, and became very large. After having been two months in town with little advantage, I tried warmer dressings, as basilicon to some parts, to see if any advantage would arise from such treatment, and it was found that these parts healed rather faster than the others; but the soreness was so great, even from the mildest dressings, that they could only be used in part. I next

next tried red precipitate mixed with the ointment; and that it might increase the pain as little as possible, I ordered only ten grains to two ounces of the ointment. This appeared to agree better with the sores than the ointment alone; and we were happy in having found a dressing which both hastened on the cure, and was easier than the former. But about the fourth or fifth dressing from beginning the use of the precipitate, she began to complain of her gums; the next day began to spit, and by the seventh or eighth day the mouth was so sore, and the spitting so considerable, that upon considering the case we began to suspect that it might proceed from the red precipitate in the dressing. The gums, inside of the cheeks, and the breath, were truly mercurial. We immediately left off this dressing, except to a small corner, and had recourse to the former dressings. In a few days the effects of the mercury abated, and the sores looked more healthy than ever, and we again began to dress part of the sores with the ointment containing precipitate, which still agreed with them. When the mouth first became affected she had not used much above one half of the ointment; and by the time we had discovered the cause about three fourths of it had been expended in dressings, so that there were not quite ten grains of precipitate applied; and although this took up seven or eight days, and the ointment must have been soon removed from the sore by the discharge, yet a considerable spitting was produced, which lasted above a month. It is hardly to be conceived that above a grain or two could really be taken into the constitution; for when we consider the particles of precipitate were covered with ointment, and a vast discharge of matter so as soon to remove this small quantity from the sore, we can hardly admit the possibility of more being absorbed; and if this idea of the quantity taken in is just, to what must we attribute the great susceptibility to the effects of the medicine? Was it the irritable state of the patient at the time? For the state of the constitution appeared to me to be that in which the locked jaw often takes place; and I often had this disease in my mind. The patient afterwards got well by the use of an ointment in which pitch was an ingredient. All this tends to show that sores and internal surfaces absorb better than the skin.

Besides the practicability of getting the medicine into the constitution in either way, it is proper to consider the easiest for the patient, each mode having it's convenience and inconvenience, which arifes from the nature of the conftitution of the parts to which it is applied, or from certain fituations of life of the patient at the time; it is therefore proper to give it in that way which fuits thefe circumftances beft.

To explain this further, we find that in many patients the bowels can hardly bear mercury at all, therefore it is to be given in the mildeft form poffible; alfo joined with fuch other medicines as will leffen or correct it's violent local effects, although not it's fpecific ones on the conftitution at large.

When it can be thrown into the conftitution with propriety by the external method, it is preferable to the internal, becaufe the fkin is not nearly fo effential to life as the ftomach, and therefore is capable in itfelf of bearing much more than the ftomach; it alfo affects the conftitution much lefs; many courfes of mercury which are abfolutely neceffary, would kill the patient if taken by the ftomach, proving hurtful both to the ftomach and inteftines, even when given in any form, and joined with the greateft correctors: on the other hand, the way of life will often not allow it to be applied externally. It is not every one that can find convenience to rub in mercury, therefore they muft take it by the mouth if poffible. To obviate the inconvenience often arifing from the vifible effects of mercury, many preparations have been invented; but any preparation of mercury producing an effect different from the fimple effects of mercury in that conftitution, fuch as fweating or an increafed difcharge of urine, muft be fuppofed either not to act as mercury, or the fubftance with which it is compounded produces this effect; but if it's peculiar effects are lefs than ufual, I fhould very much fufpect that the mercury is acting in part as a compound, and not entirely as mercury.

Mercury, like many other medicines, has two effects, one upon the conftitution and particular parts, which is according to it's mode of irritation, independent of any difeafe whatever. The other is it's fpecific effects upon a difeafed action of the whole body, or of parts, whatever the difeafe be, and which effects are only known by the difeafe gradually difappearing. The firft becomes an object of confideration for the furgeon, as it is in fome meafure meaſure by them he is to be guided in giving this medicine ſo as to have it's ſpecific effects ſufficient for the cure of the diſeaſe.

Whatever injury mercury may do to the conſtitution it is by it's viſible effects, and thence the pretended art in avoiding thoſe viſible effects has been too much the cauſe of great impoſition. The part upon which it's effects are moſt likely to fall is the part that is in moſt caſes attempted to be avoided, or guarded againſt, and that is the mouth. I believe that we are not poſſeſſed of any means of either driving the mercury to the mouth, or of preventing it from attacking that part. Cold and warmth are the two great agents mentioned by authors; we find them recommending the avoiding of cold, for fear the mercury ſhould fly to the mouth, as if warmth was a prevention; while others, and even the ſame authors, when talking of bringing the mercury to the mouth, recommend warmth, as if cold were a preventive. This being the caſe, we may reaſonably ſuppoſe that neither the one nor the other have any material effect.

In giving mercury in the venereal diſeaſe the firſt attention ſhould be to the quantity, and it's viſible effects in a given time; which when brought to a proper pitch, are only to be kept up, and the decline of the diſeaſe to be watched; for by this we judge of the inviſible or ſpecific effects of the medicine, which will often inform us that ſome variation in the quantity may be neceſſary.

The viſible effects of mercury are of two kinds, the one on the conſtitution, the other on ſome parts capable of ſecretion.

In the firſt it appears to produce univerſal irritability, making it more ſuſceptible of all impreſſions; it quickens the pulſe, alſo increaſes it's hardneſs, producing a kind of temporary fever; but in many conſtitutions it exceeds this, acting as it were as a poiſon. In ſome it produces a kind of hectic fever, that is, a ſmall quick pulſe, loſs of appetite, reſtleſſneſs, want of ſleep, and a ſallow complexion, with a number of conſequent ſymptoms; but by being a little accuſtomed to the uſe of it, theſe conſtitutional effects commonly become leſs, of which the following caſes are ſtrong inſtances.

A gentleman rubbed in mercurial ointment for the reduction of two buboes. He had only rubbed in a few times when it affected his conſtitution ſo much that it was neceſſary to leave it off. He was ſeized with feveriſh complaints of of the hectic kind, a ſmall quick pulſe, debility, loſs of appetite, no ſleep, and night ſweats. He took the bark with James's powder, and aſſes milk, and got gradually rid of theſe complaints. As the buboes were advancing, it was neceſſary to have recourſe to mercury again; and I told him that now it would not produce the ſame effects ſo quickly, nor ſo violently as before. He rubbed in a conſiderable quantity without his conſtitution or mouth being affected, but the buboes ſuppurating, made me order it to be left off a ſecond time, and when they were opened he had recourſe to the ointment again for the third time, and without producing any diſagreeable effects. The buboes took on a healing diſpoſition for a while and then became ſtationary, ſhowing that a new diſpoſition was forming. He was directed to leave off the ointment and to bathe in the ſea, which he did and the buboes began to heal. In about three weeks however it was thought neceſſary to rub in again, and when he began, which was the fourth time, it had almoſt an immediate and violent effect upon his mouth; he left off again till his mouth became a little better, and then returned to the mercury a fifth time, and was able to go on with it.

A ſtout healthy man rubbed in mercurial ointment for a bubo till it affected his mouth; it further brought on very diſagreeable conſtitutional complaints, ſuch as loſs of appetite, watchfulneſs, ſallow complexion, laſſitude from the leaſt exerciſe, and ſwelled legs; and although various means were uſed to reconcile the conſtitution to it, yet it continued to act as a poiſon.

Mercury often produces pains like thoſe of the rheumatiſm, and alſo nodes which are of a ſcrofulous nature, from thence it has been accuſed of affecting the bones, "lurking in them," as authors have expreſſed it.

It may be ſuppoſed to be unneceſſary to mention in the preſent ſtate of our knowledge, that it never gets into the bones in the form of a metal, although this has been aſſerted by men of eminence and authority in the profeſſion, and even the diſſections of dead bodies have been brought in proof of it; but my experience in anatomy has not convinced me of the reallity of ſuch appearances. Thoſe authors have been quoted by others; imaginary caſes of diſeaſe have been increaſed; the credulous, and ignorant practitioner miſled, and patients rendered miſerable.

II. OF

II. OF THE QUANTITY OF MERCURY NECESSARY TO BE GIVEN.

THE quantity of mercury to be thrown into the conſtitution for the cure of any venereal complaint muſt be proportioned to the violence of the diſeaſe. Two circumſtances are however to be ſtrictly attended to in the adminiſtration of this medicine; which are, the time in which any given quantity is to be thrown in, and the effects it has on ſome parts of the body, as the ſalivary glands, ſkin, or inteſtines. Theſe two circumſtances taken together are to guide us in the cure of the diſeaſe; for mercury may be thrown into the ſame conſtitution in very different quantities ſo as to produce the ſame ultimate effect, but the two very different quantities muſt be alſo in different times; for inſtance, one ounce of mercurial ointment rubbed in in two days will have more effect upon the conſtitution than two ounces rubbed in in ten; and to produce the ſame effect in the ten days, it may perhaps be neceſſary to rub in three ounces or more.

The effects on the conſtitution of one ounce rubbed in in two days are conſiderable, and alſo it's effects upon the diſeaſed parts; therefore a much leſs quantity in ſuch a way will have greater effects; but if theſe effects are principally local, that is, upon the glands of the mouth, the conſtitution at large not being equally ſtimulated, the effect upon the diſeaſed parts muſt alſo be leſs, which is to be determined by the local diſeaſe not giving way in proportion to the effects of the mercury on ſome particular part.

If it is given in very ſmall quantities, and increaſed gradually ſo as to ſteal inſenſibly on the conſtitution, it's viſible effects are leſs, and it is hardly conceivable how much may at laſt be thrown in, without having any viſible effect at all.[a]

[a] To give an idea of this, a gentleman had the mercury fall on his mouth upon rubbing in ten grains of the ointment a day, for ten days; the ointment was equal parts, but by leaving off and beginning anew, he at laſt rubbed in eighty grains every night for a month, without having his mouth, or any of the ſecretions viſibly affected.

These circumstances being known, it makes mercury a much more efficacious, manageable, and safe medicine, than formerly it was thought to be; but unluckily it's visible effects upon some particular parts, such as the mouth, and the intestines, are sometimes much more violent than it's general effect upon the constitution at large; therefore a certain degree of caution is necessary, not to stimulate these parts too quickly, as that will prevent the necessary quantity being given.

The constitution, or parts, are more susceptible of mercury at first than afterwards; if the mouth is made sore, and allowed to recover, a much greater quantity may be thrown in a second time, before the same soreness is produced; and indeed I have seen cases where it could not be reproduced from as much as possibly could be thrown in. Upon a renewal of the course of mercury therefore the same precautions are not necessary as at first. We are however every now and then deceived by this medicine, it being hardly possible to produce visible effects at one time; and afterwards the mouth, and intestines, shall all at once be affected.

Mercury when it falls on the mouth produces in many constitutions violent inflammation, which sometimes terminates in mortification. The constitutions in which this happens I suspect are of the erisypelatous kind, or what are called the putrid; therefore in such, greater caution is necessary. Mercury in general, that, is where it only produces it's common effects, seldom or ever does any injury to the constitution. It should seem only to act for the time, and to leave the constitution in an healthy state. But this is not always the case, for probably mercury can be made to affect every constitution very materially, being capable of producing local diseases, as has been mentioned; and also capable of retarding the cure of chancres, buboes, and certain effects of the lues venerea, after the poison has been destroyed.

III. OF THE SENSIBLE EFFECTS OF MERCURY UPON PARTS.

The sensible effects of mercury are generally an increase of some of the secretions, a swelling in the salivary glands, and increase of saliva; an increase

of

of the secretion of the bowels, which produces purging, and an increase of the secretion of the skin, producing sweat, also often an increase of the secretion of urine. Sometimes one of these secretions only is affected, sometimes more, and sometimes all of them together. But the effects upon the mouth are the most frequent.

Mercury often produces headaches, and also costiveness, when it's action on other parts becomes sensible, especially upon the glands of the mouth.

When the mercury falls upon the mouth, it does not affect all parts of it equally, sometimes attacking the gums, at other times the cheeks, which become thickened, and ulcerate, while the gums are not in the least affected, as appears by the patient being capable of biting any thing hard.

Mercury when it falls upon the mouth, and parts belonging to the mouth, not only increases the discharge of those parts, but it brings on great tumefaction, which is not of the true inflammatory kind where coagulable lymph is thrown out, but rather resembling erisypelatous tumefaction. The tongue, cheeks, and gums, swell, and the teeth become loose; all which is in proportion to the quantity of mercury given, and susceptibility of the parts for such irritation. It produces great weakness in the parts, in which ulceration easily takes place, especially if they are in the least irritated, which is often done by the teeth, and even mortification sometimes ensues. How far it produces similar effects when it falls on other parts I do not know. The saliva in such cases is generally ropy, as if principally from the glands affected. The breath acquires a particular smell.

As mercury generally produces evacuations, it was naturally imagined that it was by this means it effected a cure of the venereal disease; but experience has taught us that in curing the venereal disease by this medicine, evacuations of any kind produced by it are not at all necessary; and this might have been supposed, as similar evacuations produced by other medicines are of no service, therefore it was reasonable to imagine that these evacuations when produced by mercury, were also of no service; except we could suppose that the evacuation produced by the mercury was not the same with that produced by other medicines, but that it was a specific evacuation; that is to say, a discharge carrying off the venereal poison by it's union with the mercury; and therefore the faster the mercury went off, the sooner would the poison be carried

carried out of the conſtitution. But this is not found to be the caſe in practice; on the contrary evacuations produced by the medicine retard the cure, eſpecially if the ſecretary organs are too ſuſceptible of this ſtimulus; for then the quantity which is neceſſary, or ſufficient for the cure of the diſeaſe cannot be taken in, the effects of the medicine upon particular parts being greater than the patient can bear; and the quantity of mercury to be thrown into the conſtitution muſt be limited, and regulated according to the quantity of evacuation, and not according to the extent of the diſeaſe. On the other hand if it is given with care, ſo as to avoid violent evacuation, any quantity may be thrown in ſufficient for the cure of the diſeaſe.

Certain evacuations may be ſuppoſed to be a mark of the conſtitutional effects of mercury, but they are not to be entirely depended upon, the ſecretions being only a proof of the ſuſceptibility of ſome parts to ſuch a ſtimulus; however it is probable that in general they are a good gage of it's conſtitutional effects. Some have gone ſo far as to ſuppoſe that quantity of mercury alone, without any ſenſible effects is ſufficient for the cure of the diſeaſe; and this is in ſome degree the caſe, but not completely ſo, for we have no good proof of it's affecting the conſtitution but by its producing an increaſe of ſome of the ſecretions.

IV. OF THE ACTION OF MERCURY.

Mercury can have but two modes of action, one upon the poiſon, the the other on the conſtitution; we can hardly ſuppoſe it to act both ways. If mercury acted upon the poiſon only, it might be ſuppoſed to be in two ways, either by deſtroying it's qualities by decompoſing it, or by attracting it and carrying it out of the conſtitution. If the firſt were the action of mercury, then we might reaſonably ſuppoſe that quantity alone would be the thing to be depended upon; if the ſecond, that the quantity of evacuation would be the principal circumſtance.

But if it act upon the principle of deſtroying the diſeaſed action of the living parts, counteracting the venereal irritation by producing another of a different kind, then neither quantity alone nor evacuation will avail much; but

but it will be quantity joined with ſenſible effects that will produce the quickeſt cure, which from experience we find to be the caſe. But although the effects that mercury has upon the venereal diſeaſe are in ſome degree in proportion to it's local effects on ſome of the glands, or particular part of the body, as the mouth, ſkin, kidneys and inteſtines, yet it is not exactly in this proportion, as has been mentioned. When mercury diſagrees as it were conſtitutionally, producing great irritability and hectic ſymptoms, this action or irritation is not a counter irritation to the venereal diſeaſe, but is a conſtitutional irritation, having no effect on the diſeaſe, which continues to increaſe. Mercury loſing it's effects upon the diſeaſe by uſe, is a proof that it neither acts chymically, nor by carrying off the poiſon by evacuation, but by it's ſtimulating power.

The effects will always be in proportion to the quantity in a given time, joined with the ſuſceptibility of the conſtitution to the mercurial irritation. Theſe circumſtances require the minuteſt attention; and in order to procure it's greateſt action with ſafety, and to procure this in the moſt effectual way, it muſt be given till it produces local effects ſomewhere, but not too quickly, that we may be able to throw in a proper quantity; for local effects produced too quickly prevent the ſufficient quantity being thrown in for counteracting the venereal irritation at large. I have ſeen caſes where the mercury very readily acted locally, and yet the conſtitution was hardly affected by it, for the diſeaſe did not give way.

A gentleman had a chancre which he deſtroyed with cauſtic, and dreſſed the ſore with mercurial ointment. He had alſo a ſmall uneaſineſs in one of his groins, which went no further, but which ſhowed an abſorption of the poiſon. The chancre ſoon healed, and he rubbed in about two ounces of mercurial ointment. He began this courſe with ſmall quantities, that is, a ſcruple at each rubbing, and increaſed it; however it ſoon affected his mouth, and he ſpit for about a month. Two months after he had a venereal ulcer in one of his tonſils. Here was a conſiderable ſenſible effect from a ſmall quantity of mercury, which proved ineffectual, becauſe it's ſpecific effects, as I apprehend, were not in proportion to it's ſenſible effects; the ſalivary glands being too ſuſceptible of the mercurial irritation.

On the other hand I have ſeen caſes where quantity did not anſwer till it was given ſo quickly as to affect the conſtitution in ſuch a manner as to produce local irritation, and conſequently ſenſible evacuations, which is a proof that the local effects are often the ſign of it's ſpecific effects on the conſtitution at large, and ſhows the ſuſceptibility of the diſeaſed parts to be affected by the medicine is in proportion to the effects of it upon the mouth. It's effects are not to be imputed to evacuation, but to it's irritation, therefore mercury ſhould be given if poſſible ſo as to produce ſenſible effects upon ſome parts of the body, and in the largeſt quantity of mercury that can be given to produce theſe effects within certain bounds; and that theſe ſenſible effects ſhould be the means of determining how far the medicine may be puſhed, in order to have it's beſt effects upon the diſeaſe without endangering the conſtitution. The practice here muſt vary according to circumſtances; if the diſeaſe is in a violent degree, leſs regard muſt be had to the conſtitution, and the mercury is to be thrown in in larger quantities; but if the diſeaſe be mild it is not neceſſary to go beyond that rule, although it is better to keep up to it on purpoſe to cure the diſeaſe the ſooner.

If the diſeaſe is in the firſt order of parts a leſs quantity of mercury is neceſſary than if it were in the ſecond order of parts, and had been of long ſtanding with it's firſt appearances only cured and the venereal diſpoſition ſtill remaining in the ſecondary parts. To cure the diſeaſe, whether in the form of chancre, bubo, or lues venerea, probably the ſame quantity of mercury is neceſſary; for one ſore requires as much mercury as fifty ſores in the ſame perſon, and a ſmall ſore as much as a large one; the only difference, if there is any, muſt depend upon the nature of the parts affected, whether naturally active or indolent. If there be any material difference between the recent and conſtitutional, which I apprehend there is, it may make a difference in the quantity. I do conceive that the recent are upon the whole more difficult to cure; at leaſt they commonly require longer time, although not always.

Having thus far premiſed theſe general rules and obſervations, I ſhall now give the different methods of adminiſtering mercury.

V. OF

V. OF THE DIFFERENT METHODS OF GIVING MERCURY EXTERNALLY—INTERNALLY.

PREVIOUS to the giving of mercury it is very proper to underſtand as much as poſſible the conſtitution of the patient with regard to this medicine, which can only be known in thoſe who have already gone through a mercurial courſe; but as many of our patients are obliged to undergo this treatment more than once, it becomes no vague inquiry; for as there are many who can bear this medicine much better than others, it is very proper that this ſhould be known, as it will be a direction for our preſent practice. I think that few conſtitutions alter in this diſpoſition; although I knew one caſe which admitted of a conſiderable quantity at one time without being viſibly affected; but about a twelve month after was affected with a very little.

When mercury is given to cure the lues venerea, whatever length we mean to go in the ſenſible effects of it, we ſhould get to that length if poſſible, and we ſhould keep up to it. For we ſhall find it difficult to bring it's effects to that ſtandard again if we allow it to get below it. If the mercury ſhould get beyond what we intended, we ſhould be very much upon our guard in lowering it; and ſhould probably begin to give it again before it's effects are reduced to the intended ſtandard: for the ſame quantity now will not operate ſo powerfully as before; inſomuch that what at firſt produced greater effects than was intended, will not be ſufficient afterwards.

Mercury is beſt applied externally in form of an ointment. Unctuous ſubſtances keep it divided, attach it to ſurfaces, and do not dry; it may alſo be ſuppoſed that it becomes a vehicle for the mercury, and carries it through the abſorbents to the general circulation; for it is probable that oil is as eaſy of abſorption as watry ſubſtances.

If the ſymptoms are mild in the firſt order of parts, and the patient not accuſtomed to mercury, or it is known that he cannot bear the medicine in great quantity, and it is intended to conduct the cure by almoſt inſenſible means,

means, it is proper to begin with ſmall quantities. One ſcruple, or half a dram, of an ointment made of equal parts of quickſilver and hogs lard, rubbed in every night for four or ſix nights will be ſufficient to begin with. If the mouth is not affected the quantity may be gradually increaſed till two or three drams are rubbed in at each time; but if the firſt quantity has affected the mouth we may be almoſt certain that the glands of the mouth are very ſuſceptible of the mercurial ſtimulus; therefore it will be proper to wait two or three days till that effect begins to go off.

When we begin the ſecond time the quantity may be gradually increaſed, at leaſt a ſcruple every time, till two drams or more is rubbed in each night, which may be done without affecting the patient very conſiderably a ſecond time, as has been already obſerved.

If all the ſymptoms gradually diſappear, there is no more to be done but to continue this practice for a fortnight longer by way of ſecurity.

This method ſteadily purſued will cure moſt recent caſes of lues venerea; but it is not ſufficient if the diſeaſe has been merely kept under by ſlight courſes of mercury; a greater quantity becomes neceſſary, from a kind of habit the conſtitution has acquired, by which it is rendered leſs ſuſceptible of the mercurial ſtimulus.

If the diſeaſe ſhould return in the ſecond order of parts, we may be certain the ſame quantity of mercury will not be ſufficient to cure them, their action being ſlow under the venereal irritation, therefore require more than what had been firſt given.

I may be allowed to remark, that where the venereal ſymptoms have been ulcers in the mouth or throat, I have ſuſpected that the mercury being brought to the mouth, and the ſaliva being impregnated with it, and acting as a mercurial gargle, cured thoſe parts locally; and that the conſtitution has remained ſtill tainted; the mercurial action in it having been much inferior to what it was in the mouth. Perhaps ſomething ſimilar may take place in eruptions of the ſkin where the mercury paſſes off by ſweat; for we know that ſulphur will cure the itch by paſſing off in perſpiration. If theſe are facts, then it may in ſome degree account for the local ſymptoms in the firſt order of parts being eaſier of cure than thoſe in the ſecond.

The manner of living under a mercurial courſe need not be altered from the common, becauſe mercury has no action upon the diſeaſe which is more ſavoured favoured by one way of life than another. Let me ask any one what effect eating a hearty dinner, and drinking a bottle of wine can have over the action of mercury upon a venereal sore? Or what effect can walking in frost and snow have upon the operation of mercury, either to make it affect any part sensibly, as falling upon the glands of the mouth, or prevent it's effect upon the venereal irritation? In short I do not see why mercury should not cure the venereal disease under any mode whatever of regimen or diet.

I own however, that I can conceive cold affecting the operations of mercury upon the venereal disease; it is possible that cold may be favourable to the venereal irritation, and therefore contrary to that produced by mercury; and there is some show of reason for supposing this; for I have before asserted that cold was an encourager of the venereal irritation; and therefore keeping the patient warm may diminish the powers of the disease while under the cure.

Mercury given internally is in many cases sufficient, although in general it is not so much to be depended on as the external application; therefore I would not recommend it, or give it in cases where the disease has not been sufficiently cured by former courses of mercury. It is the most convenient way of giving this medicine, for many will swallow a pill, who do not choose to rub the body with the ointment; indeed there are many circumstances in life which make this mode of introducing it into the constitution the most convenient; but on the other hand there are many constitutions that cannot bear mercury given internally; when these two circumstances meet in the same patient it is unfortunate.

Mercury taken internally often produces very disagreeable effects upon the stomach and intestines, causing sickness in the one, and griping and purging in the other.

If it be found necessary to give it internally, and it disagree either with the stomach or intestines, or both, even in the most simple preparation, it's effects, whatever they are, must be corrected or prevented, by joining with the mercury other medicines. If it affect the stomach only, the mercury may be joined with small quantities of the essential oils, as the essential oil of cloves, or camomile flowers, which will in many cases take off that effect. If it both disagree with the stomach and bowels, which I believe arises either from the mercury meeting with an acid in the ſtomach by which part of it is diſſolved forming a ſalt, or from being given in the form of a ſalt, both of which will generally purge and become the cauſe of their own expulſion. There are two ways of obviating theſe effects; the firſt is, by preventing the ſalt from forming; the ſecond, by mitigating it's effects on the inteſtines if formed, by taking off their irritability. To prevent the ſalt from forming, the beſt way is to join the mercury with alkaline ſubſtances, either ſalts, or earths: and when given in a ſaline ſtate, it may be joined with opium, or ſome of the eſſential oils.

To prevent the formation of the ſalt, take of the preparations of mercury, ſuch as mercurius calcinatus, mercurius fuſcus, or calomel, forming them into pills with the addition of a ſmall quantity of ſoft ſoap, or any of the alkaline ſalts; the alkaline ſalt alſo prevents the pill from drying: or inſtead of theſe a calcarious earth may be joined with the mercury, ſuch as chalk or crabs eyes: upon this principle is the mercurius alkalizatus, which is crude mercury rubbed down with crabs eyes. But theſe ſubſtances add conſiderably to the bulk of the medicine, no leſs than twenty grains being neceſſary for a doſe; which contains ſeven grains and a half of crude mercury. The mercurius calcinatus rubbed with a ſmall proportion of opium makes an efficacious pill, and in general agrees well both with the ſtomach, and bowels. Opium has been long joined with mercury to cure the venereal diſeaſe. By ſome as much has been attributed to the opium as the mercury; however opium ſhould be given with care, for it is not every conſtitution with which it agrees, often producing irritability, in ſome laſſitude and debility, in others ſpaſms.

If the mercury is not given in the above manner, but in the form of a ſalt, or the ſalts are allowed to form, then it ſhould be joined with one third of opium, and a drop of the oil of cloves, or camomile, which will make it agree with the ſtomach, and prevent it's purging; or if it is found ſtill to diſagree both with the ſtomach, and bowels, compound it ſtill further, by joining with the mercury the alkaline ſalts, the opium, and ſome eſſential oil.

A grain of mercurius calcinatus made into a pill, with the addition of ſuch medicines as the ſtomach or bowels may require, may be given every night for

for a week; and if in that time it has not affected the mouth it may be repeated evening and morning; and after the patient has been accustomed to the medicine and it is found not to fall much upon the mouth, it may be increased to two grains in the evening, and one in the morning.

The same directions hold equally good either with the mercurius fuscus, or calomel; but it requires more of these last preparations of mercury to have the same medicinal effect upon the disease, than of the before mentioned; perhaps the proportion of their effects are about two, or three, to one. Why this should be the case is probably not easily accounted for, the quantity of mercury being very nearly the same in a given weight in both, for in eight grains of calomel there are seven grains of crude mercury. Three grains of these preparations appear only equal to one of the mercurius calcinatus. The crude mercury given in the same quantities with either of the former appears the least efficacious of all, for fifteen grains of crude mercury rubbed down with any mucilage, seems only equal to one or two of the mercurius calcinatus.

The corrosive sublimate, which is a salt capable of stimulating violently, is generally given in solution in water, brandy, or some of the simple waters, and has been used with the appearance of considerable success. It would appear that it removes ulcers in the mouth as soon, if not sooner than any of the other preparations; but this I suspect arises from it's application to these parts in it's passage to the stomach, acting upon them locally as a gargle; however from experience it appears not to have sufficient powers over the venereal irritation; in recent cases only removing the visible local effects, without entirely destroying the venereal action; for many more have been found to relapse after having taken this preparation, than from many of the others; which is owing to it's passing very readily off by the skin. Besides it disagrees much more with the stomach, and intestines, than any of the other preparations.

A grain of this medicine dissolved in about an ounce of some fluid, is generally the dose, and increased according as it agrees with the bowels, and according to it's effects upon the mouth, and disease.

As corrosive sublimate contains an acid, and as you must be guided by the effects of the acid on the bowels, the quantity of mercury you can give in this

this form is neceſſarily ſmaller than in the other preparations. Ward's drop containing leſs acid can be given in larger quantity, and is more efficacious on that account. Perhaps any of theſe preparations united with a ſcruple of gum guaiacum may have more effect than when given alone; an electuary is a convenient form.

This practice continued for two months will in general cure a common lues venerea; but here it is not meant that any time ſhould be ſpecified. After all the ſymptoms of the diſeaſe have diſappeared, this courſe ſhould be continued at leaſt a fortnight longer; but if the ſymptoms diſappear very ſuddenly, as they often do, perhaps within eight or ten days, probably from the medicine going off by thoſe ſurfaces where the diſeaſe appears, the medicine ſhould be continued three weeks, or perhaps a month longer, and the doſe increaſed. In ſuch caſes the viſible local effects appear to be cured, while a venereal diſpoſition remains in the parts.

Various are the preparations of mercury recommended for internal uſe, while practitioners have generally been ſatisfied with but one for external application. Every practitioner finds ſome one of the preparations anſwering better to appearance in ſome one caſe than another, which caſts the balance in favour of that medicine in his mind; or others finding the bad effects of a particular preparation at ſome one time, have generally condemned that preparation; not to mention that deceit is often practiſed in the cure of this diſeaſe. One would naturally ſuppoſe that the ſimpleſt preparation is the beſt, that which is eaſieſt diſſolved in the animal juices, does leaſt miſchief to the ſtomach, or general health, and is leaſt diſturbed or hindered in it's operations; for we can hardly ſuppoſe that any ſubſtance joined with mercury which alters either it's chymical or mechanical properties out of the body, can add to it's power in the body, except a ſubſtance which had a ſimilar power when acting alone. The preference generally given to the ointment ſhows this; and if we could find a preparation ſtill more ſimple than the ointment, that preparation ſhould be uſed in preference to the crude mercury.

VI. OF

VI. OF THE CURE OF THE DISEASE IN THE SECOND OR THIRD STAGE.

In the more advanced ſtages of the diſeaſe the mercurial courſe muſt be puſhed further. The greateſt quantity of that medicine that the patient can bear at a time is to be thrown in and continued with ſteadineſs till there is great reaſon to ſuppoſe the diſeaſe is deſtroyed. It will not be poſſible in ſuch caſes to prevent the mouth from being conſiderably affected, the quantity of mercury neceſſary to be thrown in for the cure of theſe ſtages of the diſeaſe being ſuch as will in moſt caſes produce that effect.

Before the diſeaſe has advanced ſo far, the patient moſt probably has taken mercury, and it is proper to inquire how he has been affected by it, and what quantity of it he could bear, which will in ſome degree direct us in the quantity now to be begun with. If the patient has not taken mercury for a conſiderable time, and is eaſily affected by it, which is the caſe that admits of the leaſt quantity, it will be neceſſary to begin cautiouſly, regulating the quantity according to circumſtances; but if the perſon has taken mercury lately, although eaſily affected by it, more freedom may be uſed on returning to it, becauſe it will have leſs power on his mouth, as alſo on the diſeaſe; again, if the perſon has been taking mercury very lately, and is with difficulty affected by it, which is the caſe that admits of the greateſt quantity, then it may be adminiſtered freely ſo as to affect the conſtitution in the proper time. If the mercury is brought to the mouth in ſix or eight days, and a conſiderable ſoreneſs is produced in twelve, it will in general be a good beginning. In ſuch caſes the conſtitution is if poſſible to be ſurprized by the medicine ſo as to produce it's greateſt effects, but with ſuch caution as to be able to keep up theſe effects by quantity.

Friction will anſwer better than giving it internally; for in this way we are ſurer of throwing in a larger quantity in a given time than could be taken internally without hurting the ſtomach.

The quantity of mercury applied in this way ſhould be under certain circumſtances, in an inverſe proportion to the ſurface on which it is applied, and

and the furface fhould be completely covered with the ointment; for half an ounce of mercurial ointment rubbed in upon a given furface will have nearly the fame effect as one ounce rubbed in on the fame furface; therefore one ounce to have double the effect fhould have double the furface. The quantity of ointment muft therefore be adapted to the quantity of furface, for on a certain extent of furface no more than a determined quantity of ointment can be applied fo as to be abforbed; and applying a greater quantity would be ufelefs; and if the quantity of furface is greater the fame portion of ointment cannot be diffufed fo as to employ fully all the abforbents. Every furface which is ufed may therefore have it's full quantity of ointment, but certainly fhould not have more, if we are to attribute the effects of the mercury to the quantity.

It has moft probably been always the practice to rub the mercury well in, as it is termed; but I fufpect that this arofe rather from an idea of the furface being porous like a fponge, than of abforption being performed by the action of veffels; and it is probable that this action in the veffels producing abforption may be rather difturbed than excited by friction.

How long the courfe is to be followed is not to be exactly afcertained, it may be thought proper to continue it till the local appearances, as nodes, have fubfided; but I fufpect that this is hardly neceffary, except they give way readily; for in fuch cafes the local complaints, or tumefaction, &c. generally require a longer time to be removed than the venereal action; and local applications muft be of fervice, efpecially if fuch tumefactions are obftinate.

The manner of living under fuch a fevere courfe, which is in every refpect weakening, is to be particularly attended to; the patient muft be fupported, and the local effects of the medicine in the mouth preventing his taking many kinds of nourifhment, efpecially fuch as are of a folid form; fluids muft form his only nourifhment, and thefe fhould be fuch as will become folid after they are fwallowed; milk is of this kind. An egg beat up with a little fugar, and a little wine; fago, faloop, &c. form a proper diet. In many cafes wine and bark muft be given through the whole courfe. Sugar is perhaps one of the beft reftoratives of any kind we are acquainted with, when a conftitution has been very much debilitated by long fafting, from

from whatever cauſe, whether from the want of food when in health, or in the time of diſeaſe, or where the food has not been allowed to anſwer the conſtitutional waſte, as in a courſe of mercury, and when the diſeaſe or courſe of mercury is gone, then ſugar will reſtore ſuch conſtitution probably better than any thing elſe.

Although it is not a common opinion, and therefore not a common practice to give ſugar entirely with this view, yet there are ſufficient proofs of it's nutritive qualitiy over almoſt every other ſubſtance. It is a well known fact, that all the negroes in the ſugar iſlands become extremely luſty and fat in the ſugar-cane ſeaſon; and they hardly live upon any thing-elſe. The horſes and cattle that are allowed to feed upon them all become fat. The hair of the horſe becomes fine. Birds who feed upon fruit never eat it till it become very ripe, when it has formed the greateſt quantity of ſugar, and even then only on ſuch as furniſh the largeſt quantity of ſugar. Inſects the ſame, but in this tribe we cannot have a ſtronger inſtance of this fact than in the bee. Honey is compoſed of ſugar, with ſome other juices of the plant, with a little eſſential oil; but ſugar is the principal ingredient. When we conſider that a ſwarm of bees will live a whole winter on a few pounds of honey, keep up a conſtant heat about ninety-five or ninety-ſix degrees, and the actions of the animal œconomy equal to that heat, we muſt allow that ſugar contains perhaps more real nouriſhment than any other known ſubſtance.

We ſee too that whey is extremely fattening, which is the watry part of the milk, containing neither the oil nor the coagulable matter; this ariſes principally from the ſugar it contains; for being compoſed of the watry part it holds all the ſugar of the milk in ſolution. If the milk is allowed to become ſour it is not ſo fattening, becauſe it is the ſugar which is become ſour.

Although the nutritive qualities of ſugar have not been ſo generally known as to introduce it into univerſal practice, yet they have not entirely eſcaped the notice of practitioners. Mr. Vaux, from obſerving the negroes in the Weſt Indies growing fat in the ſugar ſeaſon, has been induced to give it in very large quantities to many of his patients, and with very good effects. Honey is perhaps as good a mode of taking this ſubſtance as any:

ſweetening

fweetening every thing thet is either eat or drunk, whether by fugar in honey, or fugar alone, is probably immaterial; yet it is probable that the other ingredients in honey may add to it's nutritive quality.

VII. OF LOCAL TREATMENT.

If the local effects have gone no further than inflammation and fwelling, either of the foft or hard parts, moft probably no local treatment will be neceffary, for the treatment of the conftitution will in general remove them entirely.

It fometimes however happens that the local complaints will not give way, but the parts remain fwelled in an indolent and inactive ftate, even after there is every reafon for fuppofing the conftitution is perfectly cured. In fuch cafes the conftitutional treatment is to be affifted by local applications of mercury to the part, either in the form of a plaifter or ointment. The latter is by much the beft mode. If thefe are not fufficient, as often happens, we muft endeavour to deftroy this difpofition by producing an inflammation of another kind. I have feen a venereal node which gave excruciating pain cured by an incifion only being made down to the bone the whole length of the node; the pain has ceafed, the fwelling has decreafed, and the fore healed up kindly without taking a grain of mercury. Bliftets have been applied to nodes with fuccefs; they have removed the pains and diminifhed the fwellings; fo far furnifhing a proof that local treatment may affift mercury in many cafes.

This treatment has not only been ufed to affift mercury in thofe cafes where the medicine did not appear to be equal to the difeafe, but it has been ufed at the commencement of the cure, and even before mercury had been applied; but it was ftill thought neceffary to go through the fame mercurial courfe as if nothing had been done to the local complaints.

It may be afked, what advantage arifes from the incifion or application of the blifter? The advantage is immediate relief from violent pains; and as there are two powers acting, it is natural to fuppofe the cure will be more fpeedy.

After

After all the above trials it may happen that the local effects shall still remain, forming as it were a new disease, which mercury may increase, and therefore other methods of cure may be tried, as will be described hereafter.

VIII. OF ABSCESSES—EXFOLIATION.

When an abscess forms in a node in the periosteum the bones are generally affected and make part of the abscess. Great attention should be paid to them, for suppurations in them are not like suppurations in common abscesses, they are seldom produced from the true suppurative inflammation, and therefore are slow in their progress, rarely producing true matter, but a mucus, something resembling slime, which lies flat upon the bone. This circumstance makes it difficult to determine when suppuration has taken place, and in many cases to detect matter, even where it is formed. Another circumstance which renders the presence of matter in such cases doubtful is, that the progress of the disease is generally checked very early by the use of mercury. This matter is often reabsorbed during a mercurial course; and it is proper, particularly in an early state of the complaint, to give it this chance; but if the absorption does not take place, and the complaint is in an advanced state, it must be opened.

The surgical treatment of the parts under such circumstances is the same as in other diseases of these parts; opening with great freedom is absolutely necessary; for the more parts are exposed, the more inclinable they are in general to take on the healing state, and still more so here; for violence assists in destroying the venereal disposition. No skin covering a bone should be removed from an abscess, especially in the lower extremities.

If the abscess is opened freely, and an exfoliation takes place, which is generally the case, it is to be treated as any other exfoliation. Exfoliations succeed much better here than in many other cases, because the disease from which they proceed can generally be corrected, which is not the case in many diseases of bones where exfoliation takes place. Cases however sometimes occur in which after the venereal disposition has been corrected another diseased action takes place in the bone, the nature of which will be explained when upon the effects remaining after the diſeaſe is cured, and the diſeaſes ſometimes produced by the cure.

IX. OF NODES ON TENDONS, LIGAMENTS, AND FASCIÆ.

THE obſervations made on the nodes of the perioſteum and bones are applicable to ſwellings and ſuppurations of the ligaments and faſciæ; but it is ſtill more difficult to aſcertain the preſence of matter in them than in the former.

When a thickening only of the ligaments or faſciæ is the conſequence of the diſeaſe, it is very obſtinate, as in many caſes the diſeaſed part may be cleared of all venereal taint and ſtill the ſwellings remain. Bliſters may often be applied here with ſucceſs; but if they fail, then it will be abſolutely neceſſary to make an inciſion into the part, to excite a more vigorous action; for although the complaint has nothing venereal in it, nor is any contamination to be feared from it in future, yet as it leaves often very obſtinate and diſagreeable ſwellings, which neither give way to medicine nor time, it is proper to uſe every means for their removal.

X. OF CORRECTING SOME OF THE EFFECTS OF MERCURY.

FORMERLY when the management of mercury was not ſo well underſtood, nor it's effects in this diſeaſe ſo well known as they are at preſent, it was generally ſuppoſed to act by evacuation from the ſalivary glands, and was therefore always given till that evacuation took place; and as it's effects in the cure were imagined to be in proportion to the quantity of this evacuation, it was puſhed as far as poſſible without endangering ſuffocation. From this treatment it often happened in thoſe conſtitutions which were very ſuſceptible of the mercurial irritation, and in which the medicine produced much more violent effects on ſome particular ſecretions than could be wiſhed, that recourſe was obliged to be had to medicines correcting the effects of mercury;

as

as these effects were often an hindrance to it's being given in sufficient quantities for the cure of the disease.

I mentioned, when treating of the effects of mercury, that the sensible increase of the secretions produced by it were in the following order; first of saliva, then sweat, then urine, and often of the mucus of the intestines, producing purging; I also observed that when any of those secretions became too violent, that the hand of the surgeon was tied up till they were moderated. Attempts have been made to lessen those effects in two ways, either by the destruction of it's power on the body in general, or by it's removal, but neither of these means have succeeded. It never has once been thought necessary to attempt to lessen it's powers on the organs of secretion, so as still to retain the same quantity in the constitution, or even to throw in more, which if it could be effected would be sometimes of great service; but as we are not yet acquainted with powers sufficient for these purposes, we are obliged to observe great caution in our mode of giving the medicine.

I have endeavoured to show that this medicine need not be given with a view to procure those evacuations, and that it may be given in any quantity without increasing either of those secretions in any evident degree; however after every precaution we may be still deceived, and the medicine will every now and then produce greater effects than were intended. It is very necessary therefore to seek for a preventive of the effects of mercury, when likely to be too violent, or to remedy those effects when they have already taken place.

The common practice when mercury produced violent effects upon the intestines, was to counteract these effects; but this was not done with a view to retain the mercury in the constitution, but to relieve the bowels that were suffering by the action of the medicine: whereas the proper practice would be to stop it's progress here, as in every other outlet, that more mercury may be retained in the constitution.

Although these increased secretions arise from the constitutions being loaded with mercury, yet there is no danger in stopping them, for they do not arise from an universal disposition becoming a local, or critical one; and therefore if such an action be checked or stopped in one place, it must necessarily fall upon some other; but it is from the part being more susceptible of this irritation

irritation than any other, and the quantity now in the conftitution being equal to the fufceptibility of the part; and therefore though it's effects are ftopped here, it does not break out any where elfe, every other part being capable of fupporting this quantity, and of remaining unaffected till more is thrown in.

When the mercury attacked the falivary glands it increafed that fecretion fo much as in fome cafes to oblige practitioners to adminifter fuch medicines as were thought likely to remove this new complaint. This fufceptibility of the glands of the mouth, and the mouth in general, to be eafily put into action by this medicine, was generally fuppofed to arife from a fcorbutic conftitution, to which moft complaints of the mouth are attributed. I am of opinion that fcrofulous people, and thofe of a lax and delicate habit, are more fubject to have it fall on the mouth than thofe of a contrary temperament.

Purges were given upon a fuppofition that mercury could be carried off by the evacuation produced by them, and they were repeated according to the violence of the effects of the medicine, and the ftrength of the patient: but I can hardly fay that I ever have feen the effects of mercury upon the mouth, leffened by purging, whether it arofe fpontaneoufly, was produced by purging medicines, or even when arifing from the mercury itfelf. As this method was not found fufficient for the removal of the complaint other medicines were tried; fulphur was fuppofed to be a fpecific for the removal of the effect of mercury. Whether this idea arofe from practice or reafoning is not material;* but I think I have feen good effects from it in fome cafes. If we can fuppofe purging of any fervice, purging with fulphur would anfwer beft, as it would exert it's effects both as a purge and as a fpecific.

Sulphur certainly enters the circulation as fulphur, becaufe our fweat and urine fmell of it; if it does not combine with the mercury and deftroy it's properties as mercury, it is poffible, agreeable to the opinion of thofe who firft thought of giving it with this intention, that it may fo combine as to

* Sulphur united with any of the metals probably deftroys their folubility in the juices, or at leaft their effects in the circulation; none of the cinnabars act either as fulphur, or mercury. Crude antimony, which is regulus of antimony and fulphur, has no effect. Arfenic when joined with fulphur has no effect, nor has iron.

form

form Æthiops mineral, or something similar, for we know that the Æthiops mineral however formed does not in general salivate. It is possible too, that sulphur may act as a contrary stimulus to mercury, by counteracting the effects of it in the constitution. Sulphur has even been supposed to hinder the mercury from entering the circulation. Upon the whole, as these preparations of sulphur and mercury are still supposed to have good effects, and as I think I have seen good effects in other cases, we must either allow that they enter the circulation, or that their whole effects are on the stomach and intestines, with which the rest of the body sympathises. The good effects from sulphur in lessening or altering the immediate effects of mercury, can only take place when that medicine is really in the constitution; therefore a distinction is to be made between such as arise immediately from mercury, and one continued from habit after the mercury has been evacuated from the constitution, a case that sometimes happens, and which will be taken notice of in it's proper place.

The taste in the mouth from the use of mercury has been known to go off, and not be perceived for a fortnight, and the same taste has recurred; this I am informed has happened twice to one gentleman from the first quantity of mercury taken. To account for this is not easy; in whatever way it happens it is a curious fact.

When the mercury has fallen upon the mouth and throat, washing those parts with opium has often good effects, for opium takes off irritability, and of course the soreness, which is one means of lessening the secretion. A dram of tinctura thebaica to an ounce of water makes a good wash, or gargle.*

When the mercury falls upon the skin it is neither so disagreeable nor so dangerous as when it falls upon the mouth; however it may often happen that it will be proper to check such a discharge, both upon account of it's being troublesome and of it's lessening the effects of the medicine in the constitution by carrying it off. The bark is perhaps one of the best correctors of this increased secretion.

* My using opium in this way was from analogy, finding that opium quieted the bowels when a purging came on in consequence of mercury: I tried it by way of gargle to the mouth, and found good effects from it, but not equal to those which it produced in the bowels.

When the medicine attacks the kidneys and increafes the fecretion of thefe glands, it is not fo troublefome as when it produces fweating, though it is poffible that it may carry off the mercury too foon; but as we have but few medicines that can leffen that fecretion, in moft cafes it muft be allowed to go on. The bark may in fuch cafes be given with advantage.

When the mercury falls upon the bowels it proves often more dangerous and troublefome than in any of the former cafes, efpecially the two laft; but it is perhaps moft in our power to prevent or palliate. Opium fhould be given in fuch quantities as to overcome the complaint, and I believe will feldom fail in removing all the fymptoms.

XI. OF THE FORM OF THE DIFFERENT PREPARATIONS OF MERCURY WHEN IN THE CIRCULATION.

IT would appear from reafon, and many circumftances, that mercury muft be in the ftate of folution in the juices of the body before it can act upon the venereal difeafe, and indeed before it can act upon any other difeafe. That mercury is in a ftate of folution in our juices and not in the ftate of any preparation of mercury that we know of is very probable from the following facts.

First, crude mercury, every falt of mercury, and calx of mercury, is foluble in the fpittle, when taken into the mouth, by which means it is rendered fenfible to the tafte; from thence it muft appear that it is capable of folution in fome of our juices.

Secondly, crude mercury when divided into fmall parts by gum arabic, &c. fo as to be eafier of folution when taken into the ftomach, generally purges; but crude mercury taken without fuch divifion has no fuch powers, not being fo readily diffolved in the juices of the ftomach. The fimple calx of mercury has the fame effects, purging, and much more violently from being, I fuppofe, readier of folution in the animal juices; for if it only purged from it's union with the acid which happened to be in the ftomach it moft probably would not purge more than crude mercury; although it is very probable

bable that the calx is eafier of folution in a weak acid, than even the crude mercury.

Thirdly, every preparation of mercury producing the fame effect in the mouth, and alfo having one and the fame effect in the conftitution, fhows that they muft all undergo a change by which they are reduced to one particular form. We cannot fay what that form is, whether it is the calx, the metal, or any other that we are acquainted with; but it is probable that it is not any of them, but a new folution in the animal juices peculiar to the animal itfelf. This is rendered ftill more probable by this circumftance, that every preparation of mercury put into the mouth, undergoes the fame change, and the fpittle has the fame tafte from every one of them. If every different preparation of mercury had the fame properties in the conftitution that it poffeffes out of it, which we muft fuppofe if it enters and continues in the fame form, in that cafe the venereal poifon muft be eradicated in as many different ways as there are preparations. Crude mercury would act mechanically, by increafing the weight and momentum of the blood; the calx would act like brickduft, or any other powder that is heavy; the red precipitate would ftimulate by chymical properties in one way, while the corrofive fublimate would act in another, and the mercurius flavus in a third; this laft would moft probably vomit as ipecacuanha does, which vomits whether thrown into the ftomach or circulation.

Fourthly, all the preparations of mercury when locally applied act always in one way, that is, as mercury; but fome have alfo another mode of action, which is chymical, and which is according to the fpecific nature of the preparation. The red precipitate is a preparation of this kind, and acts in both thefe ways, it is either a ftimulant or an efcharotic.

To afcertain whether this opinion of mercury being in folution in our juices was juft, I made the following experiments upon myfelf. I put fome crude mercury into my mouth, as a ftandard, and let it ftay there working it about, fo as to render it eafier of folution, till I tafted it fenfibly; I then put into my mouth the mercurius calcinatus, and let it remain till I perceived the tafte of it, which was exactly the fame; but I obferved that it was eafier of folution than the crude mercury. I tried calomel in the fame way,

way, and alſo corroſive ſublimate, after being diluted with water, and the taſte was ſtill the ſame. It was ſome time before I perceived the taſte of the crude mercury in my mouth. I taſted the calx and calomel much ſooner. The corroſive ſublimate had at firſt a mixed taſte, but when the acid was diluted it had exactly the ſame taſte with the former; all theſe different preparations producing the ſame ſenſation or taſte in the mouth.

From the effects of theſe experiments it would appear, that the mercury in every one of them was diſſolved in the ſpittle, and reduced to the ſame preparation or ſolution.

To try whether mercury in the conſtitution would produce the ſame taſte in the mouth, I rubbed in mercurial ointment upon my thighs till my mouth was affected, and I could plainly taſte the mercury; and as far as I could rely upon my memory the taſte was exactly the ſame as in the former experiments.

I allowed ſome time for my mouth to get perfectly well and free from the taſte; I then took calomel in pills till it was affected again in the ſame way. I afterwards took mercurius calcinatus, and alſo corroſive ſublimate. All theſe experiments were attended with the ſame reſult; the mercury in every form producing the ſame taſte, which was alſo exactly the ſame as when the ſeveral preparations were put into the mouth.

From the above experiments it muſt appear, that when mercury produces evacuation by the mouth, it certainly goes off in that diſcharge; and from thence we may reaſonably conclude, that when other evacuations are produced from the medicine when in the conſtitution, as purging, ſweating, or an increaſed flow of urine, that it alſo goes off by theſe evacuations, which become outlets to the mercury.

From the above experiments it appears to be immaterial what preparation of mercury is uſed in the cure of this diſeaſe, provided it is of eaſy ſolution in our juices, the preparations eaſieſt of ſolution being always the beſt.

XII. OF

XII. OF THE OPERATION OF MERCURY ON THE POISON.

Mercury may be ſuppoſed to act in three different ways in curing the venereal diſeaſe. Firſt, it may unite with the poiſon chymically, and decompoſe it, by which means it's powers of irritation may be deſtroyed. Secondly, it may carry it out of the conſtitution by evacuation; or thirdly, it may produce an irritation in the conſtitution which counteracts the venereal and entirely deſtroys it.

It has been ſuppoſed that mercury acts ſimply by it's weight in the circulating fluids; but of this we can form no adequate idea; and if it were ſo, other ſubſtances ſhould act on this diſeaſe in proportion to their weight, and of courſe many of them ſhould cure it; but from experience we find, that ſuch bodies as have conſiderable weight, as moſt of the metals, have no effect on this diſeaſe. We have no proof of mercury acting by a decompoſition of the poiſon from any of the concomitant circumſtances.

Mercury certainly does not cure the venereal diſeaſe by uniting with the poiſon and producing an evacuation. For in thoſe caſes where mercury is given in ſuch a way as to produce conſiderable evacuations, or in thoſe conſtitutions where evacuations are eaſily excited by mercury, it's effects upon the diſeaſed action are the leaſt; and the ſame evacuations produced by any other means have not the leaſt effect on the diſeaſe.

Whether the mercury be ſuppoſed to carry off the circulating poiſon, or to decompoſe it, in neither way could it produce, when locally applied, any effect on a venereal inflammation or ſore ariſing from the conſtitution; for as long as any of the poiſon exiſted in the circulation, none of them could be healed by local applications, the circulation conſtantly carrying the poiſon to them; but we find the contrary of this to be true; for a venereal ſore ariſing from the conſtitution may be cured locally.

The laſt or third of our modes of action of mercury ſeems to me the moſt probable, and for many reaſons. Firſt, becauſe the diſeaſe can in many caſes be cured by raiſing a violent ſtimulus of another kind; and perhaps if we could raiſe ſuch a conſtitutional irritation without danger, as we often can in local cafes, we might cure the venereal difeafe in the fame manner, and in one quarter of the ufual time. Secondly, we find that mercury acts as an univerfal ftimulus, caufing great irritability in the conftitution, making the heart beat fafter, and rendering the arteries more rigid, fo as to produce a hard pulfe, as has been already obferved. It may further be faid to produce a difeafe, or a peculiar or unnatural mode of action in a certain degree. The following cafe will illuftrate this. A gentleman had electricity recommended to him for fome complaint he had. The electricity was applied, but without any vifible effect. Befides the complaint for which he ufed electricity, he had a venereal one, for which he was firft put under a courfe of mercury, and while under it the electricity was applied for the former complaint; but he had become fo irritable that he could not bear the fhocks of one half their former ftrength; but the moft curious part of the cafe was, that the fhocks had a much greater effect on the difeafe than what they had before when twice as ftrong, and he now got cured. This gave the furgeon a hint, and having another occafion to ufe electricity, alfo without effect, he put the patient under a gentle courfe of mercury, and then found the fame effects from the electricity as in the former cafe, and the patient alfo got well.

The powers of mercury upon the conftitution appear to be as the quantity of mercury and the fufceptibility of the conftitution to be affected with it, without any relation to the difeafe itfelf; and we find that the power of mercury upon the difeafe is nearly in the fame proportion. This fact gives us an idea of the irritation of mercury upon the conftitution, and confequently an idea of adminiftering it, and of the cure of any difeafe for which it is a remedy.

As we find that a given quantity of mercury produces double effects in fome conftitutions to what it does in others; alfo, that in thofe cafes it produces it's effects upon the difeafe, we are led to believe that it is this effect upon the conftitution which cures the difeafe; and therefore if it did not produce this effect it would alfo not have performed a cure. I have already obferved, that the cure does not go on exactly in proportion to the vifible effects upon the conftitution, except quantity in the medicine is joined with it; which if true would incline us to believe that there was fomething more than

than ſimply a conſtitutional ſtimulus, which moſt probably is a peculiar ſpecific effect which is not regulated entirely by it's viſible effects, either conſtitutional or local, although they appear to have ſome connection.

This fact being known obliges us to be more liberal in giving mercury in thoſe conſtitutions where it makes but little impreſſion, than in thoſe which it eaſily irritates; although in theſe laſt we muſt not be entirely regulated by it's local effects, nor depend upon a commonly ſufficient quantity, but be ruled by the ſenſibility of the conſtitution, and quantity joined; for in thoſe where the conſtitution appears to be very ſuſceptible of the mercurial irritation, where ſmall quantities produce conſiderable local effects, it is ſtill neceſſary to have quantity, although it is not ſo neceſſary to take the quantity in general that is ſuppoſed to be ſufficient. We muſt be guided by the three following circumſtances, the diſappearance of the diſeaſe, the quantity of irritation produced, and the quantity of the medicine taken.

XIII. OF GUM GUAIACUM, AND RADIX SARSAPARILLÆ IN THE VENEREAL DISEASE.

I have hitherto only recommended mercury in the cure of the venereal diſeaſe; and indeed it is the only medicine to be depended upon. However as both the guaiacum and ſarſaparilla have been recommended as powerful remedies in this complaint, I took a favourable opportunity of trying their comparative powers in the venereal diſeaſe upon the ſame perſon.

The guaiacum* I found had conſiderable ſpecific power over the diſeaſe, conſequently it may be of ſervice in ſlight caſes where it may be inconvenient or improper to give mercury on account of ſome other diſeaſe. Theſe caſes however I have not yet aſcertained; or it may be given in thoſe caſes where it is apprehended that the quantity of mercury neceſſary to ſubdue the diſeaſe would be too much for the conſtitution to bear; caſes which ſometimes occur. The ſarſaparilla appeared to have no effect at all.

* The lignum guaiaci was imported by the Spaniards from Hiſpaniola as a cure for the venereal diſeaſe, in the year 1517, having been given to one of them by a native.

I ſhall

I ſhall relate exactly the caſe in which their comparative powers were tried. A man came into St. George's Hoſpital with venereal ſores over almoſt his whole body: there were many excreſcent ſores in the armpits, ſome of which were about the ſize of an halfpenny; there were the ſame appearances about the anus, between the buttocks, along the perinæum, between the ſcrotum and thigh, where thoſe parts come in contact with one another. Thoſe upon the ſkin in general had the common appearance. I ordered a poultice of the gum guaiacum to be applied to the ſores in the right armpit; alſo a poultice of a ſtrong decoction of ſarſaparilla and oatmeal mixed, to be applied to the left armpit. Theſe poultices were changed every day for a fortnight; the excreſcent ſores in the right armpit were entirely healed, and become even with the ſkin, and covered with a natural ſkin, although ſomewhat diſcoloured; the ſores in the left armpit, which were poulticed with ſarſaparilla, were rather worſe than when the poultice was firſt applied, as indeed were all the ſores, except thoſe in the right armpit. I then ordered the poultice of guaiacum to be applied to the left armpit, which was done, and the ſores there alſo got well in a fortnight; I was now perfectly convinced that the gum guaiacum had cured theſe eruptions locally.

I next wiſhed to ſee what effect the gum guaiacum would have upon the remaining ſores when given internally, that is, thoſe about the anus, ſcrotum, and on the ſkin in general. The patient began with half a dram three times every day, which purged him; but this was prevented by joining it with opium. In about four weeks all the eruptions were cured, and he was allowed to ſtay in the hoſpital ſome time longer to ſee if he would continue well; but about a fortnight after he began to break out anew, and in a very ſhort time was almoſt as bad as ever. I began a ſecond time the gum guaiacum internally, but it had loſt all it's powers, or rather the conſtitution was no longer affected by it. He was put under a courſe of mercury and cured.

CHAPTER

CHAPTER IV.

OF THE EFFECTS REMAINING AFTER THE DISEASE IS CURED, AND OF THE DISEASES SOMETIMES PRODUCED BY THE CURE.

IN treating of the local effects of the venereal diſeaſe, the gonorrhœa and chancre, as alſo the bubo, I obſerved that after the virus was deſtroyed there remained in many caſes ſome of the ſame ſymptoms, and particularly after the gonorrhœa. It was alſo obſerved, that though all the ſymptoms were entirely cured, yet they were liable to break out again. A gleet will appear, ſometimes attended with pain, ſo as to reſemble a gonorrhœa; after chancres there will be ſores reſembling them; and buboes after the virus is gone, will not heal, but ſpread. In the lues venerea the ſame thing often happens, eſpecially if the inflammation and ſuppuration have been violent in the parts. Theſe caſes puzzle conſiderably; for it is difficult to ſay when the venereal virus is abſolutely gone. In ſuch doubtful caſes the treatment to be followed becomes more undetermined.

Such complaints are more common in the tonſils than in any other part, for we often find that while a mercurial courſe is going on, and the ulcer on the tonſils healing, or even healed, they ſhall ſwell, become excoriated, and the excoriations ſhall ſometimes ſpread over the whole palatum molle, which renders the nature of the diſeaſe doubtful. I believe theſe excoriations, as well as ſuch other appearances of diſeaſe as come on during the uſe of mercury, are ſeldom or never venereal. In all ſuch caſes I would recommend not to continue the mercury longer than what appears ſufficient for overcoming the original venereal complaints, not conſidering thoſe changes in the caſe as venereal. The bark is often of ſervice here, and may be given either with the mercury, or after the mercurial courſe is over.

It often happens that venereal abfceffes will not heal up, although they have gone a certain length towards it; for while the venereal action remained in the part, the mercury difpofed that part to heal, but under that courfe the conftitution and part had acquired another difpofition, proceeding from a venereal and mercurial irritation affecting a particular habit of body, or part, at the time, which new difpofition differs from the venereal, mercurial, and natural, being a fourth difpofition arifing out of all the three. I fufpect however that it depends chiefly on the conftitution; becaufe if it was owing to the other two, we fhould always have the fame difeafe; and what makes this opinion more probable is, that it differs in different people, at leaft it is not cured in all by the fame means. The conftitution being predifpofed, the other two become the immediate caufes of action. As foon as the venereal irritation is deftroyed by the mercury, or becomes weaker than the other two, then the effects of the others take place. While the venereal action prevails the mercury is of fervice, and the fore continues healing; but when it is leffened to a certain degree, or deftroyed, the mercury not only lofes it's powers, but becomes a poifon to the new difpofition that is formed; for if mercury is continued the fore fpreads, it fhould therefore be immediately left off.

Some of the fores formed in this way not only refift all means of cure, but often inflame, ulcerate, and form hard callous bafis, fo as to put on the appearance of a cancer, and are often fuppofed really to be fo.

We find alfo that new difeafes arife from the mercury alone. The tonfils fhall fwell where no venereal difeafe has been before, the periofteum fhall thicken, and alfo probably the bones, and the parts over them fhall become œdematous and fore to the touch; but as thefe complaints arife while under a mercurial courfe they are not to be reckoned venereal, but a new difeafe, although they are too often fuppofed to be venereal, and on that account the mercury is pufhed as far as poffible. In fuch cafes if the complaints for which the mercury was given are nearly cured, and the medicine has been continued a fufficient time after to complete the cure of thofe complaints, then of courfe it fhould be left off; and if there be any doubt it fhould be left off rather fooner than if no fuch complaint had taken place, becaufe it is probably producing a worfe difeafe than the venereal;

and

and if after the cure of thefe complaints from the mercury, the venereal difeafe begins again to come into action, mercury muft be given a fecond time, and now the conftitution will be better able to bear it, efpecially if attention has been paid to the reftoring the ftrength of it. Thofe difeafes of the tonfils and periofteum I fufpect have fomething fcrofulous in them.

Befides local complaints arifing from the combined action of the mercury, the difeafe, and the conftitution, there is fometimes a conftitutional effect, which is a weaknefs, or debility, a languor, want of appetite, frequent fweats threatning hectic; but thefe happen moftly in thofe conftitutions with which mercury difagrees. Thefe complaints, local as well as conftitutional, arife in fome meafure from weaknefs. They are difficult of cure, whether arifing from a venereal chancre, bubo, or the lues venerea. Strengthening medicines are of moft fervice: the bark is of great ufe though in general not fufficient, as it can only more or lefs remove the weaknefs, the fpecific qualities ftill remaining. What thefe are, is I believe not yet known, but I fufpect that many partake of the fcrofula, and this opinion is ftrengthened by their frequently giving way to fea-bathing.[a]

I. GENERAL OBSERVATIONS ON THE MEDICINES USUALLY GIVEN FOR THE CURE.

A decoction of the woods, among which are commonly included guaiacum and farfaparilla, is one of the firft medicines in the cure, and many of the cafes yield to it, which gives them the credit of curing the venereal difeafe, while fuch difeafes were fuppofed to be venereal. The farfaparilla was often given alone, and was found to produce nearly the fame effect. The good effects of it in one cafe eftablifhed it's reputation.[b] A diet drink difcovered

[a] In a cafe of an ulcerated rib from a venereal caufe, and five nodes on the fhin-bone, of twelve months ftanding, a deep falivation of fix months was undergone, after fruitlefs attempts by gentle friction. None of the fores were healed by the mercury, and the patient was ordered to bathe in the fea, and take the bark. In three or four months the fores all healed up very kindly; but the fide laft of all.

[b] See in London Medical Effays a cafe publifhed by Mr. Fordyce, now Sir William Fordyce.

at Lifbon was alfo of confiderable fervice; and as it cured cafes fimilar to thofe cured by the farfaparilla, it was imagined that the diet drink confifted principally of a decoction of this root. This was ftill on the fuppofition that all thofe cafes were venereal; but it was obferved at laft that thofe medicines did not cure this difeafe till mercury had been given, and in tolerably large quantity. This was fufficient to lead fome thinking minds to doubt whether they were venereal, or not; and their being cured by different medicines ought to produce a conviction of their being different from the venereal difeafe, and that they are themfelves of different kinds.

The mezereon has alfo been found to be of fervice in fome fymptoms of the lues venerea, fuch as nodes of the bones, but their being venereal was taken for granted. The mezereon is feldom given in venereal ulcers in the throat, or blotches on the fkin, which of all the venereal fymptoms are the moft certain, and the moft eafy of cure; yet it was conceived that it removed fuch fymptoms as are the moft difficult of cure; but all thofe cafes in which the mezereon has been given with fuccefs plainly appear not to have been venereal.

When the hemlock came into fafhion in this country it was given in almoft every difeafe, and of courfe was tried in fome of thofe complaints confequent to the venereal difeafe; and fome of thefe it was found to cure fo that it now ftands upon the lift of remedies. Velno's vegetable firup has had fimilar effects in fome of thefe cafes; and opium appears alfo to have many advocates. Opium, like the farfaparilla, and mezereon, was fuppofed by it's firft introducers to cure the lues venerea,[a] but like the farfaparilla, it appears to have no effect till mercury has done it's beft, or it's worft.[b] It has certainly confiderable effects in many difeafes, both in fuch as are confequent to the venereal difeafe, and others arifing from other caufes.

It has been long a favourite medicine of mine, not only as relieving pain, for that is it's common effect, but as a medicine capable of altering difeafed actions, and producing healthy ones. In all fores attended with irritability, a decoction of poppy heads made into a poultice is an excellent

[a] See Medical Communications, vol. 1, page 307.

[b] See a pamphlet publifhed by Mr. Grant.

application.

application. Bleeding sores that do not arise from weakness, but from irritability, have the bleeding stopped immediately by this application. Mr. Pott is, I believe, the first who showed the world it's use in mortifications. My first mode of applying it for the cure of diseases was locally, in which I found it had most salutary effects in some cases, and it was ordered afterwards internally upon the same principle, and it was also found to have salutary effects in this mode. In two cases that had been long suspected to be venereal, it's effects were very remarkable; and by it's having cured them it confirmed me in my opinion that they were not. But when I was informed that they cured the venereal disease in the army in America by opium, I then began to question myself, whether I had formed a right judgment of the nature of those two cases which were cured by opium. To ascertain whether opium would cure the lues venerea or not, I made the following trial at St. George's Hospital.

A woman was taken into the hospital with blotches on her skin which had arrived to the state of scabs, and with well-marked venereal ulcers on both tonsils. A grain of opium was ordered to be taken the first night, two the second, and so on, increasing a grain every night, unless something should arise to forbid it. This was closely followed till the nineteenth night, when she was ordered a dose of physic as she had become costive, and the opium was omitted. On the 20th she began again, and continued increasing the dose as before till it amounted to thirty grains, no alteration being produced in the sores, except what arose from the loss of time, whereby they were rather worse. I concluded, that if she had taken mercury to affect the constitution as much as the opium did, the venereal disease must have been nearly cured, or at least much lessened; but as that was not the case, it convinced me that the opium had no effect whatever on the venereal disease. I then put her under a course of mercury, by friction, and in a short time it affected her mouth, the sores soon began to look better, and they went on healing without interruption, till the disease was cured. I may just observe, she found very little inconvenience from the opium; it kept her quiet, but she was not particularly sleepy.

Opium for the future will be given with another view than what it has commonly been, not merely to allay pain, but to cure diseases. As those diſeaſes which opium will cure are not yet known, it will be tried in a thouſand caſes in which it will not ſucceed, and in many it will even do harm; but at laſt it will find it's place; and the doſes for ſuch purpoſes will probably far exceed what is given at preſent. But as opium is capable of doing miſchief, it ſhould always be given with great attention to it's effects. It's effects are juſt the reverſe in ſome caſes of what they are in common. In ſome conſtitutions it increaſes all the complaints, even ſuch as it commonly cures. I have known conſtitutions where opium diſagreed in every way; where it purged; where it increaſed the irritability of the bladder and urethra, producing watching, reſtleſſneſs, and extreme uneaſineſs. It in ſome caſes ſeemed to act like a poiſon: the following is a remarkable inſtance of this, and is alſo another proof of it's inefficacy in the venereal diſeaſe.

Luke Ward was admitted into St. Bartholomew's Hoſpital, January 12, 1785; his complaint was an ulcer in the throat of three months ſtanding, which both from it's appearance, and the ſymptoms which preceded it, ſeemed to be venereal. He was ordered two grains of opium twice a day, which he took a few days without any other effect than that of ſleeping better at night than uſual, when the doſe was increaſed to two grains three times a day. His throat now gave him leſs pain; but upon inſpection was not found to be at all mended. After two days the doſe was increaſed to three grains thrice a day; from this quantity he felt little or no inconvenience: he complained of being a little drowzy; his eyes were rather inflamed, and his face rather fluſhed. He continued to take this quantity for five days, and then it was increaſed to three grains four times a day. Next morning the redneſs and heat of his face was much increaſed, and had extended over his whole ſkin; he complained of pain in his head. His pulſe was full and ſtrong; he was bound in his body, and his belly was tenſe and painful. The opium was omitted, and ſuch remedies as the preſent ſymptoms ſeemed to require were given, but without effect; all his ſymptoms continuing to increaſe till he died, which was on the fourth day after; during this time the ulcer increaſed much, and the diſcharge of ſaliva was ſo great as to reſemble a ſlight ſalivation.

This

This caſe proves in the firſt place, that the opium had no effect upon the ulcer in the throat; and in the next, that it is a medicine capable of producing very violent effects in the conſtitution, requiring therefore great caution in the mode of adminiſtering it.

John Morgan was admitted into St. Bartholomew's hoſpital with an ulcerated leg. The common applications were tried for ſeven weeks, at the end of which time he was in every reſpect worſe, having no ſleep from conſtant pain, and he was ſinking very faſt. Two grains of opium were given every two hours, for twenty-three days, it made him hot and coſtive, and his pulſe became ſtrong and full, but without ſleep or abatement of pain. The doſe was increaſed to four grains every two hours in the day, and eight grains every two hours during the night. The effects were coſtiveneſs, retention of urine, loſs of appetite, an inflammatory diſpoſition, no ſleep, without any amendment of the ulcer. On the third day of taking the laſt-mentioned quantities he awoke from a ſhort ſleep delirious, and continued ſo for twelve hours, when it left him very weak, ſick at his ſtomach, and with a low pulſe. In three or four hours the delirium returned and continued forty-eight hours; the pulſe on it's return immediately roſe, and his ſtrength returned to a very great degree. When it went off he fell into a ſound ſleep for about eight hours, and awoke very tranquil, though weak; no more opium was given, and the leg in the ſpace of a month healed.

In the firſt twenty-three days he took twenty-four grains a day; for the laſt three days he took ſeventy-two grains a day. In twenty-ſix days he took ſeven hundred and ſixty-eight, which is nearly two ounces of opium.

Sarſaparilla is frequently given; but the opinions formed of it's uſe appear to be vague and undetermined. It is neither wholly allowed, nor is it abſolutely denied to have effects upon the venereal diſeaſe. It is the common opinion that ſarſaparilla does not cure, except where mercury has been given.

From the comparative experiment made with it and the guaiacum, it would appear to have no effect upon the venereal irritation itſelf, and therefore can be of no ſervice till that irritation is deſtroyed; and as mercury is the antidote for that poiſon, and becomes one of the cauſes of the com-

plaints

plaints which sarsaparilla is good for, therefore mercury is not only necessary to destroy the poison, but also assists in forming the diseases we are now treating of.

From the opinions of it's being of service in the venereal disease, it has been, and is still a common practice to give it with the mercury: whether it really is of any service, is I believe much to be doubted; but it is easy to conceive it in many cases to be of use in preventing the formation of the disease arising from mercury. When given along with the mercury it is often joined with the gum guaiacum, or the wood of the guaiacum, which we know will have some effect.

The sarsaparilla is generally given in form of a decoction, three ounces to three pints of water, boiled down slowly to a quart, and the half or whole is drank every day, generally at three different times, often at meals. It is sometimes ground to a powder and taken every day with the same effect; but I should prefer the extract made into pills, as the easiest way of taking this medicine.

In many of these cases I have seen good effects from the hemlock, of which the following is an instance; and I would further refer the reader back to the observations given of this medicine when treating of the disease produced in consequence of a bubo, page 284.

A poor woman had undergone repeated salivations, which had always relieved the most pressing symptoms; but after being afflicted more or less for three or four years, ulcers broke out in her nose, and all over her face, with what is called a true cancerous appearance. The sores became soon very deep, and gave very considerable pain. Mercury, sarsaparilla, and bark were given, without effect; the sores getting daily worse, the parts affected were ordered to be held over the steam of a decoction of hemlock every four hours, and as much extract to be taken internally as the patient could bear. She had sleep, and was free from pain the first night; and in a few days the sores put on a healing appearance. She lost her nose and one side of her mouth; but in six weeks time every part was skinned over. She remained well for three months, when the disease returned with redoubled violence and soon destroyed her: probably the hemlock should have been continued longer.

II. OF THE CONTINUANCE OF THE SPITTING.

It ſometimes happens that the ſpitting continues after there is every reaſon for ſuppoſing the mercury is entirely out of the conſtitution; for the taſte of the medicine ſhall be entirely gone: this is ſimilar to ſome of the ſymptoms of the different ſpecies of the venereal diſeaſe. As it is only a continuation of an action, or an effect of mercury when in the conſtitution, it is neceſſary to diſtinguiſh it from the original, or from the immediate effects of mercury; ſince on this diſtinction reſts the method of cure. This may be reckoned a gleet of theſe parts. Such conſtitutions have been generally ſuppoſed ſcorbutic; and where there is a great ſuſceptibility of the mercurial ſtimulus in theſe parts the ſalivation will continue for months after the mercury has been completely removed; but this medicine not being given now in quantity ſufficient to produce ſuch violent effects on the ſalivary glands, theſe caſes ſeldom occur.

In ſuch caſes I would recommend ſtrengthening diet, and ſtrengthening medicines: bark, and ſteel, are ſome of the beſt. Sea-bathing is one of the beſt reſtoratives of relaxed habits, eſpecially after mercury. Mead's tincture of cantharides is ſuppoſed to be of ſervice in thoſe caſes. I am inclined to believe that a ſolution of opium might be of ſervice as a gargle.

The alveolar proceſſes have ſometimes become dead, and exfoliations have taken place, this alone has kept up a diſcharge of ſaliva. When this happens we muſt wait till ſeparation takes place, and extract the looſe pieces, after which the ſalivation will ſubſide.

I have ſeen part of the jaw exfoliate from this cauſe. In moſt caſes the teeth are looſe; and in many they drop out.

CHAPTER V.

OF PREVENTING THE VENEREAL DISEASE.

AS diseases in general should not only be cured, but when it is possible prevented, it will not be improper to show, as far as we know, how that may be done; for in this disease we can with more certainty prevent infection, it's origin being known.

Preventives are previous or immediate applications, and may be divided into various kinds; as those that will not allow the venereal matter to come in contact with the parts; those which wash it off before it stimulates; and those which will act chymically and destroy the poison.

Oils rubbed on a dry part stick to it and prevent any thing that is watry from coming in contact with it; and as the venereal poison is mixed with a watry fluid, it is not allowed to touch the part.

Every thing which has a power of mixing with the venereal matter, and removing it from the part to which it is applied, may prove a prevention; caustic alkali is the best for this purpose, it unites with the matter, forming a soap, and is then easily washed off.

It is possible this union with the alkali may destroy the poison: the alkali must be much diluted or it will excoriate.

Lime-water would make a good wash.

If both these methods were put in practice there would be still more security.

Goulard's extract of Saturn has the power of coagulating the animal juices; how far this would answer I cannot say; for I can conceive that the matter may be coagulated and the poison not destroyed.

Corrosive sublimate in water, about a grain or two to eight ounces, has been known to prevent the catching of the disease when many other things have failed.

PART

PART VII.

CHAPTER I.

OF DISEASES RESEMBLING THE LUES VENEREA, WHICH HAVE BEEN MISTAKEN FOR IT.

THERE is probably no one diſeaſe to which ſome other may not bear a ſtrong reſemblance in ſome of it's appearances or ſymptoms, whereby they may be miſtaken for each other. The ſituation of a complaint alſo may miſlead the judgment. A lump for inſtance in the breaſt of a woman may reſemble a cancer ſo much as to be miſtaken for one, if all the diſtinguiſhing marks of cancer are not well attended to. An ulcer on the glans penis, or in the throat, and noſe, creates a ſuſpicion of the venereal diſeaſe. Even the way in which a diſeaſe is caught becomes a cauſe of ſuſpicion. The fluor albus in women ſometimes produces a gonorrhœa in men, but it is not venereal, as has been mentioned. Drinking out of the ſame cup with a venereal patient was formerly ſuppoſed to be capable of communicating the lues venerea, but this notion is I believe now exploded. Of late years a new mode of producing the venereal diſeaſe is ſuppoſed to have ariſen; this is by the tranſplanting of a tooth, from the mouth of one perſon into the mouth of another. That ſuch practice has produced diſeaſe is undoubted, but how far it has been venereal remains to be conſidered.

Diſeaſes which reſemble others, ſeldom do it in more than one or two of the ſymptoms; therefore whenever the nature of a diſeaſe is ſuſpected the whole of the ſymptoms ſhould be well inveſtigated, to ſee whether it agrees in all of them with the diſeaſe it is ſuſpected to be, or only in part. This obſervation ſeems to be more applicable to the venereal diſeaſe than any other; for

for there is hardly any diſorder that has more diſeaſes reſembling it in all it's different forms than the venereal diſeaſe; and when a diſeaſe reſembles the venereal in ſome of it's ſymptoms, but not at all in others, then thoſe other ſymptoms are to be ſet down as the ſpecific or leading ones of the diſeaſe to which it belongs; the reſembling ſymptoms to the venereal being only the common ones. But if a diſeaſe is ſuſpected to be venereal, though it is not perfectly marked, yet if it reſembles the venereal in moſt of it's ſymptoms, it muſt be ſuppoſed to be venereal, that being the moſt probable, although it is by no means certain; for probably the venereal can hardly be demonſtrated in any caſe, eſpecially in the form of the lues venerea, from it's not having the power of contamination.

Although the venereal diſeaſe keeps it's ſpecific properties diſtinct in it's ſeveral forms, yet it's ſymptoms are in appearance common to many other diſeaſes, and in that light it cannot be ſaid to have any one ſymptom peculiar to itſelf. For inſtance, every ſymptom of the venereal diſeaſe, in form of a gonorrhœa, may be produced by any other viſible irritating cauſe; and often without any cauſe that can be aſſigned; even buboes and ſwelled teſticles, which are ſymptoms of this diſeaſe, have followed both ſtimulating injections and bougies, when applied to the urethra of a ſound perſon; and indeed theſe two ſymptoms when they do ariſe from a venereal cauſe in many caſes are only ſymptomatic, not ſpecific, but more eſpecially the ſwelled teſticle.

Sores on the glans penis, prepuce, &c. in form of chancres, may, and do ariſe without any venereal infection; although we may obſerve that they are in general a conſequence of former venereal ſores which have been perfectly cured.

The ſymptoms produced from the infection when in the conſtitution are ſuch as are common to many other diſeaſes; viz. blotches on the ſkin, are common to what is called ſcorbutic habits; pains common to rheumatiſm, ſwellings of the bones, perioſteum, faſciæ, &c. to many bad habits, perhaps of the ſcrofulous and rheumatic kind. Thus moſt of the ſymptoms of the venereal diſeaſe in all it's forms are common to many other diſeaſes; therefore we are led back to the original cauſe, to a number of leading circumſtances, as dates, and it's effects upon others from connection when only local,

local, joined with the present appearances and symptoms before we can determine absolutely what the disease truly is; for all three taken together may be such as can attend no other disease. However with all our knowledge, and with all the application of that knowledge to suspicious symptoms of this disease, we are often mistaken, often calling it venereal when it is not; and sometimes supposing it to be some other disease when it is venereal.

Rheumatism in many of it's symptoms, in some constitutions, resembles the lues venerea; the nocturnal pains, swelling of the tendons, ligaments, and periosteum, and pain in those swellings are symptoms both of the rheumatism and the venereal disease when it attacks these parts: I do not know that I ever saw the lues venerea attack the joints, though many rheumatic complaints of those parts are cured by mercury, and therefore supposed to be venereal.

Mercury given without caution often produces the same symptoms as rheumatism; and I have seen even such supposed to be venereal and the medicine continued.

Other diseases shall not only resemble the venereal in appearance but in the mode of contamination, proving themselves to be poisons by affecting the part of contact, and from thence producing immediate consequences similar to buboes; also remote consequences similar to the lues venerea.

As errors in forming a judgment of a disease lead to errors in the cure, it becomes almost of as much consequence to avoid a mistake in the one as in the other; for it is nearly as dangerous in many constitutions to give mercury where the disease is not venereal, as to omit it in those which are; for we may observe, that many of the constitutions which put on some of the venereal symptoms, when the disease is not present, are those with which mercury seldom agrees, and commonly does harm. I have seen mercury given in a supposed venereal ulcer of the tonsils produce a mortification of those glands, and the patient has been nearly destroyed.

When treating of the lues venerea and giving the symptoms and general appearances of the disease, I related some cases which appeared to be venereal, though they really were not; and I shall now refer the reader to these, as it will be unnecessary to give them again here, although if they had not been formerly taken notice of this would have been a very proper place.

As the diseases in question are various, and not to be reduced to any system or order that I am acquainted with, I shall content myself with relating the cases, and thereby put it in the power of others to judge for themselves, if they should not be inclined to adopt the conclusions I have drawn from them.

On the 28th of July 1776, a gentleman, then in the West Indies, scratched the end of his finger with a thorn. On the 31st he opened an abscess on the shoulder of a negro woman who had the yaws, and had been long subject to such abscesses in different parts of the body, and to incurable ulcerations afterwards. At the instant after the operation, he perceived a little of the matter upon the scratch, and exclaimed that he was inoculated. On the 2nd of August, he amputated a boys finger of thirteen years of age, for a sore resembling worm-eaten wood. The scratch on his finger did not heal, but from time to time threw off whitish scales: this appearance alarmed him, and he rubbed in mercurial ointment very freely. Notwithstanding this, in the month of September, a painful inflamed tumor appeared on the second joint of the finger, which was soon followed by several others on the back of the hand, in the course of the metacarpal bone of the forefinger. He still continued the mercurial friction, but without effect, for the tumors daily multiplied; and by the month of November extended to within a small distance of the axilla. They did not go on to suppuration at this time. About the end of November he began to be affected with severe nocturnal pains in different parts of the body, but especially along the tibia and fibula, with frequent severe headachs, which continued to increase to an almost intolerable degree for five months, though he used mercurial friction, with decoction of sarsaparilla every day in great quantity.

In the month of May 1777, a scabby eruption appeared in different parts of the body, especially the legs and thighs, and the before mentioned tumors ulcerated; but this was followed by a remission of the nocturnal pains.

He never could bring on a salivation, though his mouth was constantly tender, even for months. The ulcerations became daily worse, and a voyage to England was thought the only resource. He arrived in London the 1st of August, and by the advice of Dr. William Hunter and Sir John Pringle he began again a course of mercury and sarsaparilla, with a milk diet. I was called

called in, and judging that two thirds of a grain of mercurius calcinatus every day was too ſmall a doſe, if it were judged to be venereal, it was ordered to be gradually increaſed to five grains; and he continued this courſe till November, when all the ſores were perfectly healed.

He now diſcontinued the mercury, and remained free from all ſymptoms of the diſorder, except ſome nodes on the tibia, and rheumatic pains on expoſure to cold, until about twelve months ago he began to have an uneaſineſs in ſwallowing, a rawneſs in the throat, and a diſcharge of viſcid mucus from that and the poſterior noſtrils, all of which ſtill continue.

The following obſervations may be made on the above caſe.

There can be little doubt that the diſeaſe was the yaws. The yaws is a diſeaſe that reſembles the venereal in ſeveral of it's ſymptoms as well as in the manner in which it is moſt commonly communicated. It differs however in ſome eſſential particulars. The yaws have a regular progreſs, after going through which they leave the conſtitution in an healthy ſtate, at leaſt free from that diſeaſe: it being ſufficient for the cure that the patient be put in a ſtate favourable to general health. Thus, a negro labouring under the diſeaſe muſt do little or no work, be kept clean, and have a better diet than uſual. Under theſe circumſtances, he commonly gets well in from four to nine months; although the unſavourable caſes will continue much longer. Various medicines are given for the cure, but it is not clear that any of them do good. Mercury has conſiderable power over the diſeaſe, without being a ſpecific for it. If given early it will either check the progreſs of the diſeaſe or perhaps even heal up all the ſores on the ſkin: but nothing is gained by this, for the diſeaſe ſoon breaks out anew. Some practitioners of medicine in the Weſt Indies, are of opinion that interrupting the courſe of the diſeaſe by mercury is productive of no other evils than thoſe of loſs of time, and an imperfect cure; others affirm, that it is often the cauſe of what they call the bone-ach. Towards the end of the diſeaſe it is generally allowed that mercury may be given ſafely and even with advantage. It is probable the long continuance of the diſeaſe being above fourteen months, and alſo the pains in the bones in the preſent caſe, were owing to the very early and free uſe of mercury. It may be allowable to add, that the yaws do not differ more from

from the venereal difeafe in curing themfelves, than in this circumftance, that like the fmallpox they affect none a fecond time.

A gentleman applied to me for the cure of chancres, fituated on the attachment of the prepuce to the penis, and alfo on the frænum. Mercury was ufed chiefly by friction, in order to affect the conftitution; it was alfo applied to the fores, in order to affect them locally. The cure of the chancres went on gradually and without interruption, and in about five weeks they were perfectly healed. He almoft immediately had connection with a woman, and long before we could fuppofe the mercury had all got out of his conftitution. In a very few days after the firft connection the prepuce began to be chopped all round on the edge of it's reflection. He continued his connections, and upon it's growing worfe he applied to me, and I found the chops very deep and the prepuce there fo tight and fore that he could not bring it back upon the penis. The queftion now was, whether this was venereal or not? The fores themfelves did not appear to be fo, but more was to be taken into the account than fimply appearances. It was firft to be confidered, whether it might poffibly be a return of his former complaint. This could not be the cafe, becaufe they were not in the fame parts. It was next to be queftioned, was it poffible for this part of the prepuce to have been contaminated at the fame time with the former, without having come into action till now, having been prevented by the courfe of mercury, which had not cured the difpofition, and being now left off it had come into action? This could not be well anfwered, although not probable, becaufe it appeared to come too foon into action after the leaving off of the medicine, for I did fuppofe there was ftill a great deal of mercury in the conftitution. Was it then poffible for him to have caught it from the woman? This I fuppofed could not have been the caufe of thefe chops, whatever effect this connection might have to render them venereal hereafter, for they appeared too foon after it, efpecially as he had mercury in his conftitution at the time, and as the parts had been accuftomed to the application of venereal matter but a very little time before. Although from all circumftances taken together I was convinced it was not venereal, yet an apprehenfion arofe in his mind concerning the poffibility of having given it to the lady, as he had connection after their firft appearance. I was equally

equally convinced of the impoſſibility of the one as of the other, therefore deſired him to reſt eaſy on that head. He went immediately into the country, and without doing any thing for thoſe chops they got perfectly well. In leſs than a fortnight after this connection the lady became a little indiſpoſed with a ſlight fever, and a ſwelling came in one of her groins. I watched the progreſs of this ſwelling, which was ſlow, and I did not believe it to be venereal. It at laſt formed matter and broke, and a poultice was applied to it. Inſtead of ulcerating or ſpreading, it rather took on a healing diſpoſition, and in about ſix weeks it was perfectly well. While it was healing, ſcurfy eruptions came out on the ſkin, ſome on the face and thighs, but more eſpecially on the hands and feet, where the cuticle peeled off. Upon the firſt appearance of theſe, I was a little ſtaggered, but as the ſore was healing I was unwilling to give credit to the appearance, and therefore begged that nothing might be done, and they all got well.

From the general outline of theſe caſes, one would naturally have ſaid they were venereal, but the particular circumſtances being all inveſtigated, and the whole taken together, led me to ſuppoſe that they were not, and the event proved that to be the caſe.

The following caſe was communicated by Mr. French of Harpur-ſtreet.

"June the 9th, 1782, a gentleman applied to me for an ulcer which was ſeated on the glans penis, attended with exceſſive pain. Knowing him to be an intemperate man, and learning from himſelf that during a ſtate of intoxication he had been connected with a woman, I judged the complaint to be venereal. He was now in a feveriſh ſtate and unfit for the exhibition of mercury, I therefore preſcribed for him decoction of bark with elixir of vitriol and tinctura thebaica proportioned to his pain. I directed him to abſtain from every kind of fermented liquor, to live chiefly upon milk, and to waſh the ulcer with a liniment compoſed of equal parts of oil of almonds and aqua ſapphirina.

About the 17th of the ſame month, ſome check having been given to the fever, the ſore looking cleaner, and his pain having abated, I ordered him ſmall doſes of the argentum vivum and extract of hemlock.

July the 4th, finding the mercurial courſe diſagree, I ordered three grains of the extract of hemlock to be taken two or three times a day, and the decoction of bark to be taken as before, with twenty drops of tinctura thebaica, which was gradually increased to sixty, at bed-time.

The ulcer had spread very much during the mercurial course, and had now destroyed half the glans penis.

October 1st, Mr. Hunter was consulted, and ordered the patient to add the powder of sarsaparilla to the decoction of bark, to take laudanum freely, and wash the sores with tinctura thebaica. Soon after beginning this course the remainder of the glans penis sloughed off, the parts gradually healed, and health was restored.

There were two other symptoms in this case which deserve to be taken notice of, a considerable enlargement of the scalp on the right side of the os frontis, and on the left parietal bone, attended with excessive pain, and vibices resembling the sea-scurvy on the inside of the left tibia, both of which disappeared in the course of the cure.

Some months after, the tumor in the head returned, and several abscesses were formed which were opened, and the cranium found carious to a great extent. On account of the pain, he has for some months past taken two hundred and forty drops of laudanum, and six grains of opium daily. These sores healed up and others broke out in different parts of the head, which also got well, and in June 1785 there was only one large ulcer in the angle of the right eye."

A lady was delivered of a child on the 30th of September 1776, the infant being weakly and the quantity of milk in the mother's breasts abundant, it was judged proper to procure the child of a person in the neighbourhood to assist in keeping the breasts in a proper state. It is worthy of remarking, that the lady kept her own child to the right breast, the stranger to the left. In about six weeks the nipple of the left breast began to inflame, and the glands of the axilla to swell. A few days after several small ulcers were formed about the nipple, which spreading rapidly soon communicated and became one ulcer, and at last the whole nipple was destroyed. The tumor in the axilla subsided, and the ulcer in the breast healed in about three months from it's first appearance. On inquiry, about this time the child of the stranger was short breathed, had the thrush, and died tabid, with many sores on different parts of the body. The patient now complained of shooting

pains

pains in different parts of the body, which were succeeded by an eruption on the arms, legs and thighs, many of which became ulcers.

She was now put under a mercurial course, with a decoction of sarsaparilla. Mercury was tried in a variety of forms, in solution, in pills internally, and externally in the form of ointment. It could not be continued above a few days at a time, as it always brought on fever or purging, with extreme pain in the bowels. In this state she remained till March 16, 1779, when she was delivered of another child in a diseased state. This child was committed to the care of a wetnurse, and lived about nine weeks; the cuticle peeling off in various parts, and a scabby eruption covering the whole body; the child died.

Soon after the death of the child the nurse complained of headach and sore throat, together with ulceration of the breasts. Various remedies were given to her, but she determined to go into a public hospital, where she was salivated, and after some months she was discharged, although not cured of the disease. The bones of the nose and palate exfoliated, and in a few months she also died tabid.

Of the various remedies tried by the lady herself, none succeeded so well as sea-bathing. About the month of May she began a course of the Lisbon diet-drink, and continued it with regularity about a month, dressing the sores with laudanum, by which treatment the sores healed up; and in September she was delivered of another child, free from external marks of disease, but very sickly; and it died in the course of the month.

About a twelvemonth after the sore broke out again, and although mercurial dressings and internal medicines were given, remained for a twelvemonth, when they began again to heal up.

The following cases being all derived from one stock, they show as much as possible, that new poisons are rising up every day, and also very similar to the venereal in many respects, although not in all; therefore it is the want of similarity that becomes the criterion to judge by, and not the similarity. The parents of the child, who was the subject of the following history, were and are to all appearance healthy people. The child was weakly when born; and the mother having little or no milk, when it was three weeks old she gave it to a nurse whose milk was then seven months old,

old, and was giving ſuck to her own child. The foſter-mother allowed her own to ſuck the right breaſt while the other ſucked the left.

The nurſe obſerved that the ſkin of the foſter-child began to peel off; but no rawneſs or ſoreneſs took place except about the anus, where it looked as if ſcalded. The ſame kind of peeling took place on the lips, but they did not appear to be ſore, although the people in the country ſaid it was the thruſh. The inner ſurface of the mouth and tongue appeared ſound. In a fortnight after her receiving the child it died, and then ſhe allowed her own child to ſuck both breaſts for three weeks; at the end of which ſhe came to town to nurſe a gentleman's child.

She gave ſuck to this ſecond child; but after being in town about ten or eleven days, ſhe did not feel herſelf perfectly well; which made them ſuppoſe that the new mode of life, confinement in town, and probably better living, might not agree with her, and ſhe went into the country and took the gentleman's child with her. About three or four days after ſhe went to the country, for inſtance, about a fortnight after ſhe took this child, and five weeks after the death of the firſt child, her left nipple, which the firſt nurſed child had always ſucked, began to be ſore, ſo that ſhe could not let the child ſuck it. This ulcer on the nipple became extremely painful, and in a day or two eruptions came out on her face, which were ſoon followed by the ſame over her whole body, but moſt on her legs and thighs; they continued coming out for about a fortnight, and had at firſt very much the appearance of the eruptions of the ſmallpox, on the third day of their eruption attended with fever, univerſal uneaſineſs, and great pain. The ſalt of wormwood mixture, with the teſtaceous powders, was given every four hours, with ſome opening medicines, as the infuſion of ſena, ſoluble tartar, &c. every ſecond or third day, but without effect, the complaints increaſing.

Two or three days after the eruption on the ſkin appeared, one of the glands of the armpit began to ſwell, and formed matter, and was opened within a fortnight after it's firſt appearance, and healed almoſt directly. Some of the eruptions increaſed faſt and become very broad ſores, nearly of the ſize of a half-crown, eſpecially on the legs and thighs, and were covered with a broad ſcab; many remained ſmall and only appeared like pimples.

pimples. About a fortnight after the first appearance of the eruption, some began to die away, becoming less sore; and about four weeks after this appearance a foul ulcer attacked the left tonsil.

The surgeon in the country, from all these circumstances, finding he could not get any ground by the before mentioned treatment, determined to give her the solution of the corrosive sublimate, of which he gave half a grain in solution night and morning; in about a week there seemed to be a stop put to the spreading of the ulcers, and the discharge to be lessened something, the ulcer in the throat putting on a better appearance.

It was at this period I first saw her, which was about six weeks after the first appearance of the eruption, and a fortnight after the appearance of the ulcer in the tonsil. The eruptions were then very much as before described; but the ulcer in the tonsil was clean and healing. From the history of the case I did conceive it not to be venereal; I therefore desired that all medicines might be left off, which medicines could only have been taken for a fortnight at most, because it was after the appearance of the ulcer on the tonsil the mercury was given, which was only of a fortnight's standing when I saw her. She soon after recovered.

After being well for some time, she again applied to the surgeon in the country, an abscess having formed where the complaint first began in the breast, attended with fresh eruptions on the face.

The abscess was opened, and it healed up in a few days, and upon taking some cooling physic the eruptions disappeared. She has continued very well ever since without any other bad effect than the total loss of her nipple. This case was certainly understood to be venereal.

About five days after the appearance of the eruption on the nurse, the gentleman's child was taken away and given to a healthy woman of a florid complexion, aged twenty-four years, and who had lain in with her first child eleven months when she became wet nurse to this child. After a few days she observed eruptions on the child's head, not unlike those already described on the first nurse which it had sucked. It's mouth soon after became excoriated, so that it sucked with difficulty. After a short time those eruptions on the head became dry and peeled off, others appeared on the face, knees and feet, but wholly unlike the former, as the first matu-

 rated,

rated, while the latter appeared only cutaneous, peeling off and leaving a circumfcribed fpot of a light dun color, which continued increafing for five weeks. Thefe eruptions continued nearly three months from their commencement, at which period the child was extremely emaciated, but no particular treatment was indicated, fo no medicine was exhibited, and in a few weeks after it came to London and got perfectly well.

The fecond nurfe a few days after giving fuck to the child, had blotches appear on her left breaft, precifely the fame with thofe on the firft nurfe; with this difference only, that they were fewer in number, and attended with a greater degree of phlegmonous inflammation. They continued, and increafed in fize for feven or eight days; then the nipple of the fame breaft became ulcerated; the ulceration fpreading fo much as to endanger the lofs of it; her thighs now became difeafed, and afterwards her legs.

She fuckled this child about twelve weeks. The difeafe feemed no longer to increafe, and in twelve or fourteen days after this entirely difappeared without her taking any medicine, except a few ounces of the decoction of the bark. The only application to the breaft was unguentum fimplex.

The milk at this time became fo fmall in quantity, that they were under the neceffity of providing a third wetnurfe for the child, and the fecond returned to the country. Her own child being weaned fhe had no further occafion for the milk, and in a few days it wholly difappeared; but by way of amufing the child when peevifh, fhe allowed it to take the nipple, which had been difeafed, in it's mouth; the confequence was, that in a few days this child alfo became difeafed in like manner with the former. She now applied to an eminent furgeon for affiftance, who not being acquainted with the hiftory, fuppofed it venereal, and ordered a colourlefs medicine, fuppofed from circumftances to be the folution of fublimate, fixteen grains to half a pint of water; the dofe a table-fpoonful. She took this medicine as directed, and alfo gave it to her hufband and child; the child a tea-fpoonful only at a time. While taking this medicine fhe got well.

The third wetnurfe, like the former, was in a fhort time affected, but the blotches in this cafe were ftill fewer in number, the difeafe appearing to

lofe

lofe confiderably in it's power, as each frefh infection became lefs malignant than the former. She got well without taking any medicine.

I. OF DISEASES SUPPOSED TO BE VENEREAL PRODUCED BY TRANSPLANTED TEETH.

SINCE the operation of tranfplanting teeth has been practifed in London, fome cafes have occured in which the venereal infection has been fuppofed to be communicated in this way; and they have been treated accordingly; nor has the method of cure tended to weaken the fufpicion: yet when all the circumftances attending them, both in the mode of catching the difeafe, and in the cure when treated as venereal, are confidered, there is fomething in them all which is not exactly fimilar to the ufual appearance of the venereal difeafe when caught in the common way; efpecially too when it is confidered that fome of the cafes were not treated as venereal and yet got well, and therefore the cures of the others which appeared to be from mercury are not clear proofs of their having been venereal.*

I believe that I have feen moft if not all the cafes of this kind which have occured, and have attended fome of them. In all of them the time of local affection after the infertion of the tooth has been almoft regularly a month, which is too long for the venereal to take effect at a medium; and where they have produced conftitutional fymptoms thofe again have either followed the local too clofe for the venereal or too regular as to time. But it may be advanced that a difeafe has been produced probably as bad in it's confequences as the venereal. That a difeafe has been formed in this way is certain.

The firft cafe of this kind which came under my care, was a lady who had one of the bicufpidati tranfplanted. The tranfplanted tooth faftened

* It is to be remarked here, that I do not in the prefent cafe lay any ftrefs at all on my opinion of the lues venerea not having the power of contamination; and I believe we muft allow if thefe are venereal it muft have been the lues venerea in the perfon from whom the tooth was taken; for chancres are not common in the mouth, and they would be feen on examination. I believe few difcharges fimilar to gonorrhœa take place there.

very

very well. About a month after she danced till five or six o'clock in the morning, caught cold, and had a fever in consequence, which lasted near six weeks. In this time ulceration in the gum and jaw took place, though it was then not known. And when she was beginning to recover, it was found that not only the gum and socket of this tooth were diseased, but also those of the teeth next to it. The two teeth were taken out, and the sockets of both afterwards exfoliated, but the parts were very backward in healing. This backwardness gave rise to various opinions, the principal of which was, that it was venereal. In the mean time a rising appeared upon one of the legs, which was of the indolent node kind, this was also suspected by some to be venereal, or rather was a corroborating circumstance of the former opinion; but I gave it as my opinion that it was not. I desired she might go to the sea and bathe, which she did, and got perfectly well, both in the jaw and leg, and has continued so ever since.

The second case of this kind I have seen was also in a young lady: the transplanted tooth fastened extremely well, and continued so for about a month, when the gum began to ulcerate, leaving the tooth and socket bare. The ulcer continued, and blotches appeared upon the skin, and ulcers also in the throat. The disease was treated as venereal, the complaints gave way to this course, but they recurred several times after very severe courses of mercury: however she at last got well.

The only observation I can make on this case is, that the symptoms recurred after continued courses of mercury, much oftener than is usual in venereal cases; and I had my suspicions all along that it was scrofulous.

The third case was of a gentleman, where the transplanted tooth remained, without giving the least disturbance, for about a month, when the edge of the gum began to ulcerate, and the ulceration went on till the tooth dropped out. Some time after, spots appeared almost every where on the skin; they had not the truly venereal appearance, but were redder, or more transparent, and more circumscribed. He had also a tendency to a hectic fever, such as restlessness, want of sleep, loss of appetite, and headach. After trying several things and not finding relief, he was put under a course of mercury, and all disease disappeared according to the common course of the cure of the venereal disease, and we thought him well; but some time after,

after, the same appearances returned, with the addition of swelling in the bones of the metacarpus. He was now put under another course of mercury more severe than the former, and in the usual time all the symptoms again disappeared. Several months after, the same eruptions came out again, but not in so great a degree as before, and without any other attendant symptoms. He a third time took mercury, but it was only ten grains of corrosive sublimate in the whole, and he got quite well. The time between his first taking mercury and his being cured was a space of three years.

Query: Could this case be venereal? The two first courses of mercury removing the eruptions, would seem to prove it was; but the third course also removing them, which consisted of only ten grains of corrosive sublimate, would seem to prove that it could not be venereal; for if it had, the appearances which returned after the second course, in which a considerable quantity of mercury had been given, would not have yielded to ten grains.

The fourth case was that of a young lady who had a tooth transplanted, and about the same distance of time after it, as mentioned in the former cases, the gum began to ulcerate, and the ulceration was making considerable progress. The surgeon who was first consulted desired mercury to be given immediately. I was afterwards desired to see her, and advised that mercury should not be had recourse to, that we might ascertain the nature of the case; for if she took mercury and got well, it would be adding one more to the number of the supposed venereal cases arising from such a cause. I recommended drawing the tooth, that we might see what effects would be produced by the removal of the first cause.

The tooth was drawn, and the gum healed up as fast as any common ulcer, and has ever since continued well.

This case requires no comment. I may however be allowed to observe, that if the lady had gone through a course of mercury, she would have in all probability also got well; for the tooth, in the time necessary for compleating the course of mercury, would have dropped out; and if this had really happened, we need not hesitate in affirming, that it would have been considered as venereal.

The fifth case was that of a young lady, eighteen years of age, who had one of the incisores transplanted, which fastened very well; but six or seven weeks after the operation, an ulceration of the gum took place, the tooth was immediately ordered to be removed, and the bark was given without any other medicine being had recourſe to, and ſhe got well in a few weeks.

The ſixth caſe was that of a gentleman, aged twenty-three, a native of one of the Weſt India iſlands, who had the two front inciſores tranſplanted; and about the ſame time after the operation, as in the former caſes, an ulceration of the gums took place, which increaſed to a very great degree, and the edges of the gum ſloughed off. An eminent ſurgeon was conſulted, who ordered the bark, and the patient without taking any other medicine got well, in nearly the ſame time as the lady in caſes four, and five, who had the teeth taken out. The gums recovered themſelves perfectly, but were conſiderably ſhorter.

If we take ſome of the above caſes and conſider them as they at firſt appeared, we ſhall almoſt pronounce them to have been venereal. If we take the others, we ſhall pronounce them abſolutely not to be venereal; and if we conſider every circumſtance relating to thoſe probably venereal, we ſhall as far as reaſoning goes, conclude that they were not venereal. The firſt caſe that appeared at the time to be venereal, is the ſecond of thoſe before related; but as I did not attend the lady through the whole of the cure, I can ſay leſs upon it; ſhe certainly had the ſymptoms recur oftner than they do in venereal caſes in common, where the diſeaſe is attended with no ambiguity, and took more than the uſual quantity of mercury; there is therefore in this caſe ſomething not clearly underſtood, becauſe it does not exactly agree with venereal caſes in general in all it's parts.

The fourth caſe was ſimilar in it's recurring, and in the quantity of mercury that appeared to be neceſſary to remove the ſymptoms.

The moſt ſerious effects of the tranſplanting of a tooth happened to a young lady, and which is related in the Medical Tranſactions by Dr. Watſon.

The dentiſt being alarmed at the firſt appearance, deſired me to go and ſee her upon his own account. The edge of the gum was juſt then begun to ulcerate. As I did not know well what was beſt to be done, I deſired him to make a ſtrong ſolution of corroſive ſublimate, and let the mouth be often waſhed with it, alſo ſome lint ſoaked in it and applyed to the

part;

part; but as this did not ſtop it's progreſs, ſhe applyed to Dr. Watſon, to whoſe account of the caſe I muſt refer the reader, and from that account I muſt take my materials to reaſon upon. However I may remark, that the caſe appears to have been ſuppoſed at laſt to have been venereal, whatever might have been the firſt opinion, and for the two following reaſons; firſt, from the mode of catching the diſeaſe being poſſible; and ſecondly, from it's not giving way to medicines which are of no ſervice in the venereal diſeaſe; and this opinion appears to have been confirmed by the diſeaſe giving way to mercury. But the caſe itſelf abſtracted from the mode of catching it, and even the mode of cure, does not perfectly agree with the common attending circumſtances of the venereal, nor has that attention been paid to the neceſſary circumſtances ſufficient to determine it to be venereal.

The progreſs of the ulceration in the mouth, which was the firſt ſymptom, was by much too rapid for a venereal ulcer in common; for it muſt be conſidered, if venereal, ſimply as a chancre, or local affection.

Now let us trace the progreſs of the diſeaſe into the conſtitution. "About this time" viz. when the local diſeaſe was making ſuch rapid progreſs "blotches appeared in her face, neck, and various parts of the body; ſeveral of theſe became ulcerated painful ſores".* Now this date of the conſtitutional affections following the local, is by much too ſoon to be venereal; we know if a lues venerea ariſes either from a gonorrhœa or chancre, it does not appear in common till about ſix weeks, often much later, but ſeldom ſooner. I ſhall leave the circumſtance of there being no ſwelling of the lymphatic glands of the neck, forming buboes, as that is not a conſtant ſymptom attending the venereal matter getting into the circulation, although it ſhould be allowed to have ſome weight, eſpecially where other circumſtances do not perfectly agree. The appearances from the conſtitution when they did take place, were much more violent and rapid in their progreſs than any venereal blotches I ever ſaw: we know in the lues venerea that they are months before they arrive at the ſtage of ſcabs; alſo the pain attending thoſe ſores did not in the leaſt correſpond with the lues venerea. Venereal blotches hardly give any ſenſation, or at leaſt

* Medical Tranſactions, vol. 3, page 328.

very

very little; but after all, mercury cured this diſeaſe whatever it was: twenty-eight grains of calomel made into fourteen pills was taken, probably, in ten or twelve days; for it was directed ſhe ſhould take one or two each day, as the bowels would allow; but although tinctura thebaica was given, they purged ſo much as made it neceſſary to give no more in this way; but although ſo little mercury was taken, and had alſo run off conſiderably by the bowels, yet " During the taking of theſe, however, the ulceration of her mouth and cheeks did not ſpread, but were leſs painful and of a milder appearance; the blotches in her face and body grew paler, and ſuch of them as had ulcerated healed apace and no new ones appeared." " Unguent cæruleum fortius" was therefore directed " to be well rubbed into her legs and thighs twice a day, in ſmall doſes," leaſt it ſhould be determined to the bowels. " In about ten or twelve days her griping and purging returned with violence, the ointment was therefore diſcontinued; at this time the blotches were all gone; the ulceration in her face and body were completely healed, and thoſe of her mouth nearly ſo."

The only remark I have to make on the cure is, that the quantity of mercury was not ſufficient to cure chancres on the penis, making ſuch rapid progreſs as thoſe did in her mouth; nor could the ſame quantity of mercury cure venereal ſores on the ſkin, which had made ſuch rapid progreſs as they did in this caſe; and if we take in the effect this had upon her health, with the termination of the whole, I think we ſhould pronounce it not venereal; for the ſpecific circumſtances, if it was venereal, were juſt as uncommon as the mode of catching it.

Many of theſe caſes, ſuſpected of being venereal, I have ſeen occaſionally, and although the patients recovered while under a courſe of mercury, yet on account of the want of attention in the practitioners to the very circumſtances that would decide the diſeaſe to be either venereal or not, I paſs them over unnoticed.

After having conſidered the caſes themſelves of thoſe who had the teeth tranſplanted, let us alſo conſider the perſons from whom the teeth were taken; for I cannot help thinking that this will throw ſome light upon the ſubject. Let me ſuppoſe that the young girls from whom the teeth were taken really had the lues venerea, and that the teeth were of courſe alſo infected,

fected, which is a ſuppoſition moſt unfavourable to my real opinion, it appears to me that even in this caſe there can be no difference between the gums of the girl from whom the tooth was taken, and the gums of the perſon who received it: if the ulceration took place in the laſt from contamination, would not the ſocket in the girl from whom the tooth was taken likewiſe have ulcerated? But this did not happen in any of them. I have here ſuppoſed the teeth capable of being contaminated; although I believe we have never yet ſeen them have this diſeaſe primarily, but only in conſequence of it's breaking out ſomewhere elſe, in the mouth, throat, or noſe, and ſpreading to them; but ſtill, if they are capable of having the diſeaſe, and communicating it to others, it becomes very extraordinary that theſe people ſhould have hit upon the only ſuch teeth that probably were ever ſo contaminated.

When we conſider that the girls from whom the teeth were taken, had not the leaſt appearance of diſeaſe at the time, and had none when the diſeaſe broke out in the perſon who received the teeth, it becomes ſtrange that it ſhould break out in the receivers, and not in the giver.

It is alſo ſingular that an ambiguity ſhould follow this diſeaſe in all it's ſtages; in the mode of it's being caught, the appearance, and the cure.

Let us ſum up all the arguments in favor of the diſeaſe not being venereal. Firſt; two patients whoſe caſes were ſimilar to the others in their origin, recovered without medicine.

Secondly; they who ſeemed to be cured by mercury had not a treatment exactly ſimilar to thoſe who were indiſputably poxed.

Thirdly; I conſider it as impoſſible for parts to have the power of contaminating, which have not themſelves aſſumed the diſeaſed action.

Fourthly; the parts contaminating were never known to have been contaminated themſelves.

But it muſt be nearly the ſame thing to thoſe who want to have teeth tranſplanted, whether my reaſoning is juſt or not; for a diſeaſe in conſequence of the operation moſt certainly has taken place; and in ſome caſes this has been worſe, or cured with more difficulty, than the lues venerea in common; and whatever the diſeaſe may be, I yet know of no mode of

 prevention,

prevention, except the drawing of the tooth early, and that has been tried in one case only, and in that case was succefsful.

From this account many may be deterred from having this operation performed; in that light no evil can arife, except being mortified that no means of relief can be had recourfe to in cafes of bad teeth; but it is to be remembered, that this is a publication of all the unfuccefsful cafes, which is the very reverfe of what is generally practifed in medical books; and they are mentioned upon no other principle than that the difeafe, when it happens, may not be improperly managed.

It may be afked, what is this difeafe? That may be with more difficulty anfwered, than what it is not. I fhould fay that a found tooth tranfplanted may occafion fuch an irritation as fhall produce a fpecies of difeafe which may be followed by the local complaints above mentioned.

I cannot conclude without intimating that undefcribed difeafes refembling the venereal are very numerous; and that what I have faid is rather to be confidered as hints for others to profecute this inquiry further, than as a complete account of the fubject.

THE END.

11.1.61

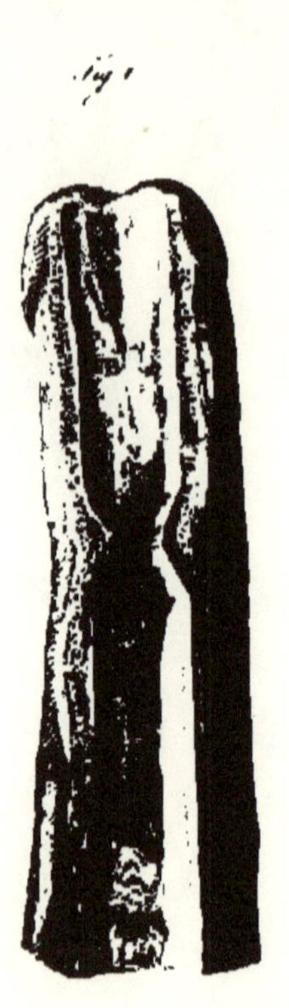
Fig 1

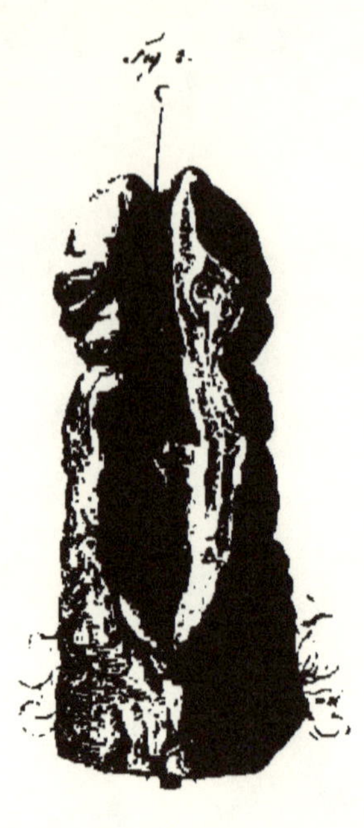
Fig 2.

EXPLANATION

OF THE

PLATES.

PLATE I.

FIGURE I.

THE penis slit open, showing a stricture in the urethra, about two inches from the glans; the stricture is but slight.

AA. The cut surface of the corpus spongiosum urethræ.

BB. The canal of the urethra in which may be observed the orifices of the lacunæ.

C. The stricture.

FIGURE II.

The penis slit open for about three inches, to show the lacunæ, which become occasionally an obstruction to the passage of the bougie.

AA. The Corpus spongiosum urethra.

BB. The internal surface of the canal of the urethra pointing to the orifice of two of the lacunæ.

C. A bristle introduced into a lacuna.

D. The end of the bougie introduced into the remaining part of the urethra.

11.1.61

407

ogl.

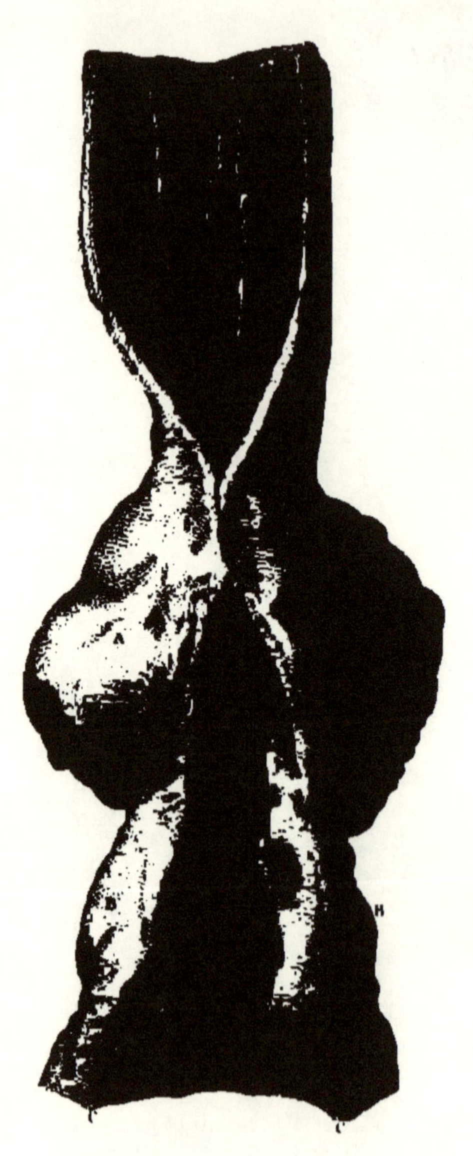
A
H

EXPLANATION

OF

PLATE II.

THE urethra opened in two different places, one before the ſtricture, the other behind: the one before, is through the body of the penis; the other behind, is upon the anterior ſurface of the membraneous part, and a bougie paſſes from the one opening to the other.

AA. The crura penis and bulbous part of the urethra all blended together by inflammation and ſuppuration, which has taken place in many parts.

BB. The proſtate gland in a diſeaſed ſtate.

CC. The cut edges of the bladder.

D. The urethra behind the ſtricture very much enlarged, irregular on the ſurface in conſequence of ulceration.

EE. The cut ſurface of the corpus cavernoſum penis.

FF. The cut ſurface of the corpus ſpongioſum urethræ.

GG. The bougie paſſing from the ſound to the unſound part of the urethra.

H. A ſmall bougie in the new paſſage.

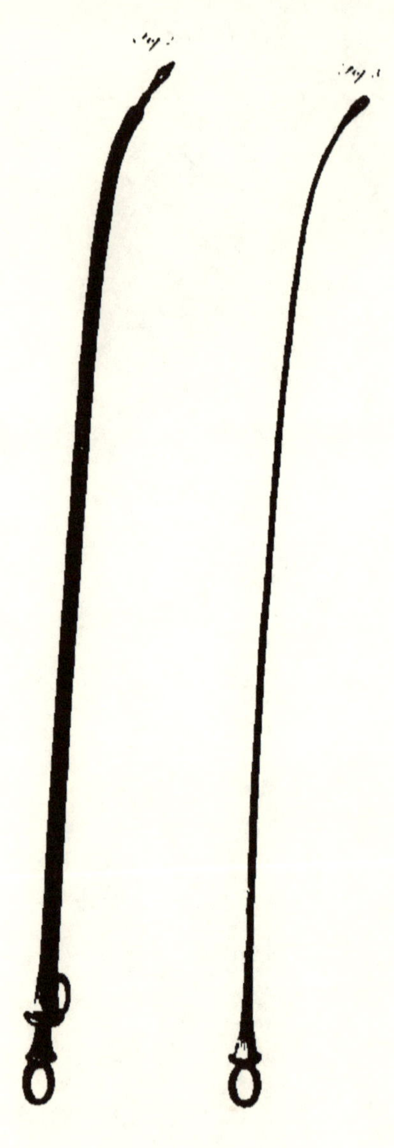

EXPLANATION

OF

PLATE III.

TWO canulas for applying caustic to strictures in the urethra.

FIGURE I.

A straight silver canula with the plug projecting beyond the termination of the canula, making a rounded end; at the other end of the wire is a small port-crayon in which is represented a piece of caustic.

FIGURE II.

A flexible canula for applying the caustic to strictures in the bend of the urethra. The wire with the small port-crayon is pushed out beyond it's end.

FIGURE III.

A piece of silver wire with the plug at the end to be introduced into the canula, as in Figure I.

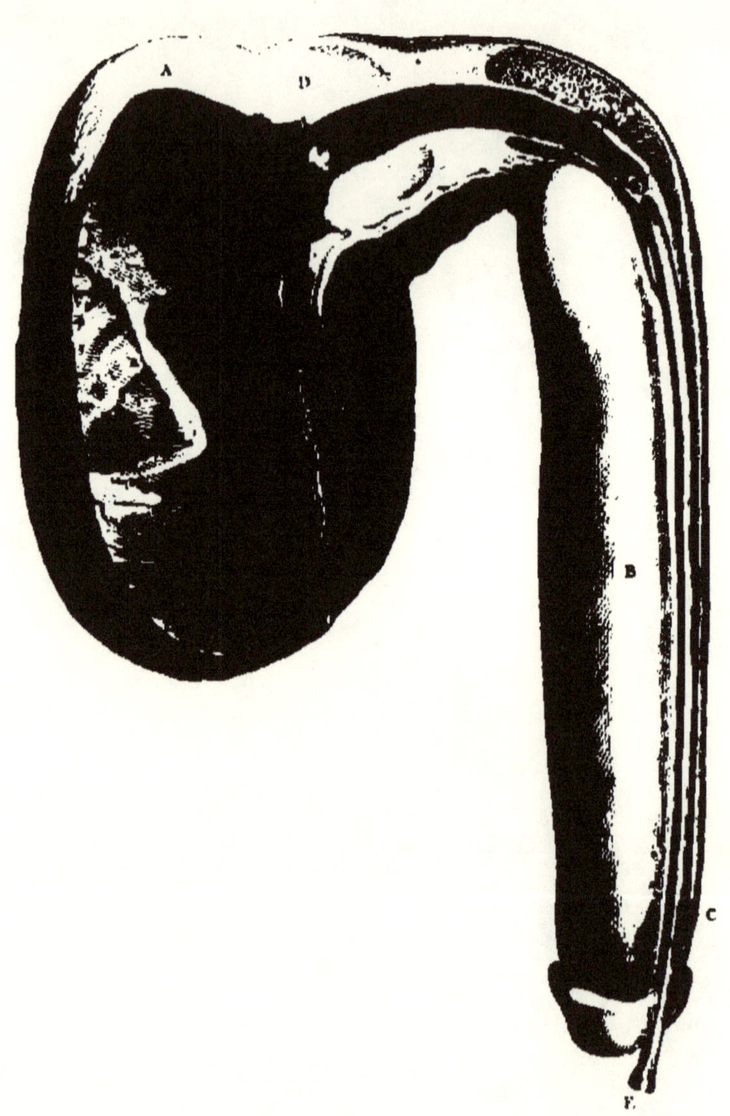
A
D
B
C
E

EXPLANATION

OF

PLATE IV.

THE bladder and penis of a perſon who died of a mortification of the bladder in conſequence of a ſtricture and ſtone in the urethra. In this plate not only the ſtricture is repreſented, but the thickened coats and faſciculated inner ſurface of the bladder; as alſo the ſmall ſtone which acted as a valve, or plug; beſides which a canula is introduced from the glans down to the ſtricture, ſhowing the practicability of deſtroying it with cauſtic.

AA. The bladder cut open, ſhowing it's coats a little thickened, and it's inner ſurface faſciculated.

B. The body of the penis.

CC. The corpus ſpongioſum urethræ cut open through it's whole length, expoſing the urethra.

D. The proſtate gland divided.

E. A ſilver canula introduced into the urethra through which the cauſtic is paſſed on to the ſtricture.

F. Points out the ſtricture with the ſtone laying above it, ſo as entirely to prevent the paſſage of urine.

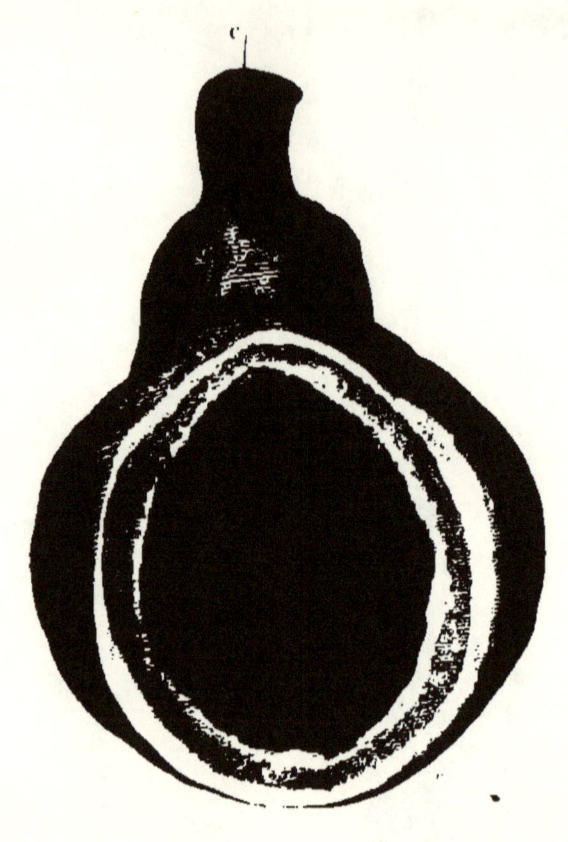
c

EXPLANATION

OF

PLATE V.

AN enlarged proſtate gland, particularly the valvular proceſs, which has increaſed inwards into the bladder in form of a tumor, in conſequence of which the water paſſed with difficulty, which became the cauſe of the increaſed thickneſs of the bladder.

A. The proſtate gland.
B. The projecting part paſſing into the cavity of the bladder.
CC. A briſtle in the urethra to ſhow it is above this tumor.
D. The cut edge of the bladder, which ſhows it's increaſed thickneſs.*

* The preparation from which this drawing was made I was favoured with by Mr. Gunning, and which is in his poſſeſſion.

11.1.61

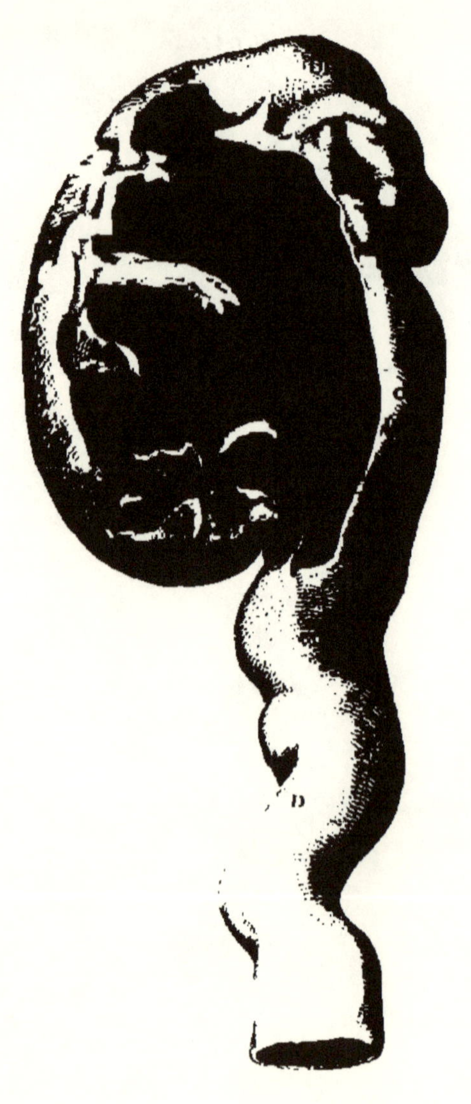
D

EXPLANATION

OF

PLATE VI.

A Kidney whose ureter, pelvis, and infundibula, are very considerably enlarged in consequence of a stricture in the urethra.

A. The substance of the kidney, which is become very thin.
BB. The infundibula much enlarged.
C. The pelvis very much enlarged.
D. The ureter increased more than ten times it's natural size.

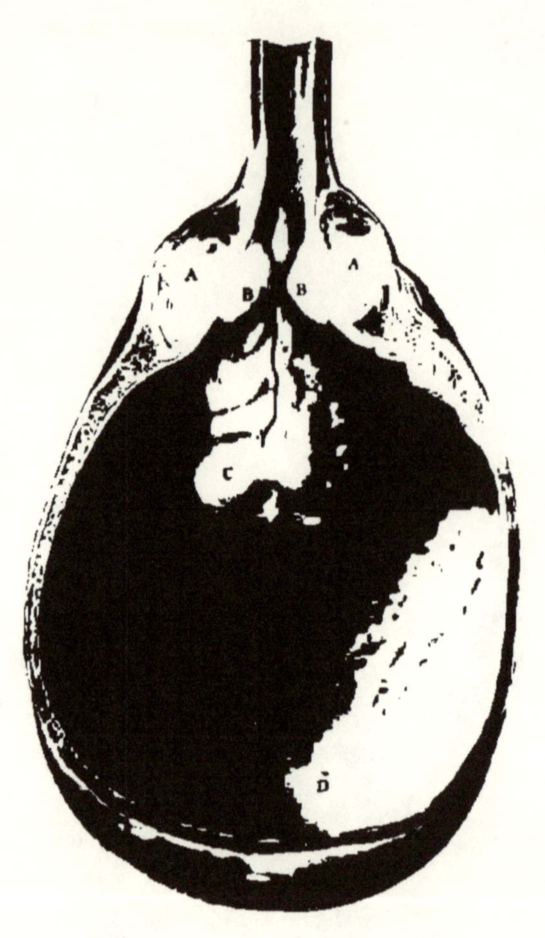
A
B
B
A
C
D

EXPLANATION

OF

PLATE VII.

THE valvular part of the bladder ſo increaſed as to form a conſiderable tumor, projecting into the cavity of the bladder. The proſtate is alſo enlarged. This tumor had been the occaſion of ſeveral ſevere ſuppreſſions of urine, and had often been the cauſe of a failure in drawing off the water with the catheter, by that inſtrument moſt probably paſſing into it's ſubſtance ſo deep as to hinder the urine entering it's openings. The dark line paſſing along the tumor from the urethra was probably made by this means, but now collapſed.

AA. The cut ſurface of the proſtate gland.
BB. The inner ſides of the proſtate gland projecting inwards.
C. The tumor.
D. The cavity of the bladder.

INDEX.

I N D E X.

A.

B.

C.

Case

INDEX.

complaints

Chord,

D.

E.

F.

G.

I N D E X.

H.

I.

Ipecacuanha,

L.

M.

N.

O.

P.

S.

Scrofula,

T.

V.

I N D E X.

V.

U.

W.

Y.